Microinjection and Organelle Transplantation Techniques

Microinjection and Organelle Transplantation Techniques

methods and applications

edited by

J. E. Celis
Division of Biostructural Chemistry,
Department of Chemistry,
Aarhus University,
Aarhus, Denmark

A. Graessmann
Institute of Molecular Biology,
and Biochemistry,
Freie University,
Berlin,
Federal Republic of Germany

A. Loyter
Department of Biological Chemistry,
Institute of Life Sciences,
The Hebrew University of Jerusalem,
Jerusalem, Israel

1986

ACADEMIC PRESS
Harcourt Brace Jovanovich, Publishers

London Orlando San Diego New York Austin
Montreal Sydney Tokyo Toronto

ACADEMIC PRESS INC. (LONDON) LTD.
24/28 Oval Road, London NW1 7DX

United States Edition published by
ACADEMIC PRESS, INC.
Orlando, Florida 32887

British Library Cataloguing in Publication Data

Microinjection and organelle transplantation techniques:
methods and applications.
1. Cytology—Technique
I. Celis, J. E. II. Graessmann, A. III. Loyter, A.
574.87′028 QH583

ISBN 0-12-164722-6
ISBN 0-12-164723-4 Pbk

Phototypeset by
Paston Press, Norwich

Printed in Great Britain by
St Edmundsbury Press, Bury St Edmunds, Suffolk

Contributors

R. S. Bhatt, *Department of Molecular Genetics, Roche Research Center, Nutley, New Jersey 07110, USA*

*J. E. Celis, *Division of Biostructural Chemistry, Department of Chemistry, Aarhus University, Langelandsgade 140, DK-8000 Aarhus C, Denmark*

N. Chejanovsky, *Department of Biological Chemistry, Institute of Life Sciences, The Hebrew University of Jerusalem, 91904 Jerusalem, Israel*

S. J. Degudicibus, *Roche Institute of Molecular Biology, Roche Research Center, Nutley, New Jersey 07110, USA*

J. R. Feramisco, *Cold Spring Harbor Laboratory, Cold Spring Harbor, New York 11724, USA*

D. Fernig, *Department of Biochemistry, University of Nottingham Medical School, Queen's Medical Centre, Nottingham NG7 2UH, UK*

B. Gentile, *Department of Molecular Genetics, Roche Research Center, Nutley, New Jersey 07110, USA*

A. G. Gitman, *Department of Biological Chemistry, Institute of Life Sciences, The Hebrew University of Jerusalem, 91904 Jerusalem, Israel*

J. W. Gordon, *Department of Obstetrics, Gynecology and Reproductive Science, Mount Sinai School of Medicine, One Gustave L. Levy Place, New York, NY 10029, USA*

A. Graessmann, *Institut für Molekularbiologie und Biochemie, Freie Universität Berlin, Arnimallee 22, D-1000 Berlin 33, West Germany*

M. Graessmann, *Institut für Molekularbiologie und Biochemie, Freie Universität Berlin, Arnimallee 22, D-1000 Berlin 33, West Germany*

F. L. Graham, *Departments of Biology and Pathology, McMaster University, 1280 Main Street W, Hamilton, Ontario L8S 4K1, Canada*

G. Gregoriadis, *Medical Research Council Group, Academic Department of Medicine, Royal Free Hospital School of Medicine, Pond Street, London NW3 2QG, UK*

H. Grosjean, *Université Libre de Bruxelles, Laboratoire de Chimie Biologique, 67 rue des Chevaux, B-1640 Rhode St-Genèse, Belgium*

J. B. Gurdon, *CRC Molecular Embrology Unit, Department of Zoology, University of Cambridge, Downing Street, Cambridge CB2 3EJ, UK*

* *Present affiliation:* Department of Medical Biochemistry, Ole Worms Alle, Building 170, University Park, Aarhus University, DK-8000 Aarhus C, Denmark.

G. Huez, *Université Libre de Bruxelles, Département de Biologie Moléculaire, Laboratoire de Chimie Biologique, Rue des Chevaux 67, 1640 Rhode St-Genèse, Belgium*

E. Kubli, *Universität Zürich-Irchel, Zoologisches Institut, Winterthurerstrasse 190, CH-8057 Zürich, Switzerland*

A. Loyter, *Department of Biological Chemistry, Institute of Life Sciences, The Hebrew University of Jerusalem, 91904 Jerusalem, Israel*

R. D. McKinnon, *Research Institute of Scripps Clinic, 10666 N. Torrey Pines Road, La Jolla, CA 92037, USA*

C. Marbaix, *Université Libre de Bruxelles, Département de Biologie Moléculaire, Laboratoire de Chimie Biologique, Rue des Chevaux 67, 1640 Rhode St-Genèse, Belgium*

R. J. Mayer, *Department of Biochemistry, University of Nottingham Medical School, Queen's Medical Centre, Nottingham NG7 2UH, UK*

C. Nicolau, *Centre de Biophysique Moléculaire, C.N.R.S., 1A avenue de la Recherche Scientifique, 45045 Orléans Cédex, France*

O. Nussbaum, *Department of Biological Chemistry, Institute of Life Sciences, The Hebrew University of Jerusalem, 91904 Jerusalem, Israel*

D. Papahadjopoulos, *Cancer Research Institute, M-1282, University of California San Francisco, San Francisco, California 94143, USA*

M. S. Poonian, *Department of Molecular Genetics, Roche Research Center, Nutley, New Jersey 07110, USA*

M. C. Rechsteiner, *Department of Biology, University of Utah, Salt Lake City, Utah 84112, USA*

D. Röhme, *Institute of Genetics, University of Lund, Sölvegatan 29, S-223 62 Lund, Sweden*

R. A. Schlegel, *Molecular and Cell Biology Program, The Pennsylvania State University, University Park, PA 16802, USA*

J. Senior, *Medical Research Council Group, Academic Department of Medicine, Royal Free Hospital School of Medicine, Pond Street, London NW3 2QG, UK*

D. W. Stacey, *Roche Institute of Molecular Biology, Roche Research Center, Nutley, New Jersey 07110, USA*

R. M. Straubinger, *Cancer Research Institute, M-1282, University of California San Francisco, San Francisco, California 94143, USA*

L. Wakefield, *CRC Molecular Embryology Unit, Department of Zoology, University of Cambridge, Downing Street, Cambridge, CB2 3EJ, UK*

W. J. Welch, *Cold Spring Harbor Laboratory, Cold Spring Harbor, New York 11724, USA*

B. Wolff, *Medical Research Council Group, Academic Department of Medicine, Royal Free Hospital School of Medicine, Pond Street, London NW3 2QG, UK*

Preface

The development of techniques to introduce macromolecules and organelles into somatic cells, oocytes and eggs has opened up the possibility of using the cell as a test tube in which to study complex biological phenomena that are not amenable to experimentation using conventional *in vitro* systems. Refinements of the various techniques to the point at which they are accessible to any laboratory ensure that they will enjoy widespread application in all areas of biology. This volume attempts to present an overview of current procedures and to review a few areas of research in which these techniques are currently being applied.

The book has been divided into two sections—Part I: Transfer of Cell Constituents into Somatic Cells and Part II: Transfer of Macromolecules and Organelles into Oocytes and Eggs. The transfer of cell constituents into somatic cells can be brought about in a variety of ways, namely (i) by direct microinjection using glass capillaries, (ii) by vehicle-mediated transfer (erythrocyte, liposomes, reconstituted Sendai virus envelopes) and (iii) by the use of facilitators (calcium phosphate, DEAE dextran, etc.). A step-by-step guide to these techniques and details of their most commonly encountered applications are given in Part I. The potential of liposomes and reconstituted Sendai virus envelopes to deliver genes and drugs to whole organisms is discussed in this section, and chapters on fusion of cell fragments and microdissection of metaphase chromosomes for gene transfer are also included. Part II is dedicated mainly to microinjection and manipulation of amphibian oocytes and eggs. Particular emphasis is given to studies on nuclear transfer, gene injection, mRNA translation and functional aspects of microinjected tRNAs. The technology for transferring genes into mouse embryos is also described in this section.

We would like to thank the authors for their readiness to contribute to this volume. Our gratitude is also due to the staff of Academic Press for their help and cooperation with the completion of this work.

November 1985

J. E. Celis
A. Graessmann
A. Loyter

Contents

Part I

Transfer of Cell Constituents into Somatic Cells

1

Microinjection of Tissue Culture Cells using Glass Capillaries: Methods

M. Graessmann and A. Graessmann

I. INTRODUCTION

Microinjection of macromolecules into culture cells provides an efficient method of studying the biological activity and the fate of molecules in their native environment, the living cell. In 1971 it was shown for the first time that macromolecules are biologically active in microinjected cells. mRNA isolated from Harding Passey Melanoma cells was translated after injection into rat myotubes. Subsequently translation of rat haemoglobin mRNA was demonstrated in microinjected frog oocytes by Lane *et al.* (1971), and Gurdon *et al.* (1971).

Of the different transfer techniques available, direct microinjection is the most efficient (see also Chapter 12). Up to 100% of the recipient cells support expression of the injected material and transformed cell lines can be isolated with a frequency of 20–30% after microinjection of DNA (Graessmann *et al.*, 1979a; Capecchi, 1980). Furthermore, biochemical studies can be performed on a small number of injected cells (Celis *et al.*, 1980; Graessmann and Graessmann, 1982), and injected material can be reisolated and analysed by standard procedures such as blot analysis or electron microscopy using less than 100 injected cells (Graessmann *et al.*, 1983, 1985).

In this chapter we describe some technical aspects of the procedure. The direct microinjection technique is based on the use of small glass capillaries which allows the transfer of almost any type of test material (virus particles, DNA, RNA, protein, etc.) into the cytoplasma or the nuclei of culture cells. This technique has no cell type restriction and suspension culture cells can also be injected after binding the cells to the culture dish by a suitable linker (Graessmann *et al.*, 1980).

Microinjection and Organelle Transplantation Techniques

ISBN: 0-12-164722-6
ISBN: 0-12-164723-4 Pbk

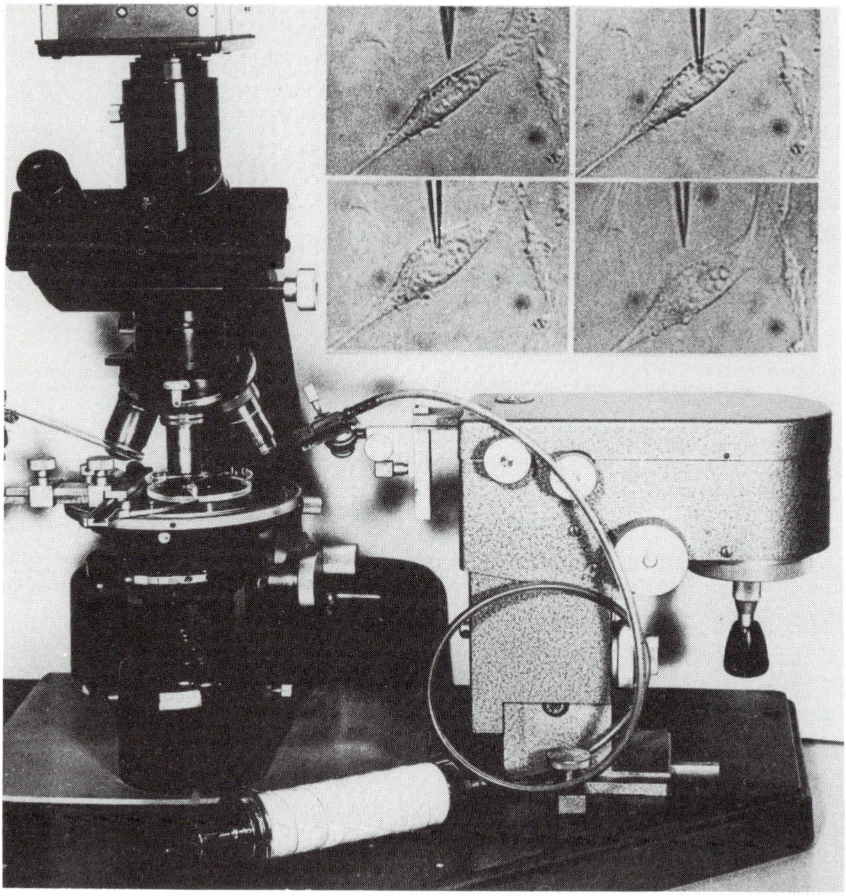

Fig. 1. Assembled instruments for microinjection. The inset photographs show four steps of the microinjection procedure.

II. PROCEDURES

A. General

Microinjection is performed under a phase-contrast microscope (Fig. 1): a glass microcapillary, pre-filled from the tip with the biological sample, is directed into the cells to be injected with the aid of a micromanipulator, and an appropriate sample volume is transferred by gentle air pressure exerted by a syringe connected to the capillary. Recipient cells are grown on glass slides imprinted with numbered squares for convenient localization of the cells injected.

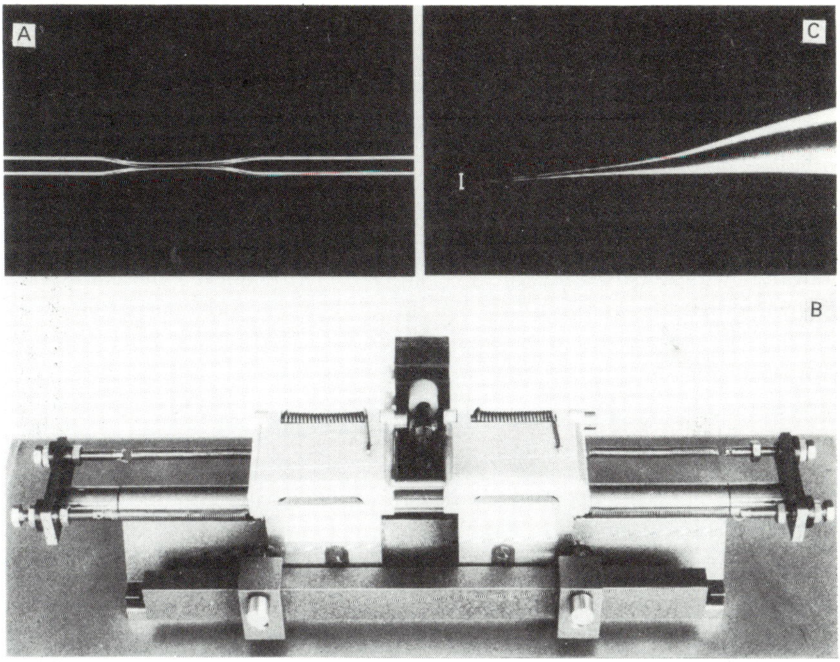

Fig. 2. Pulling of the glass microcapillaries. (A) Glass tube with constriction, (B) partial view of the drawing apparatus; (C) microcapillary tip. Bar = 10 μm.

B. Preparation of glass microcapillaries

Glass tubes of 1.2 mm inner and 1.5 mm outer diameter (SGA Scientific, Inc., Bloomfield, New Jersey, USA) are broken into pieces about 30 cm in length and cleaned by treatment with a mixture of one-third concentrated H_2SO_4 and two-thirds concentrated HNO_3 (v/v) for 24 h and by extensive washings with tap water, double distilled water, and ethanol (p.a.). Glass tubes pre-treated in this way and air-dried at 120°C for 24 h were kept in a closed container until use.

Before pulling the capillary, a constriction is introduced at the middle of the glass tube. This is done by hand, using the flame of a Bunsen burner. The glass is softened in the flame, and the ends are pulled apart, resulting in a constriction 8–15 mm in length and 0.3–0.5 mm in diameter (Fig. 2A). The glass tube is then clamped into a capillary puller, the middle of the constriction being surrounded by the heating wire (Fig. 2B). The shape of the capillary to be obtained is shown in Fig. 2C; the tip should be rigid and open, with an outer diameter of about 0.5 μm. Conditions for the mechanical pulling must be optimized by varying the temperature of the heating wire and the pulling forces at the carriage. The puller shown in Fig. 2B was built in our workshop.

The capillary tips are further treated by connecting the capillary to a 50 ml syringe, dipping the tip into 1–5% HF for 1 s, and then serially washing it by suction and pressure exerted by the syringe with double distilled water, ethanol (p.a.), tetrahydrofuran (p.a.), 0.5% dichlorodimethylsilane in tetrahydrofuran (v/v), and again with tetrahydrofuran and ethanol. This treatment produces a smooth capillary tip, but for most purposes it may be omitted without affecting the microinjection procedure. Capillaries are conveniently stored upright (tip end up) by inserting them into fitting holes pierced into a perspex block. The block is placed into a Petri dish and covered with a beaker. Capillaries are then air-dried at 120°C for 4 h.

C. Preparation of glass slides

Glass slides (5 × 1 cm) are coated on both sides with a melted mixture of one-third beeswax and two-thirds stearine (w/w) using a cotton plug, resulting in a thin, supple film. This film is then scored (squares of 1 or 4 mm^2) and numbered (Fig. 3) with a steel needle; the glass is etched with a paste made from CaF_2 (precipitated) and 40% HF, which is spread over the slide and left there for 10–15 min. The slides are held under running tap water overnight to split off the wax. Finally the slides are treated with a mixture of one-third concentrated HNO_3 (v/v), washed with running tap water for 24 h, followed by washings with double distilled water and ethanol (p.a.). They are air-dried, wrapped in aluminium foil, sterilized in an oven at 200°C for 24 h, and stored until use.

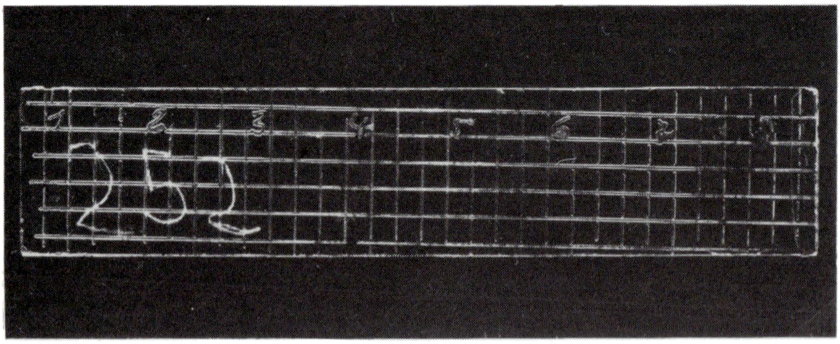

Fig. 3. Scored and numbered glass slides.

D. Cells

Cells are grown on plastic dishes or slides (Fig. 3) under standard conditions. Cells growing in suspension culture become accessible to microinjection after they have been bound to a substrate by suitable linkers (e.g. concanavalin A, phytohaemagglutinin P, poly(L-lysine), pockweed mitogen, IgG).

Figure 4 shows Friend leukemia cells unattached (Fig. 4A) and attached to the plastic surface of a Petri dish via concanavalin A (Fig. 4B). For this, a 60 mm Petri dish was incubated for 2 h with 2.5 ml of 2.5% glutaraldehyde at room temperature, washed four times with sterile water, covered with 200 μl of concanavalin A (100 μg/ml), and kept for 1–2 h at 37°C in an incubator. After drying, the dish was washed with PBS without Mg^{2+} and Ca^{2+}, and the cells were plated.

E. Sample

Whenever feasible, the material to be injected is dissolved in injection buffer (0.048 M K_2HPO_4, 0.014 M NaH_2PO_4, 0.0045 M KH_2PO_4, pH 7.2), but other compositions, such as 0.01–0.1 M Tris-HCl, pH 7.2, will be tolerated by the cells. Concentrations up to 1 mg of DNA, 5–10 mg of RNA, or 10–20 mg of protein per ml of injection solution can be handled. The sample is centrifuged (Eppendorf) for 10 min directly before microinjection and then transferred as a small drop to a 60 mm plastic Petri dish furnished with a moistened filter paper. The drop is placed on a small sheet of Parafilm, a volume of 2 μl being sufficient. The sample dish is kept on ice. We normally fill the needle under the microscope from the tip. This has the advantage that dust particles inside move away with the meniscus. Backfilling brings the particles down to the tip, very often blocking the needle. Only glass material without an inner filament is used.

F. Microinjection

A Leitz Ortholux microscope with phase-contrast equipment (Phaco 10/0.25 objective lens, Periplan GF 16 × oculars) and a Leitz micromanipulator (Fig. 1) are employed for microinjection in our laboratory. These instruments are placed vibration-free in a room reserved for the purpose, which can be UV-sterilized for long-term experiments. The microcapillary is fixed to the instrument holder of the manipulator, and the tip is focused under the microscope. Next, the sample drop is brought into the plane of focus and the needle is filled by capillary attraction forces supported by negative pressure exerted by the syringe. The capillary tip is slightly raised by turning the

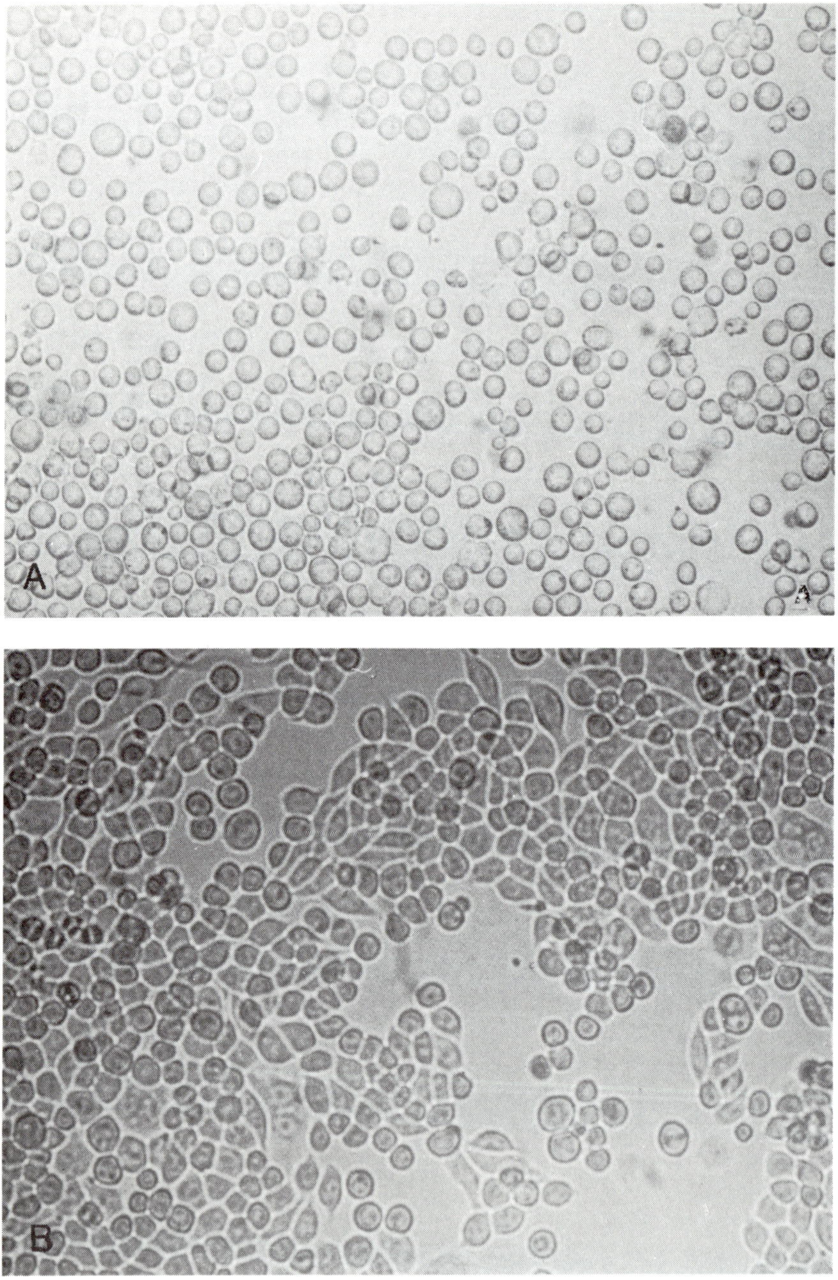

Fig. 4. Friend leukemia cells. (A) Unattached; (B) attached to the Petri dish.

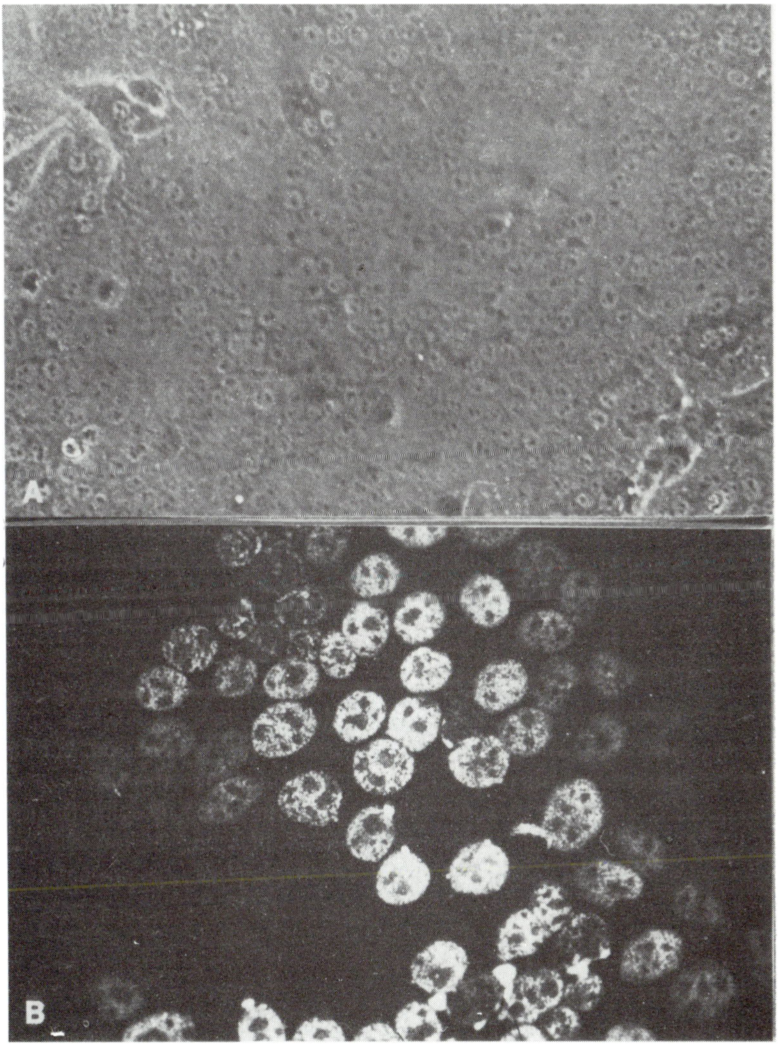

Fig. 5. (A) Partial view of fused HeLa cells with several hundred nuclei. (B) T antigen positive nuclei of fused HeLa cells, fixed and stained 24 h after injection of SV40 DNA. The nuclei are located in different planes, therefore some are out of focus.

vertical adjustment knob of the manipulator, and the cells (immersed in medium in an open 60 mm Petri dish) are placed on the microscope stage. A gentle stream of CO_2 maintains the optimum pH. Cells are brought into focus, and a distinct field is chosen for injection. The capillary is now lowered until it is almost in focus, and an individual cell is approached by operating the manipulator lever for horizontal movements. The cell is injected by further lowering the capillary tip once it is directly above the cells. Both movements of the capillary are controlled by one hand (the right), while the other hand exerts a gentle pressure on the syringe. A dent is seen on the cell surface when the capillary touches the cell. Microinjection itself is marked by a slight enlargement (swelling) of the cell, and the nucleus gains in contrast. Either the nucleus or the cytoplasm can be injected. After transfer of the sample, the capillary tip is raised just above the plane of the cell layer and moved to the next cell. About 150–200 cells can be injected within 10 min with some practice. After microinjection, cells are maintained as usual, checked at appropriate intervals for possible cytotoxic effects of the sample, and finally processed for evaluation.

The volume injected per cell can be estimated by measuring the distance covered by the meniscus within the pipette after microinjection of a certain number of cells and by determining the inner diameter of the capillary. By this method, we determined a mean injection volume of between 1×10^{-11} and 2×10^{-11} ml per fibroblast culture cell, but up to 10^{-10} ml can be transferred. Another approach is to microinject a radiolabelled compound of high specific activity.

The injection volume per cell can be enlarged by a factor of 10^4–10^5 using as recipients multinucleated giant cells generated by the fusion of tissue culture cells with appropriate agents (Fig. 5) (Graessmann *et al.*, 1979b).

Optimal fusion conditions must be tested for each individual cell line. Variables are (a) the choice of the fusion agent, e.g. polyethylene glycol 1000 or 6000, inactivated Sendai virus; (b) concentration and time of action of the fusion agent; (c) density of cells before fusion; and (d) mode of washing the cells after fusion.

III. GENERAL FEATURES OF THE DIRECT MICROINJECTION TECHNIQUE

For a comparison with related techniques developed for the transfer of biomaterials into eukaryotic cells, the following list of general features of the direct microinjection system (see also Table I) may be helpful (see also Chapter 12).

1. Every tissue culture cell line tested so far has proved to be suitable for microinjection; suspension culture cells, e.g. lymphocytes, are prepared for microinjection by binding them to a substrate via suitable linkers.

2. Virtually no limitations exist regarding the material to be transferred. Intact virions, DNAs, RNAs, and proteins as well as small metabolites or substances unrelated to cellular metabolism can be introduced in purified form without the involvement of helper macromolecules or chemical treatment. The number of molecules transferred is directly correlated to the concentration of the injection solution and to the volume transferred per cell. Even intact cell organelles, e.g. cell nuclei, can be implanted into culture cells by microinjection (Graessmann, 1970).

3. The site of inoculation within the recipient cell — nucleus or cytoplasm — can be chosen by the investigator. This allows studies on intracellular transport and compartmentalization, compartment-dependent modification steps, etc.

4. A sample volume of about 2 μl is sufficient for microinjection; most of this material is retained for other experiments.

5. The number and localization of recipient cells are known.

6. Injected cells respond efficiently and remain as viable as their uninjected neighbours provided that the material transferred has no cytopathic effects.

Table I. General features of the direct microinjection technique.

	Single adherent tissue culture cells	Suspension culture cells, fixed to dish	Fused cells; PEG-1000 as fusion agent
Recipient cells	Primary or secondary cells; all permanent cell lines	Lymphocytes	Permanent cell lines: lymphocytes
Material transferable	Cell organelles, viruses, DNA, RNA, proteins, etc.	Viruses, DNA, RNA, proteins, etc.	Viruses, DNA, RNA, proteins, etc.
Site of application	Nucleus/ cytoplasm	Nucleus/ cytoplasm	Cytoplasm
Injection volume per cell (ml)	10^{-10}–10^{-11}	10^{-11}	10^{-6}–10^{-5}
Method of analysis	Biological/ biochemical	Biological/ biochemical	Biochemical/ biological
Efficiency (%)	90–100	90–100	70–90

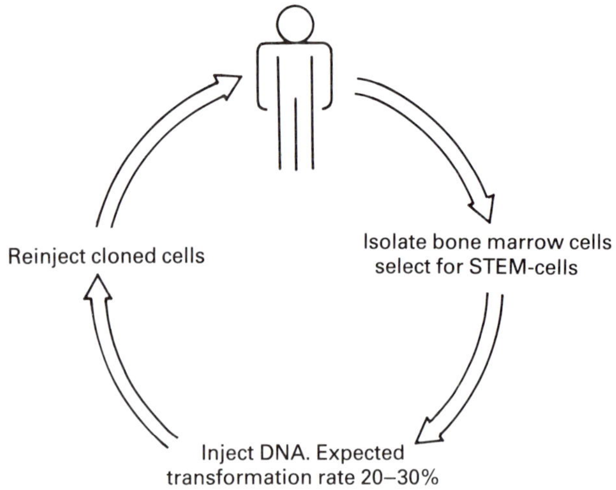

Fig. 6. Possible application of the direct microinjection technique.

The direct microinjection technique is restricted, however, to the use of cultured cells as recipients; it is not applicable to intact organisms. Yet it is conceivable that we could isolate cells from individuals (e.g. bone marrow cells), passage them *in vitro*, and clone out lines from injected cells. The donor individual could then be the recipient for these cells (Fig. 6).

ACKNOWLEDGEMENTS

This work was supported by the Deutsche Forschungsgemeinschaft, Grants Gr.384/5-9 and Gr.599-3 and by the Verband der Chemischen Industrie eV, 1428.

REFERENCES

Celis, J. E., Graessmann, A. and Loyter, A., eds. (1980). "Transfer of Cell Constituents into Eukaryotic Cells". Plenum Press, New York.

Capecchi, M. R. (1980). *Cell* **22**, 479–488.

Graessmann, A. (1970). *Exp. Cell Res.* **60**, 373–382.

Graessmann, A. and Graessmann, M. (1971). *Hoppe-Seyler's Z. Physiol. Chem.* **352**, 527–532.

Graessmann, A., Graessmann, M., Topp, W. C. and Botchan, M. (1979a). *J. Virol.* **32**, 989–994.

Graessmann, A., Graessmann, M. and Mueller, C. (1979b). *Biochem. Biophys. Res. Commun.* **88**, 428–432.

Graessmann, A., Wolf, H. and Bornkamm, G. W. (1980). *Proc. Natl. Acad. Sci. USA* **77**, 433–436.

Graessmann, M. and Graessmann, A. (1982). *EMBO J.* **1**, 1081–1088.

Graessmann, M., Graessmann, A. and Westphal, H. (1983). *J. Virol.* **48**, 296–299.

Graessmann, A., Bumke-Vogt, C., Buschhausen, G., Bauer, M. and Graessmann, M. (1985). *FEBS Lett.*, **179**, 41–45.

Gurdon, J. B., Lane, C. D., Woodland, H. R. and Marbaix, G. (1971). *Nature* **253**, 177–182.

Lane, C. D., Marbaix, G., Gurdon, J. B. (1971). *J. Mol. Biol.* **61**, 73–91.

2

Transformation Capacity of SV40 DNA and Subgenomic DNA Fragments

M. Graessmann and A. Graessmann

I. INTRODUCTION

Oncogenic cell transformation is efficiently induced by direct microinjection of SV40 DNA or DNA fragments. On average, between 15 and 30% of the injected cells are converted into transformed cell lines (A. Graessmann *et al.*, 1979; Capecchi, 1980; A. Graessmann *et al.*, 1981). Induction and maintenance of the transformed state require expression of the early genome part. The genome region encodes for two related proteins, the large tumour (T) antigen and the small t antigen (for review see Tooze, 1980). Experiments with small t antigen negative mutants have shown that synthesis of the large T antigen is sufficient to cause cell transformation (Lewis and Martin, 1979; Seif and Martin, 1979; Topp and Rifkin, 1980). In the meantime many details about the T antigen have become known, but it is still unclear which of the T antigen specific functions is responsible for the viral oncogenicity. This matter is complicated by the fact that the T antigen is a pleiotropic effector with multiple biological and biochemical functions. To name only a few, T antigen is a DNA binding protein with an inherent ATPase and an associated protein kinase activity; it induces cellular and viral DNA replication, stimulates cellular RNA and protein synthesis and carries out a helper function for adenovirus in monkey cells (Rabson *et al.*, 1964; Friedmann *et al.*, 1970; Martin and Chou, 1975; M. Graessmann and A. Graessmann, 1976; Tjian, 1978; Mueller *et al.*, 1978; Tjian and Robins, 1979; Galanti *et al.*, 1981; A. Graessmann *et al.*, 1981; McKay, 1981). Some of these functions were mapped by microinjection of different early SV40 DNA fragments (A. Graessmann *et al.*, 1976; Mueller *et al.*, 1978;

Microinjection and Organelle Transplantation Techniques

ISBN: 0-12-164722-6
ISBN: 0-12-164723-4 Pbk

M. Graessmann *et al.*, 1980; Soprano *et al.*, 1981). In these experiments only transient expression of the injected DNA fragments was tested.

To learn if the SV40 transformation activity can be attributed to one of the two "T antigen exons", the biological functions and transformation capacities of the PstI A-DNA fragment (m.p. 0.039–0.272) and of the TaqI/BamHI fragment (m.p. 0.566–0.144) were analysed in this investigation. The Pst fragment contains the intact coding region for the small t antigen, the first large T antigen exon and about 70% of the second T antigen exon (see Fig. 1). Permanent expression of this fragment required coinjection of a polyadenylation signal containing DNA segment (polyoma virus Pst D-DNA fragment m.p. 0.168–0.331). The TaqI/BamH1 DNA fragment codes only for the intact second T antigen exon. Expression of this fragment was possible by coinjection of the early SV40 promotor/enhancer-HpaII/BglI DNA fragment (m.p. 0.725–0.661, see Fig. 7).

Cell lines isolated from cells injected with Pst DNA fragments exhibit different parameters of wild type transformed cells, but do not grow in soft agar. In contrast, maximally transformed cell lines with a high rate of anchorage independent growth were obtained after injection of the HpaII/BglI and Taq/Bam SV40 DNA fragments.

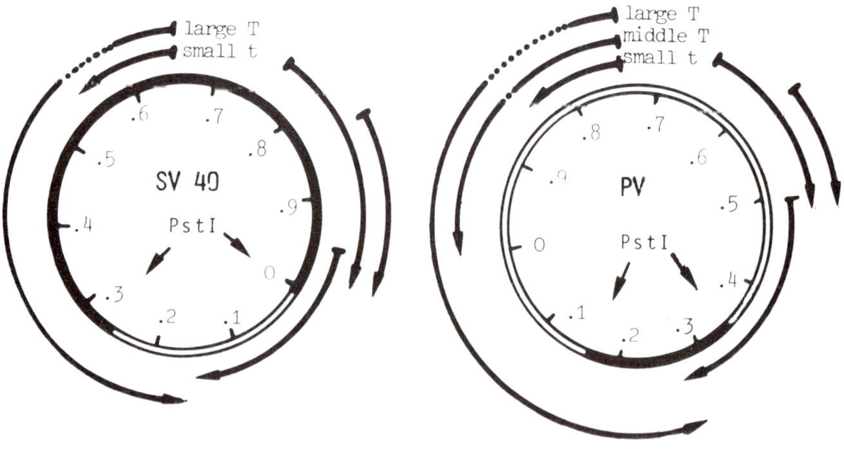

Fig. 1. Assignment of the SV40 PstI A fragment (m.p. 0.272–0.039; nucleotides 3187–1971, filled part of the circle) and of the PV PstI D fragment (m.p. 0.168–0.331, nucleotides 2451–3313) to the physical maps of the SV40 and PV genomes. Arrayed around the outside of the circle are the positions of the early and late viral coded proteins (Tooze, 1980).

Table I. Biological activity of early SV40 fragments and cRNA.

	Antigenicity*			DNA synthesis†		Helper function of AD2 virus in TC7 cells	Reduction of‡ actin cables
	T	N	C	Cellular	Viral		
SV40 DNA I	+	+	+	+	N.D.	+	+
Pst-A-fragment	+	+	−	+	−	−	+
Taq/Bam fragment	−	−	−	N.D.		N.D.	N.D.
Taq/Bam-cRNA	+	−	+	+	−	+	−
HpaII/BglI fragment	−	−	−				
Taq/Bam + HpaII/BglI fragments	+	−	+	+	−	N.D.	−

* Antigenicity was tested by the indirect immunofluorescence staining technique.

† Stimulation of cellular DNA synthesis was tested on cultures of primary mouse kidney cells as described (M. Graessmann and A. Graessmann, 1976). To analyse viral DNA replication, TC7 cells were microinjected with the test material, then infected with tsA 58 virus and further cultivated at the non-permissive temperature of 41.5°C. One day later, cells were fixed and stained for V antigen.

‡ Change of the cytoskeleton structure was demonstrated by double staining the cells with fluorescein-conjugated anti-T serum and rhodamine B-conjugated anti-actin serum (kindly provided by K. Weber).

N.D. = not determined.

II. BIOLOGICAL ACTIVITY OF THE SV40 Pst DNA FRAGMENT

The map position of the SV40 Pst A DNA fragment (m.p. 0.27 to 0.03) is shown in Fig. 1. By microinjection into tissue culture cells, different T antigen-specific functions were attributed to the early SV40 DNA segment as summarized in Table I. Since maintenance of the transformed state requires permanent expression of the early SV40 genome region (Martin and Chou, 1975; Osborn and Weber, 1975; Tegtmeyer, 1975), the time-course of T antigen synthesis in cells injected with Pst A DNA fragment was analysed. Ref 52 cells (Fisher rat embryo fibroblasts provided by W.C. Topp, Cold Spring Harbor) were microinjected into the nuclei with a multiplicity of 200 to 400 DNA fragment molecules per cell. At different times after injection, cells were fixed and stained for T antigen by the indirect immunofluorescence technique. These experiments have shown that T antigen synthesis is demonstrable only up until 100 to 120 h after injection. At later times, the recipient cells always stained negative for T antigen

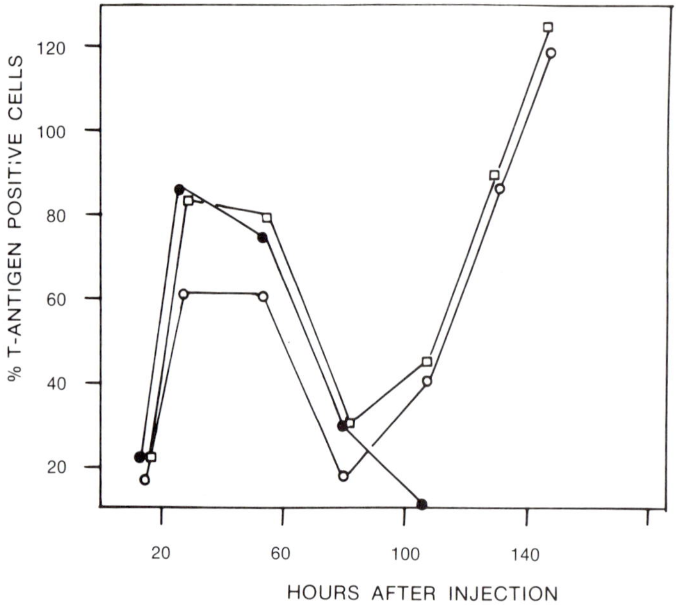

Fig. 2. Time-course of T antigen synthesis in Ref 52 cells after microinjection of: (●) SV40 Pst A DNA fragment; (○) HpaII/BglI and Taq/Bam SV40 DNA fragment mixture; and (□) SV40 Pst A DNA fragment and the PV Pst D DNA fragment. Cells were fixed and stained with anti-T serum isolated from tumour-bearing hamster by the indirect immunofluorescence technique at the time points indicated.

(Fig. 2). Similar results were obtained with an antiserum specific for the first eight amino residues of the N terminus of T antigen (N antigenicity). The cells always stained negative after treatment with an antiserum specific for the last 11 amino acid residues of the C terminus of T antigen (C antigenicity). These antisera were kindly provided by G. Walter (Walter *et al.*, 1980). To determine whether the transient expression of the Pst DNA fragment is correlated with the loss of the injected Pst fragment, we coinjected the Pst fragment with the HSV I thymidine kinase gene into the TK minus rat 2 cells. One day after injection, cells were transferred into HAT medium supplemented with 5% fetal calf serum. Based on the number of injected cells, TK positive clones were isolated with a frequency of between 1 and 5%. Cellular DNA was extracted from two randomly chosen T antigen negative lines, and analysed by the Southern blotting technique (Southern, 1975; Botchan *et al.*, 1976). These experiments showed that the DNA of both T antigen negative cell lines contain multiple SV40 Pst fragment insertions (data not shown). We have not tested whether these cells synthesize SV40 RNA.

III. TRANSFORMATION CAPACITY OF THE SV40 Pst DNA FRAGMENT

Permanent expression of the SV40 Pst fragment was obtained after coinjection with a DNA segment containing the putative polyadenylation signal (A–A–T–A–A–A). For this purpose the PV Pst D fragment was chosen (m.p. 0.168–0.331). This PV DNA segment has the same cohesive ends as the SV40 Pst fragment, and contains the A–A–T–A–A–A sequence in both possible ligation orientations (Fig. 1) (Soeda *et al.*, 1980). Both fragments were microinjected into the nuclei of Ref 52 cells without prior ligation *in vitro*. The concentration of each fragment was 0.1 mg per ml of injection buffer. Under these conditions, the number of T antigen positive cells increased again about 80 to 120 h after injection (Fig. 2). The T antigen positive cells appeared in clusters.

To obtain cell lines that permanently express the Pst DNA fragment, 200 Ref 52 cells were microinjected in groups of 25 with the DNA fragment mixture. The Ref 52 cells were chosen for these experiments, as Ref 52 is an exceptionally untransformed established rat line, which in our hands has not shown any spontaneous colony formation in soft agar. Recipient cells were grown on glass slides subdivided into numbered squares 2 mm × 2 mm. One week after injection cells within these squares were isolated and cultivated further in microwells (M. Graessmann and A. Graessmann, 1983). After the second passage in 60 mm dishes, control slides with the cells were stained for T antigen. From the eight independent isolates obtained, six contained T antigen positive cells. Further enrichment of T antigen positive cells was obtained by mild trypsinization and serial dilution. Between passage number 5 to 8, the lines contained, on average, 90 to 95% T antigen positive cells. Selective pressure, e.g. low serum concentration, was not applied. These lines were designated Ref-Pst lines 1 to 6. To test the state of the SV40 and PV Pst DNA fragments, DNA was extracted from the Ref-Pst line 6 cells. Following the restriction of the DNA with different restriction endonucleases, duplicate blots were prepared. One was hybridized with nick-translated SV40 DNA and the other with nick-translated PV DNA.

As shown in Fig. 3A, lane 3, the DNA of the Ref-Pst line 6 cells carries one prominent SV40 DNA insertion. The cellular DNA in this lane was restricted with the BglII endonuclease, an enzyme that does not cut the SV40 or the PV DNA fragments. Part B of the blot hybridized with PV DNA shows one insertion in lane 3 (see Fig. 3B), which is in the same position as the strong SV40 DNA band. After digestion of the cellular DNA with endonuclease EcoRI, two SV40-specific bands were obtained, the upper still connected to the PV DNA (lanes 1). The EcoRI enzyme cleaves the SV40 DNA at map position 00, but does not cut the PV DNA fragment. Digestion

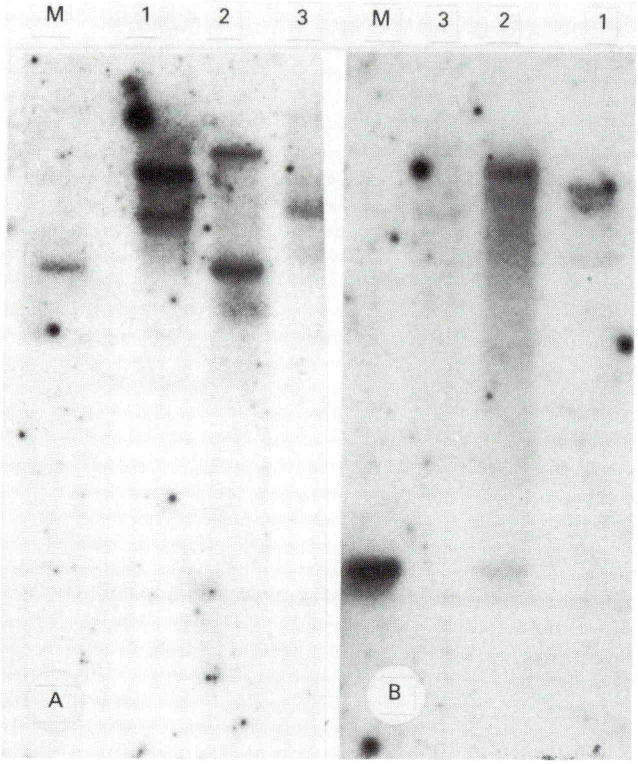

Fig. 3. Southern blotting analysis of the Ref-Pst line 6. The restriction endonuclease digests of 5–10 μg genomic DNA were fractionated by electrophoresis on a 1% agarose gel and transferred to one nitrocellulose sheet which was divided into two parts. Part A was hybridized with nick-translated ^{32}P-SV40 DNA, and part B with nick-translated ^{32}P-PV DNA. M contains as marker a mixture of the fragments SV40 Pst A DNA and PV Pst D DNA. High relative molecular mass cellular DNA of Ref-Pst line 6 restricted in lane 1 with $EcoR_I$, in lane 2 with PstI and in lane 3 with BglII.

of the cellular DNA with endonuclease PstI separated a portion of the SV40 from the PV fragment insertion and generated both viral DNA fragments of the original size (lanes 2). These results support the assumption that the SV40 and PV fragments are cointegrated directly in a tandem array in the Ref-Pst line 6 cell DNA. DNA re-extraction experiments and blot analysis have shown that oligomerization of the DNA fragments by end-to-end ligation starts as early as one to three minutes after intranuclear microinjection in the recipient cells (Graessmann *et al.*, unpub. res.). The cells of all six Ref-Pst lines permanently synthesize the intact small t antigen and a truncated large T antigen (Pst T antigen). The relative molecular mass of this Pst T antigen as deduced from the DNA sequence should be about 66×10^3.

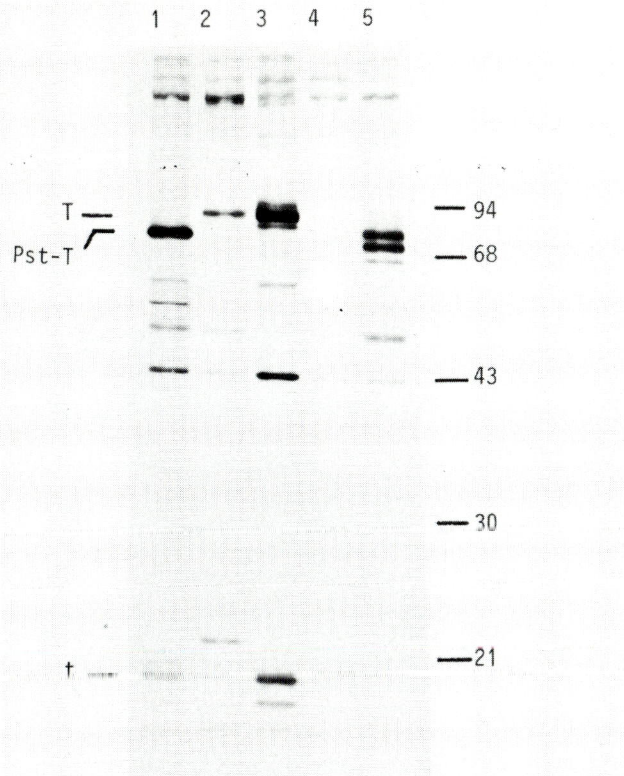

Fig. 4. Fluorogram of a SDS-polyacrylamide gel (7–15%) of proteins immunoprecipitated with anti-T serum. Immunoprecipitates of the following cell lines: lane 1, Ref-Pst line 6; lane 2, Ref-wt; lane 3, cos 7; lane 4, Ref 52; lane 5, Ref-Taq/Bam line 5.

However, on sodium dodecyl sulphate/polyacrylamide gels, this polypeptide migrates more slowly than expected (Fig. 4, lane 1). A Pst T antigen polypeptide with the same mobility was also synthesized in Ref 52 cells after microinjection of the SV40 Pst cRNA. RNA complementary to this particular SV40 DNA segment was obtained by transcription *in vitro* with *Escherichia coli* DNA-dependent RNA polymerase (M. Graessmann and A. Graessmann, 1976). Under similar experimental conditions, the intact large wild-type T antigen also migrated more slowly than expected. Calculated from the amino acid composition of T antigen, this protein has a relative moleculary mass of 82×10^3 but it migrates on SDS-containing gels as a 92×10^3 protein (Fig. 4, lane 2).

There is no obvious explanation for the difference between calculated size and mobility on SDS/polyacrylamide gels, but this is generally observed with

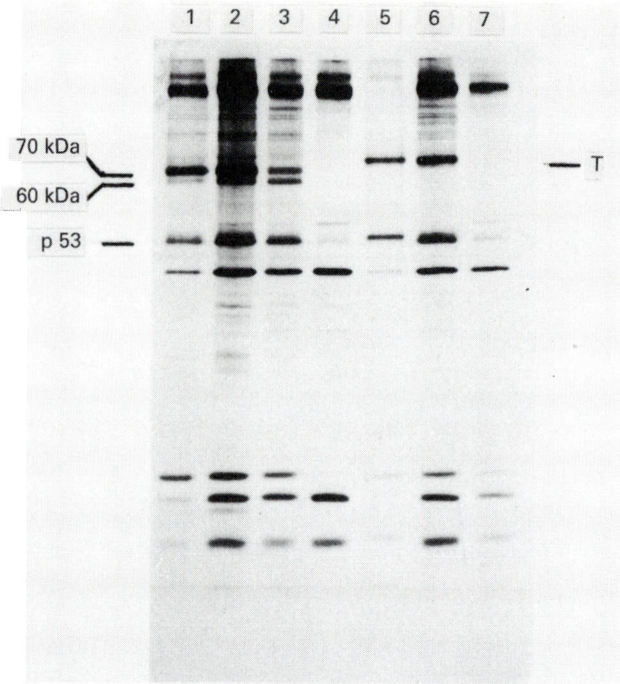

Fig. 5. Fluorogram of a SDS-polyacrylamide gel (7–15%) of proteins immunoprecipitated with anti-p53 serum (kindly provided by E. Gurney) from the following cells: Lane 1, Ref-Taq/Bam line 5_{agar}; lane 2, Ref-Taq/Bam line 5; lane 3, Ref-Taq/Bam line 4; lane 4, Ref-Pst line 6; lane 5, Ref-wt; lane 6, Cos 7; lane 7, Ref 52.

T antigen synthesized both *in vivo* and *in vitro* (Pauscha *et al.*, 1978; M. Graessmann and A. Graessmann, 1982; Rawlins *et al.*, 1983). So far, we cannot exclude that the Pst T antigen is a fusion protein that contains also some amino acids coded by the PV Pst DNA fragment. Fingerprint analysis of T antigen should give an answer to this question. A large range of different tumour cell types, including SV40-transformed rat cells, contain the cellular p53 protein at elevated concentrations (Levine, 1982). We tested the p53 concentration in the Ref-Pst cells by immunofluorescence staining (serum was kindly provided by E. Gurney) and gel electrophoresis. Both methods have shown that all Ref-Pst cells contain the p53 protein at the same concentration as the parental Ref 52 cells (Fig. 5, lanes 4 and 7). To analyse the transformation capacity of the SV40 Pst fragment, different parameters specific for SV40-transformed rat cells were tested (Pollack *et al.*, 1974). These included the reduction of the cytoplasmic actin cable structure, pericellular matrix change (fibronectin), secretion of plasminogen activators and serum requirement. All these criteria were found to be associated with

Table II. Transformation parameters of the Ref 52 transformed cell lines.

Cell type	Antigenicity				Fibronectin*	Growth at low serum concentration	Secretion of plasminogen activator	Growth in soft agar
	T	N	C	p53				
Ref 52	−	−	−	−	+++	−	+	−
Ref-wt	+	+	+	+	+	+	+++	+++
Ref-Pst line 6	+	+	−	−	++	+	++	−
Ref-Taq/Bam line 5	+	−	+	+	+	+	+++	++
Ref-Taq/Bam line 7	+	−	+	+	+++	+	++	−

* The pericellular fibronectin content was tested on formaldehyde fixed cells with anti fibronectin serum, kindly provided by R. Hynes. Observations qualified on follows: +++ > ++ > +.

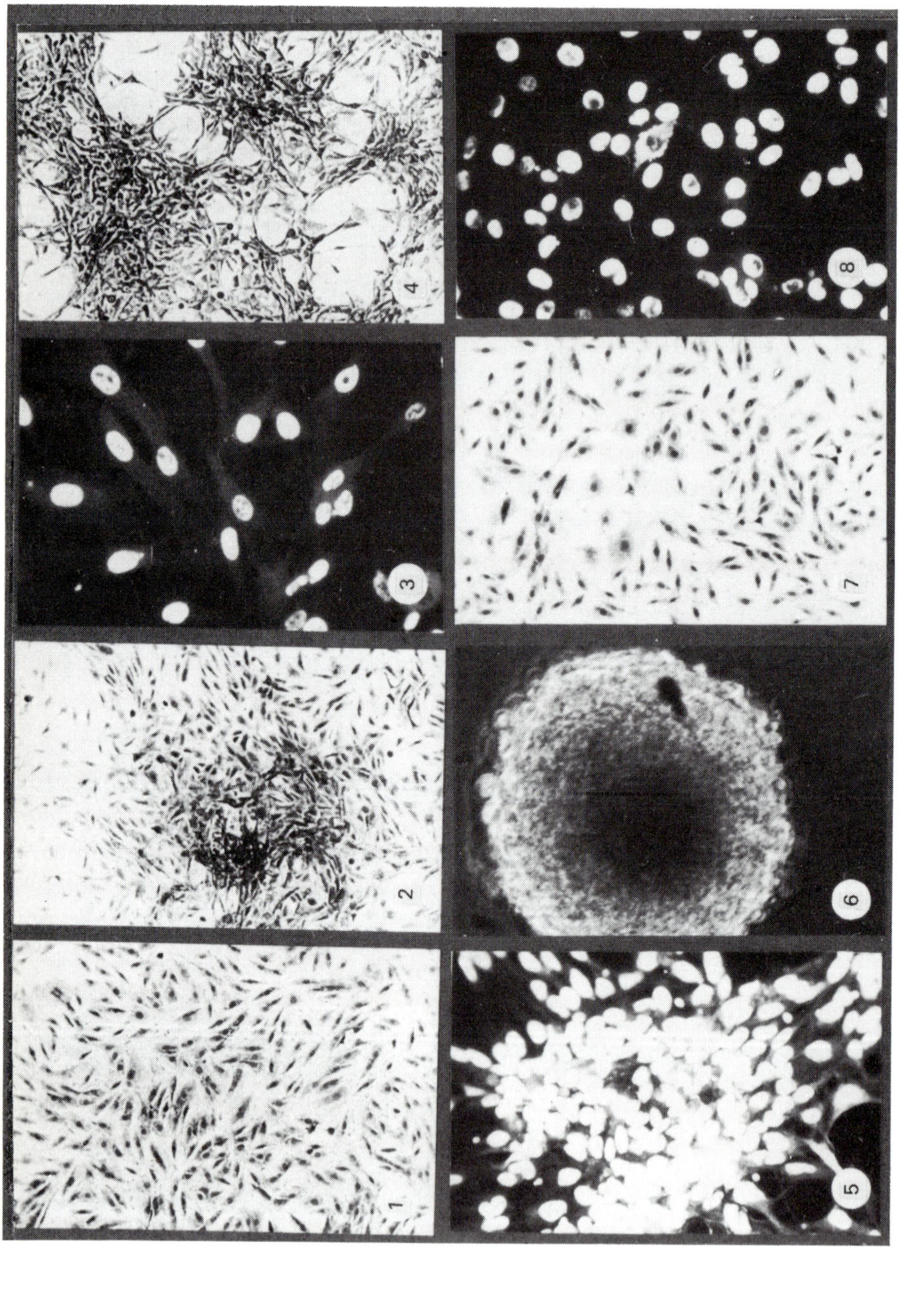

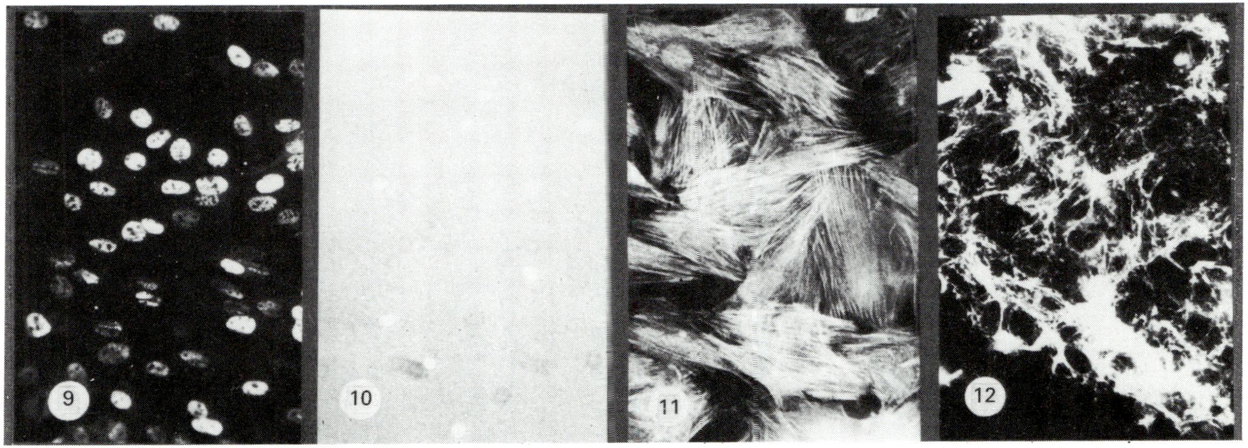

Fig. 6. Morphology of SV40 DNA fragment transformed cells. (1) Phase contrast picture of confluent Ref 52 cells; (2) the Ref-Pst line 6 cells; (3) T antigen positive Ref-Pst line 6 cells; (4) Ref-Taq/Bam line 5 cells; (5) T antigen positive Ref-Taq/Bam line 5 cells; (6) a clone of a Ref-Taq/Bam line 5, 2 weeks after plating into soft agar; (7) (×320) Ref-Taq/Bam line 7 cells; (8) T antigen positive Ref-Taq/Bam line 7 cells; (9) Ref-Taq/Bam line 7 cells stained with anti p53 serum; (10) Ref-Taq/Bam line 7 cells, 2 weeks after plating into soft agar; (11) Ref-Taq/Bam line 7 cells stained with anti-actin serum; (12) Ref-Taq/Bam cells stained with anti-fibronectin (kindly provided by R. Hynes).

Table III. Colony formation in soft agar (in % of the input cells) at different passage numbers.

Cell type	Passage number		
	10–15	20–25	50–60
Ref 52	N.D.	0	0
Ref-wt	1–2	30–40	40–50
Ref-Pst line 6	0.0	0.0	0.0
Ref-Taq/Bam line 5	0.05–0.1	0.1–0.2	1–2
Ref-Taq/Bam line 5_{agar}	60–80	60–80	N.D.
Ref-Taq/Bam line 7	0.0	0.0	0.0

Anchorage-independent growth was tested by colony formation in soft agar. Colonies were counted 15–18 days after plating. N.D. = not determined.

the Ref-Pst cells to an extent typical for wild-type SV40-transformed cells (Ref-wt: Table II). Also the morphology and the growth characteristic of the Ref-Pst cells resembled that of the Ref-wt cells. The Ref-Pst cells are smaller than the parental cells, reach a high cell density and overgrow the Ref 52 cells (Fig. 6). However, anchorage-independent growth, the major criterion *in vitro* for fully transformed cells, was not demonstrable (Pollack *et al.*, 1974; Risser and Pollack, 1974). Following plating into agar or agarose with different concentrations of fetal calf serum (5%, 10% and 20% final), the Ref-Pst cells always remained as single cells for at least three weeks. Under similar conditions, Ref-wt cells formed large colonies with an efficiency of 40 to 50% of the input cells (Table III).

IV. BIOLOGICAL ACTIVITY OF THE SECOND LARGE SV40 T ANTIGEN EXON

In order to test the biological activity of the second large T antigen exon exclusively, SV40 DNA I was cleaved with endonucleases TaqI and BamHI. As shown in Fig. 7, the Taq/Bam DNA B fragment (m.p. 0.566–0.144) codes only for this part of the T antigen. After preparation and ligation of SalI linkers, the Taq/Bam fragment was inserted into the Sal site of the pBR322 DNA and cloned in *E. coli* (Mueller *et al.*, 1978). To test the biological activity, the Taq/Bam DNA fragment was liberated from the plasmid by treatment with SalI, purified by agarose gel electrophoresis, and microinjected into the nuclei of TC7 (a subline of the African green monkey kidney cells CV1) and Ref 52 cells. As expected, the promotor minus DNA fragment was biologically inactive. None of the recipient cells synthesized T

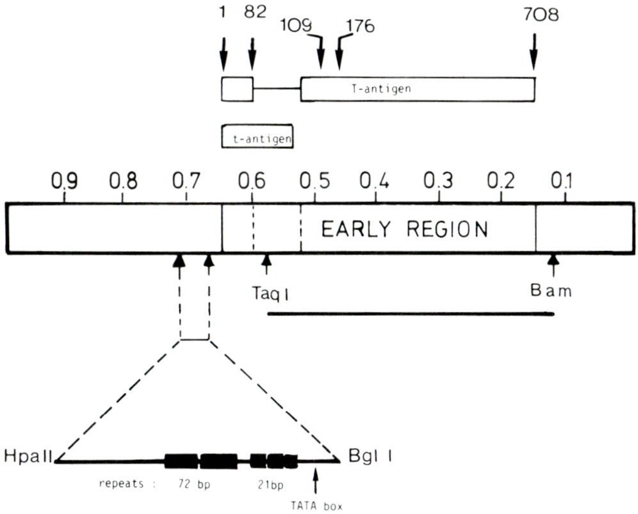

Fig. 7. Assignment of the HpaII/BglI (nucleotides 5218–329) and TaqI/Bam H_1 (nucleotides 2516–4722) DNA fragments to the physical map of the SV40 genome (Tooze, 1980). On the left at the bottom of the figure is an amplification of the HpaII/BglI fragment with the positions of 72 bp and 21 bp repeats and the TATA box. The bars at the top indicate the positions of small t antigen and of the two large T antigen exons. Arrows numbered 109 and 176 above the bar indicate the positions of the first two methionine residues of the second T antigen exon

antigen in detectable amounts. In order to test whether RNA specific for the Taq/Bam DNA fragment is translatable, we transcribed the fragment *in vitro* with *E. coli* DNA-dependent RNA polymerase, and injected the cRNA into TC7 and Ref 52 cells (cRNA concentration 0.5 mg/ml; M. Graessmann and A. Graessmann,, 1976). The recipient cells were fixed and stained for T antigen at different times after injection. Intranuclear T antigen accumulation was first demonstrable 2 to 3 h after injection, and about 50% of the cells stained positive for T antigen 20 h later. The same pattern of fluorescence was obtained with the anti-C serum but not with the anti-N serum (Table I). These experiments have shown that a second T antigen exon specific RNA can be translated *in vivo*, although this RNA does not have the authentic 5′ end of the early SV40 mRNA. To test further if the second large T antigen exon *per se* is biologically active, two T antigen specific functions were analysed; namely, stimulation of cell DNA synthesis and helper function for adenovirus serotype 2 (AD2) in monkey cells (Tjian *et al.*, 1978). Stimulation of cell DNA synthesis was tested in confluent cultures of primary mouse kidney cells. After cRNA injection, (^{3}H)-thymidine (final concentration 0.1 μCi/ml) was added to the culture medium for 20 h. Thereafter, cells were fixed and stained for T antigen and processed for autoradiography. These experiments have shown that the Taq/Bam cRNA has the capability of inducing cell DNA synthesis. About 80% of T antigen positive cells incorporated thymidine (mock-injected cells only 5%). The Taq/Bam cRNA also acts as helper for AD2 in monkey cells. TC7 cells, pre-injected with the cRNA and infected with the virus (5–10 pfu/cell), synthesized the adenovirus fibre protein as tested by immunofluorescence staining (Table I). Synthesis of this protein is an indirect marker for AD2 DNA replication and hence for helper activity.

V. TRANSFORMATION CAPACITY OF THE SECOND LARGE SV40 T ANTIGEN EXON

Further, we asked whether expression of the Taq/Bam fragment can be obtained by coinjection with the SV40 HpaII/BglI fragment (m.p. 0.725 to 0.666). As shown in Fig. 7, this DNA fragment contains the early SV40 promotor region, the 72 bp enhancer repeats and the TATA box. The 5′ end of the early SV40 19S mRNA is distal to the BglI site. The HpaII/BglI fragment was also cloned in the SalI site of pBR322. Without prior ligation *in vitro*, the isolated TaqI/BamH1 and the HpaII/BglI fragments were microinjected at a concentration of 0.1 mg/ml each into the nuclei of Ref 52 cells. The time-course of T antigen synthesis in these cells is shown in Fig. 2. About 60% of the injected Ref 52 cells exhibited a strong intranuclear T antigen fluorescence 20 to 40 h after injection. The cytoplasmic fluorescence did not exceed the background staining of the uninjected control cells. The decline of T antigen positive cells around 60 h after injection was followed by an increase in the number of positive cells 80 to 120 h later. These T antigen positive cells appeared in a clonal fashion. Similar results were obtained using TC7 cells as recipients. Replication of the injected fragments was not demonstrable. This was tested by blot analysis of the re-extracted DNA fragments (data not shown).

To obtain T antigen positive cell lines, 300 Ref 52 cells were injected in groups of 25 and isolated as described above. In this way, seven permanent T antigen positive lines were isolated (Ref-Taq/Bam lines 1 to 7). To characterize the Taq/Bam T antigen polypeptides synthesized in these lines, cells were labelled with (^{35}S)methionine for two hours, and the immunoprecipitates were analysed by discontinuous SDS/polyacrylamide gel electrophoresis (7 to 15%). According to the T antigen polypeptides synthesized in these cells, two categories of cell lines were obtained. Cells of the Ref-Taq/Bam lines 1 to 5 synthesized two T antigen-related polypeptides (Taq/Bam T_1 and Taq/Bam T_2) not demonstrable in the Ref-wt cells. Cells of the Ref-Taq/Bam line 6 and 7 synthesized only the low molecular mass

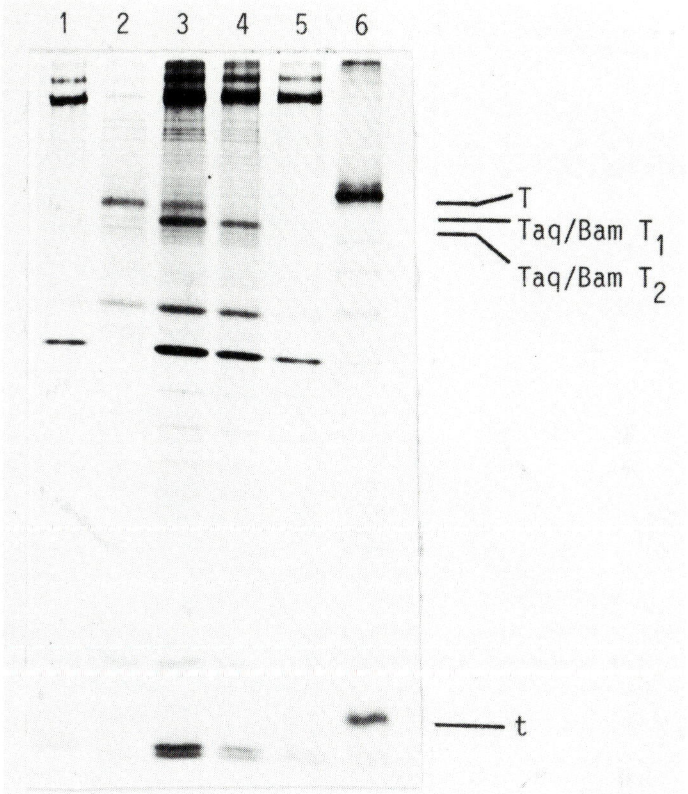

Fig. 8. Fluorogram of a SDS polyacrylamide gel (7–15%) of the anti-T immunoprecipitates from the following cells: lane 1, Ref 52; lane 2, Ref-Taq/Bam line 5_{agar}; lane 3, Ref-Taq/Bam line 5; lane 4, Ref-Taq/Bam line 7; lane 5, Ref 52; lane 6, Cos 7.

Taq/Bam T_2 polypeptides form (Fig. 8). Both polypeptides are also precipitable by the anti-C serum. This indicates that the two Taq/Bam polypeptides differ in their amino-terminal portion. As deduced from the DNA sequence, the Taq/Bam fragment codes for a polypeptide of maximum relative molecular mass 70×10^3, however on SDS/polyacrylamide gels, the Taq/Bam T antigens migrated more slowly than predicted. The same phenomenon was described above for the Pst T antigen and the intact T antigen.

Enhanced concentration of the cellular p53 protein was demonstrated in all Ref-Taq/Bam lines by both immunofluorescence staining and by electrophoresis of the p53 immunoprecipitates (Fig. 5). Figure 5 shows further that both Taq/Bam T antigens form a stable complex with the p53 protein, which allows coprecipitation of these polypeptides by anti-p53 serum treatment.

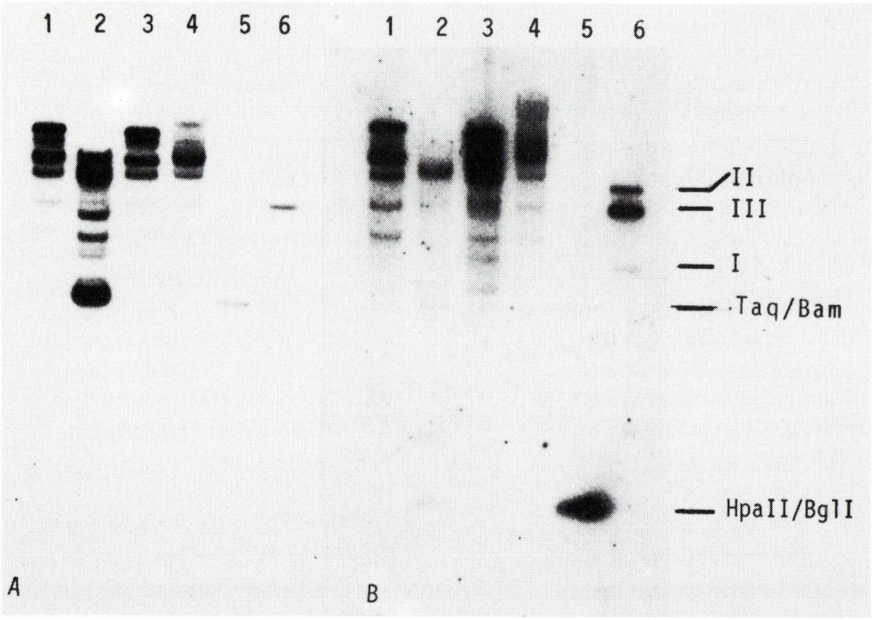

Fig. 9. Southern blotting analysis of the Ref-Taq/Bam line 5. Following extraction of the cellular DNA and digestion with different restriction endonucleases, one blot was prepared and divided in two parts for hybridization. Part A was hybridized with nick-translated ^{32}P-Taq/Bam SV40 DNA fragment, and part B with ^{32}P-HpaII/BglI SV40 DNA fragment. The lanes 1–4 contain 8 μg high relative molecular mass DNA restricted with the following endonucleases: lanes 1, BglII and Bam H1; lanes 2, BglII and SalI; lanes 3, BglII and EcoRI; lanes 4, BglII. Lanes 5 contain a mixture of the SV40 DNA fragments HpaII/BglI and Taq/Bam, and lanes 6 contain marker DNAs I, II and III.

To analyse the state of the Taq/Bam and the HpaII/BglI DNA fragments in the transformed cells, cellular DNA was extracted from the Ref-Taq/Bam line 5 and Ref-Taq/Bam line 7 cells. Following digestion of the DNA with different restriction endonucleases, two blots were prepared. One was hybridized with the nick-translated Taq/Bam DNA fragment and the other with the nick-translated HpaII/BglI SV40 fragment. Figure 9A shows the blot of the Taq/Bam line 5 DNA hybridized with the nick-translated Taq/Bam DNA fragment. Lane 1 contains the cellular DNA digested with endonucleases BglII and BamHI. These enzymes do not cut the SV40 DNA fragments (the cloned Taq/Bam DNA fragment does not contain the intact BamHI site). Six independent bands are demonstrable. The blot hybridized with the HpaII/BglI fragment (Fig. 9B) contains five strong HpaII/BglI specific bands in lane 1, all at the same position as the Taq/Bam DNA fragment. Direct cointegration of both types of SV40 DNA fragments was demonstrated after further digestion of the cellular DNA with the SalI enzyme. This treatment separated most of the common integrations and generated SV40 DNA fragments of the original size (lane 2). The Taq/Bam and HpaII/BglI DNA fragments could also be rescued from the cellular DNA of the Taq/Bam line 7 by treatment with SalI (data not shown). To analyse the transformation capacity of the Taq/Bam DNA fragment, we monitored the morphology and anchorage-independent growth of the Taq/Bam cell lines 1 to 7 for a period of about 1.5 years. Lines with about 95% T antigen positive cells were obtained between passage numbers 5 to 10. At this point in time the morphology of the cells was close to the parental Ref 52 cells. With continuous further cultivation the shape of the line 1 to 5 cells changed gradually from normal to the morphology of fully SV40-transformed rat cells. The cells became smaller, exhibited a reduced cytoplasmic actin cable network, a change in the pericellular matrix, an increase in plasminogen activator secretion and a low serum requirement, but anchorage-independent growth did not correlate directly with these alterations (Table II). At passage numbers 20 to 25, when the morphology of the Taq/Bam cell lines 1 to 5 was close to the morphology of the Ref-wt cells, only 0.1 to 0.2% of these cells formed colonies in soft agar. At passage numbers 50 to 60, the rate was still only 1 to 2%. This observation indicates that under standard conditions the cells with anchorage growth characteristics do not have a significant growth advantage over the rest of the cell population. Furthermore, it was not possible to select these cells by means other than soft agar (e.g. low serum concentration, mild trypsinization). However, once isolated from soft agar, these cells exhibited a high efficiency in colony formation (60–80%) after replating into semi-solid media (agar or agarose), as shown exemplarily for the Ref-Taq/Bam line 5_{agar} cells (Table III).

With increased passage numbers, the cells of the Ref-Taq/Bam lines 6 and 7 did not change their cell morphology or growth behaviour significantly. As shown in Fig. 6 the morphology of these cells was still close to the morphology of the parental Ref 52 cells, and the cells still contained their well-developed actin cable structure after a continuous culture period of 1.5 years (Fig. 6).

From the transformation criteria tested, the line 6 and 7 cells exhibited only a low serum requirement (Fig. 10), but growth in soft agar or in agarose was not demonstrable (Fig. 6, Table II). We also considered whether the change from anchorage-dependent to anchorage-independent growth could be associated with an alteration in the pattern of T antigen synthesis. For this reason, T antigen was extracted from the Ref-Taq/Bam line 5 cells at low and high passage number (15 to 65) and analysed by gel electrophoresis. Synthesis of the two Taq/Bam polypeptides was demonstrable at low and high passage numbers (Fig. 8, lane 3; Fig. 4, lane 5). However, most of the

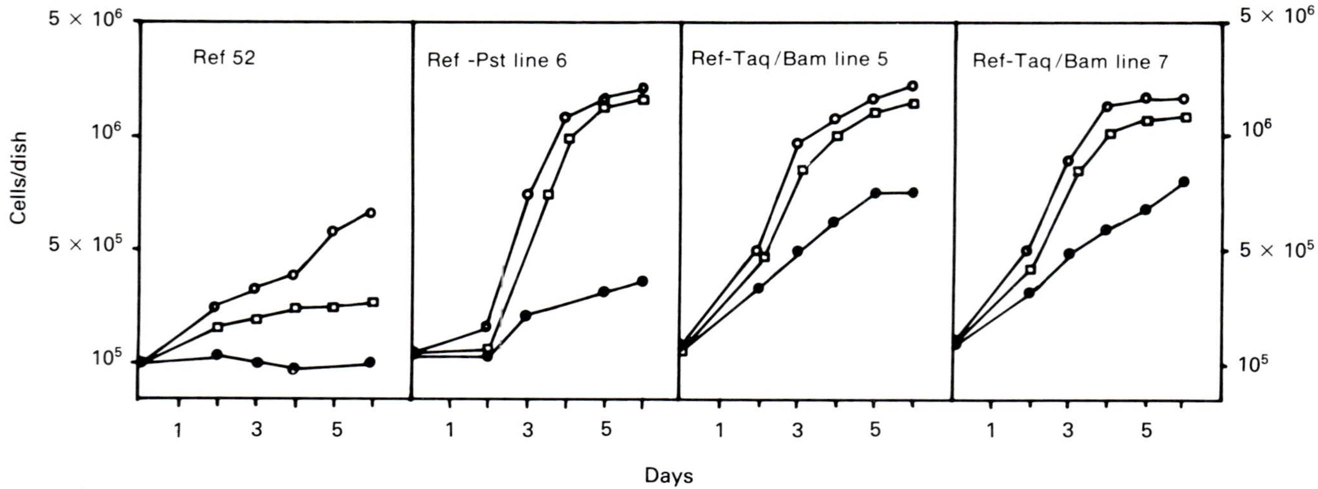

Fig. 10. Serum requirement of the Ref 52 cells and the transformed cell lines. Cells were plated at a density of 10^5 cells/60 mm dish in medium supplemented with 5% FCS. On the next day after plating, medium was removed and new medium with (○) 5%, (□) 1% or (●) 0% fetal calf serum was added to the cells. At the time points indicated cells were trypsinized and counted.

soft agar isolates (e.g. Ref-Taq/Bam line 5_{agar}) synthesized mainly the Taq/Bam T_1 polypeptide (Fig. 8, lane 2). Cells of the Ref-Taq/Bam lines 6 and 7 synthesized exclusively the Taq/Bam T_2 polypeptide (Fig. 8, lane 4) over the whole period monitored.

The ultimate goal of the fragment injection experiments is to determine the minimum early SV40 DNA sequence required for cell transformation, thus learning somewhat more about the T antigen specific function(s) crucial for the viral oncogenicity. In this investigation it was shown that the early SV40 Taq/Bam DNA fragment (m.p. 0.566–0.144), which codes exclusively for the second large T antigen exon, has the capability to transform the Ref 52 cells fully. Expression of this promotor minus SV40 DNA segment was possible by coinjection with the early SV40 promotor/enhancer HpaII/BglI DNA fragment (m.p. 0.72–0.66) (Mueller *et al.*, 1978; Benoist and Chambon, 1981). Ligation of the two fragments *in vitro* was not required because coligation occurred inside the recipient cells. DNA re-extraction experiments and Southern blot analysis have shown that formation of polymers by end-to-end ligation started as early as one to two minutes after injection. This oligomerization process was certainly facilitated by the fact that the DNA fragments had the same overlapping ends (SalI linker). However, fragments with different or blunt ends were also coligated, although with a lower efficiency (Graessmann *et al.*, unpub. res.). Comparable results have been reported by other groups (Folger *et al.*, 1982, Wilson *et al.*, 1982). Stable T antigen positive cell lines were isolated with a frequency of 1 to 5%. This remarkably high transformation rate was observed only after intranuclear and not after cytoplasmic injection of the fragment mixture. Rapid degradation of the DNA fragments inside the cytoplasm is responsible, at least partly, for this lower efficiency (Graessmann *et al.*, unpub. res.). The Ref Taq/Bam lines fall into two distinct categories of cells, namely, into maximal and into minimal transformed cells (Pollack *et al.*, 1974). The maximal transformants show, among other things, anchorage-independent growth, low serum requirement, loss of actin cable structure and alteration of the perinuclear matrix (fibronectin). The only transformation parameter attributable to the minimal transformants (Ref-Taq/Bam lines 6 and 7) is the reduced serum requirement (Fig. 10). Cells of the first category synthesize two second T antigen exon-specific polypeptides (Taq/Bam T_1 and T_2). Some of the soft agar isolates synthesize mainly the high relative molecular mass Taq/Bam T_1 polypeptide (e.g. Ref-Taq/Bam line 5_{agar}). We have not tested whether translation of the Taq/Bam mRNA or cRNA starts with AUG. If it does, the triplets coding for the T antigen amino acid residues 109 and 176 are the potential initiation signals. These are the first two AUG triplets of the second T antigen exon in the reading frame of the wild-type protein (Fig. 7).

The predicted relative molecular masses of these polypeptides would be 68×10^3 and 62×10^3 (Tooze, 1980). The conflict between the calculated size and mobility of T antigen and T antigen-related polypeptides on SDS/polyacrylamide gels is addressed above and elsewhere (Pauscha *et al.*, 1978; M. Graessmann and A. Graessmann, 1982; Sompayrac and Danna, 1983).

The two minimally transformed Taq/Bam cell lines 6 and 7 synthesize only the Taq/Bam T_2 polypeptide. This observation implies that the amino acid sequence 82 to 176 of large T antigen is important for maximal cell transformation (see Fig. 7). It has been shown that the amino acid sequence 82 to 130 is part of the specific DNA binding domain of the T antigen (Morrison *et al.*, 1983); however, these results cannot be considered as proof that this T antigen activity is essential for anchorage-independent growth. It has not even been established that the nuclear localization of the T antigen is essential for cell transformation. It is known that small amounts of T antigen are also associated with cell membrane (Deppert and Henning, 1979; Soule and Butel, 1979). To allow intranuclear accumulation, amino acid 128 of the T antigen seems to be of certain importance. Point mutation or substitution at this particular T antigen coding region cause T antigen to be located in cytoplasm. The altered T antigen molecules still have the capacity to induce anchorage-independent growth. Underphosphorylation of the T antigen has been mentioned as a possible reason for this atypical localization (Jarvis *et al.*, 1984; Scheidtmann *et al.*, 1984; A. E. Smith, pers. commun.). It will be of interest to discover whether the Taq/Bam T_2 polypeptide has phosphorylation characteristic of the nuclear or of the cytoplasmic T antigen.

The SV40 Pst fragment injection experiments have further shown that the 20% at the C-terminal part of T antigen (168 amino acid residues) is also required to fully transform the Ref 52 cells. The T antigen specific functions attributed to the Pst fragment include stimulation of cellular DNA and RNA synthesis, change of the cytoskeleton, secretion of plasminogen activator and immortalization of cells (for a review, see A. Graessmann *et al.*, 1981). It is likely that these functions are involved in cell transformation but they are not sufficient to transform the Ref 52 cells fully. The only biological function attributed to the very C-terminal end of T antigen so far is the helper activity for Ad2 in monkey cells, a mechanism not understood at its molecular biological level (Tjian *et al.*, 1978). The transformation capacity of the SV40 Pst DNA fragment is a controversial subject. Different laboratories have obtained fully transformed rat cells by transfection of SV40 DNA fragments with an even lower coding capacity than the SV40 Pst fragment (Clayton *et al.*, 1982; Colby and Shenk, 1982; Sompayrac and Danna, 1983). Shenk's group has transformed primary rat cells with a recombinant DNA plasmid (pSV8) that contains only the early SV40 coding sequence between m.p. 0.65 and 0.37. The type of transformants isolated ranged from normal to fully transformed cells (Colby and Shenk, 1982). The same authors failed to transform the Ref 52 cells with this DNA. One difference between our Ref 52-Pst lines and PSV8-transformed cells concerns the cellular p53 protein. All Ref-Pst line cells contain this protein at the same concentration as the parental Ref 52 cells, while the pSV8-transformed cells have this protein at the level of wild-type virus-transformed cells. Elevated concentrations of the p53 protein and its complex formation with T antigen, however, are not sufficient for maximal cell transformation. The minimally transformed Ref-Taq/Bam line cells contain the p53 protein in the same amount as the fully transformed cells (Fig. 5). The Taq/Bam DNA fragment injection experiments have shown that the first T antigen exon and small t antigen are not essential for maximal transformation of Ref 52 cells. However, the long latency period required for the cells to acquire anchorage-independent growth was striking. There is increasing evidence that maximal cell transformation is a multi-step process, and that the SV40-specific oncogenicity is a combined effect of the large and small T antigen (Topp *et al.*, 1979; Land *et al.*, 1983). In this team effort, the small t antigen accelerates initiation of cell transformation but functions of the second large T antigen exon are essential if the cells are to achieve the fully transformed state. This assumption is in accordance with the observation that small t antigen negative SV40 deletion mutants (e.g. dl884) have a lower transformation efficiency than the wild-type virus, and a long latency period for manifestation of anchorage-independent growth (Sleigh *et al.*, 1978; Rubin *et al.*, 1982; Graessmann, *pers. obs.*).

ACKNOWLEDGEMENTS

We thank J. Fuhrhop, E. Guhl, and C. Ziechmann for their excellent technical assistance, and I. Beuker for typing the manuscript. This work was supported by the Deutsche Forschungsgemeinschaft (Gr 384/8 and Gr 599/4-2) and the Verband der Chemischen Industrie (1498).

REFERENCES

Benoist, C. and Chambon, P. (1981). *Nature* **290**, 304–310.
Botchan, M., Topp, W. C. and Sambrook, J. (1976). *Cell* **9**, 269–287.
Capecchi, M. R. (1980). *Cell* **22**, 479–488.
Clayton, C. E., Murphy, D., Lovett, M. and Rigby, P. W. J. (1982). *Nature* **229**, 59–61.
Colby, W. W. and Shenk, T. (1982). *Proc. Natl. Acad. Sci. USA* **79**, 5189–5193.

Deppert, W. and Henning, R. (1979). *Cold Spring Harbor Symp. Quant. Biol.* **44**, 225–243.
Folger, K. R., Wong, E. A., Wahl, G. and Capecchi, M. (1982). *Mol. Cell Biol.* **2**, 1372–1387.
Friedman, M. P., Lyons, M. J. and Ginsberg, H. S. (1970). *J. Virol.* **5**, 568–579.
Galanti, N., Jonak, G. J., Soprano, K. J., Floros, J., Kaczmarek, L., Weissmann, S. M., Reedy, V. B., Tilghman, S. M. and Baserga, R. (1981). *J. Biol. Chem.* **256**, 6469–6474.
Goldberg, A. R. (1974). *Cell* **2**, 95–102.
Graessmann, A. and Graessmann, M. (1971). *Hoppe-Seyler's Z. Physiol. Chem.* **352**, 527–532.
Graessmann, A., Graessmann, M., Bobrik, R., Hoffmann, E., Lauppe, F. and Mueller, C. (1976). *FEBS Lett.* **61**, 81–84.
Graessmann, A., Graessmann, M., Topp, W. C. and Botchan, M. (1979). *J. Virol.* **32**, 989–994.
Graessmann, A., Graessmann, M. and Mueller, C. (1981). *Adv. Cancer Res.* **35**, 111–146.
Graessmann, M. and Graessmann, A. (1976). *Proc. Natl. Acad. Sci. USA* **73**, 366–370.
Graessmann, M. and Graessmann, A. (1982). *EMBO J.* **1**, 1081–1088.
Graessmann, M. and Graessmann, A. (1983). *Methods Enzymol.* **101**, 482–492.
Graessmann, M., Graessmann, A. and Mueller, C. (1980). *Cold Spring Harbor Symp. Quant. Biol.* **44**, 605–610.
Graham, F. L. and van der Ebb, A. J. (1973). *Virology* **52**, 456.
Jarvis, D. J., Lanford, R. E. and Butel, J. S. (1984). *Virology* **134**, 168–176.
Land, H., Parada, L. F. and Weinberg, R. A. (1983). *Nature* **304**, 596–602.
Levine, A. (1982). *In* "Advances in Cancer Research", Vol. 37 (G. Klein and S. Weinhouse, eds). pp. 75–104. Academic Press, New York and London.
Lewis Jr., A. M. and Martin, R. G. (1979). *Proc. Natl. Acad. Sci. USA* **76**, 4299–4302.
Loyter, A., Vainstein, A., Graessmann, M. and Graessmann, A. (1983). *Exp. Cell Res.* **143**, 415.
Martin, R. G. and Chou, J. Y. (1975). *J. Virol.* **15**, 599–612.
McKay, R. (1981). *J. Mol. Biol.* **145**, 471–488.
Morrison, B., Kress, M., Khoury, G. and Jay, G. (1983). *J. Virol.* **47**, 106–114.
Mueller, C., Graessmann, A. and Graessmann, M. (1978). *Cell* **15**, 579–589.
Osborn, M. and Weber, K. (1975). *J. Virol.* **15**, 636–644.
Pauscha, E., Harvey, R. and Smith, A. (1978). *J. Virol.* **28**, 154–170.
Pollack, R., Risser, R., Conlon, S. R. and Rifkin, D. (1974). *Proc. Natl. Acad. Sci. USA* **71**, 4792–4796.
Rabson, A. S., O'Conor, G. T., Berezesky, I. K. and Paul, F. J. (1964). *Proc. Soc. Exp. Biol. Med.* **116**, 187–190.
Rawlins, D. R., Collins, P. and Muzyczka, N. (1983). *J. Virol.* **47**, 202–216.
Risser, R. and Pollack, P. (1974). *Cold Spring Harbor Symp. Quant. Biol.* **38**, 317–324.
Rubin, H., Figge, J., Bladon, M. T., Bo Chen, L., Ellmann, M., Bikel, I., Farrell, M. and Livingston, D. M. (1982). *Cell* **30**, 469–480.
Scheidtmann, K. H., Schickedanz, J., Walter, G., Lanford, R. E. and Butel, J. S. (1984). *J. Virol.* **50**, 636–640.
Seif, R. and Martin, R. G. (1979). *J. Virol.* **32**, 979–988.

Sleigh, M. J., Topp, W. C., Hanich, R. and Sambrook, J. F. (1978). *Cell* **14**, 79–88.
Soeda, E., Arrand, J. R., Smolar, N., Walsh, J. E. and Griffin, B. E. (1980). *Nature* **283**, 445–453.
Sompayrac, L. and Danna, K. J. (1983). *J. Virol.* **46**, 475–480.
Soprano, K. J., Jonak, G. J., Galanti, N., Floros, J. and Baserga, R. (1981). *Virology* **109**, 127–136.
Soule, H. R. and Butel, J. S. (1979). *J. Virol.* **30**, 523–532.
Southern, E. M. (1975). *J. Mol. Biol.* **98**, 503–518.
Stocker, M. (1968). *Nature* **218**, 234–238.
Tegtmeyer, P. (1975). *J. Virol.* **15**, 613–618.
Tjian, R. (1978). *Cell* **3**, 165–179.
Tjian, R., Fey, G. and Graessmann, A. (1978). *Proc. Natl. Acad. Sci. USA* **75**, 1279–1283.
Tjian, R. and Robins, A. (1979). *Proc. Natl. Acad. Sci. USA* **76**, 610–614.
Tooze, J., ed. (1980). "DNA Tumor Viruses", Cold Spring Harbor Laboratory, Cold Spring Harbor, NY.
Topp, W. C. and Rifkin, D. B. (1980). *Virology* **106**, 282–291.
Topp, W. C., Rifkin, D., Graessmann, A., Chang, C. M. and Sleigh, M. J. (1979). Cold Spring Harbor Conference on Cell Proliferation **6**, pp. 361–370.
Walter, G., Scheidtmann, K. H., Carbone, A., Laudano, A. P. and Doolittle, R. F. (1980). *Proc. Natl. Acad. Sci. USA* **77**, 5197–5200.
Wilson, J. H., Berget, P. B. and Pipas, J. (1982). *Mol. Cell Biol.* **2**, 1258–1269.

3

Modulation of Cellular Activities via Microinjection into Living Cells

J. R. Feramisco and W. J. Welch

I. INTRODUCTION

The technique of direct microinjection provides a powerful addition to the many other experimental methods available to the biochemist, cell biologist and molecular biologist. Many of the current experimental designs involving microinjection techniques have involved the introduction into living cells of defined genes and/or cDNAs, mRNAs or anti-sense RNAs, functional proteins (either fluorescently labelled to facilitate localization studies or unlabelled to assess biological responses), and finally antibodies specific for defined proteins. Microinjection studies involving DNA and RNA are covered in other chapters in this volume. In the present chapter (as well as in several others presented in this volume), we will attempt to cover part of the field describing studies in which particular proteins or antibodies are introduced into living cells via direct microinjection.

A major problem for the cell biologist studying somatic cells is the lack of genetic analysis to complement biochemical and cellular studies. Hence, the method of microinjection of macromolecules into living cells provides the investigator with another powerful tool by which to examine specific proteins and their possible function within the cell. For example, we and others have used microinjection techniques to examine the effects of purified proteins introduced into the living cell, or to directly inactivate particular proteins by the introduction of specific antibodies. Some pertinent examples of experiments utilizing these approaches include the microinjection of the SV40 large T antigen (Tjian *et al.*, 1978) or the human *ras* oncogene protein (Feramisco *et al.*, 1984). In both cases, the injected proteins were observed to result in a stimulation of DNA synthesis and in the case of the *ras* protein a subsequent stimulation of cell proliferation. In another study, Cleveland *et*

Microinjection and Organelle Transplantation Techniques

ISBN: 0-12-164722-6
ISBN: 0-12-164723-4 Pbk

al. (1983) demonstrated that introduction of 6S tubulin into living cells resulted in the diminished synthesis of endogenous α- and β-tubulin, thereby confirming previous suggestions that the level of free 6S tubulin in the cell acts to regulate its own synthesis.

Experiments in which specific antibodies against particular proteins have been introduced into living cells via microinjection have also proven to be most useful. Some examples include the disruption and aggregation of the intermediate filaments following injection of a monoclonal antibody specific for intermediate filament associated proteins (Klymkowski, 1981; Lin and Feramisco, 1981), inhibition of DNA synthesis via injection and inactivation of the large T antigen in SV40 infected cells by anti-large T antibodies (Antman and Livingston, 1980), inactivation of the proliferative effects induced by the *ras* oncogene protein using the anti-*ras* antibody (Feramisco *et al.*, 1985), inhibition of junctional communication between cells caused by the microinjection of antibodies to gap-junction protein (Warner *et al.*, 1984), and disruption of focal adhesion plaques following introduction of anti-vinculin antibodies (Kreis and Birchmeier, 1981). In the case of following the fate of fluorescently labelled purified proteins introduced into living cells, considerable success has been realized with respect to various cytoskeletal proteins. Examples of cytoskeletal proteins injected into cells and which became incorporated into their proper cellular locale include actin (Kreis *et al.*, 1979), α-actinin (Feramisco, 1979; Feramisco and Blose, 1980), vinculin (Burridge and Feramisco, 1980), tropomyosin (Wehland and Weber, 1980), and tubulin (Keith *et al.*, 1981). These sorts of experiments involving injection of cytoskeletal proteins or antibodies against cytoskeletal components have been and will continue to be invaluable in studying the dynamics and organization of the cytoskeleton in the living cell.

In this chapter we will present different microinjection approaches we have utilized to study the structure and function of various macromolecules in our laboratory. Specifically, we will summarize our data concerning proteins involved in cytoskeletal organization, transformation, and the heat-shock response.

II. MICROINJECTION OF CYTOSKELETAL PROTEINS INTO LIVING FIBROBLASTS: INCORPORATION INTO DYNAMIC STRUCTURES AND EFFECTS ON PROTEIN SYNTHESIS

Studies in our laboratory several years ago were aimed, in part, on understanding how various cytoskeletal systems are assembled in the living cell. One approach to this problem was to examine the effects of introducing into living cells purified cytoskeletal proteins, covalently tagged with fluorescent chromophores, and to determine whether the cells would both recognize the injected proteins and subsequently incorporate them into the same structures as that found for the cells' endogenous cytoskeletal proteins. This approach provides a way to observe the dynamic distribution of a particular protein within cells in a manner that avoids the potential problems associated with fixation, extraction, and immunological cross-reactivities and/or accessibility often encountered during indirect immunofluorescence analyses using specific antibodies. An example of the microinjection approach is presented in Fig. 1. Here, the two cytoskeletal proteins, vinculin and α-actinin, were purified from chicken smooth muscle, the purified proteins conjugated with either fluorescein or rhodamine, respectively, and the proteins coinjected into living gerbil fibroma cells growing on glass coverslips. Following a 3 h incubation at 37°C the living cells were photographed using phase-contrast and epifluorescence microscopy. In the case of the fluorescently labelled α-actinin, the injected protein localized along the actin-containing stress fibres and appeared prominent at many sites where the stress fibres appear to terminate near the cell periphery (Fig. 1B and E). This distribution of the microinjected protein appears identical to that observed for the endogenous gerbil fibroma alpha-actinin protein as determined by indirect immunofluorescence (data not shown). Similarly, the distribution of the injected vinculin protein appeared identical to the distribution of the endogenous protein observed after indirect immunofluorescence analysis. For example, the majority of the fluorescence was observed to localize prominently as bright focal patches near the bottom of the injected cells (Fig. 1C and F). Some of the injected vinculin protein also distributed at the leading edge of the cells, the site of active membrane ruffling. Finally, some fluorescence was visible toward the cortex of the cell, in what appeared to be the uppermost portion of the cell. These studies along with those of Geiger (1979) established that the bright focal patches of vinculin found near the bottom of the cells actually corresponded to so-called adhesion plaques, sites where cells make a firm contact with the underlying substratum. Using microinjection and indirect immunofluorescence analysis, it was shown that the vinculin-containing adhesion plaques also represented sites at which many of the actin filaments terminated and where much of the extracellular fibronectin was deposited. Consequently, this colocalization of these different structures and/or macromolecules has prompted the suggestion that adhesion plaques themselves may in fact serve in linking the actin cytoskeleton to the plasma membrane and/or proteins of the cell surface or extracellular matrix. These results examining the distribution of microinjected proteins into living cells illustrate a number of important points that will be discussed throughout this chapter: First, microinjection studies provide a method to assay the "nativeness" of

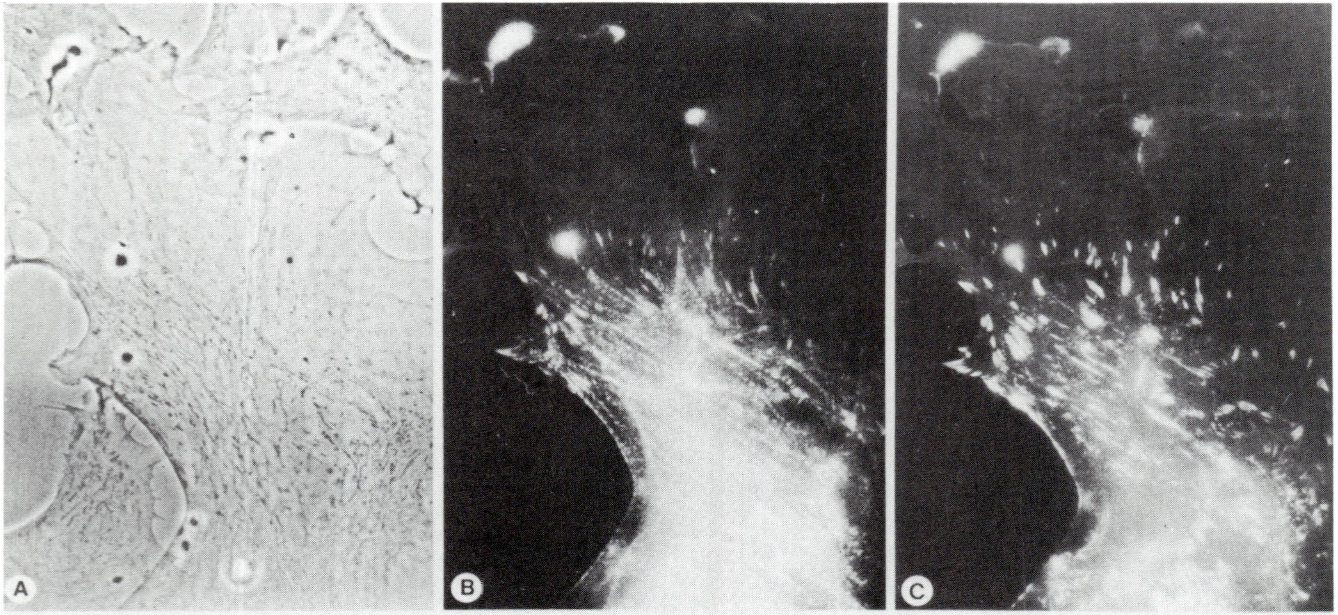
A
B
C

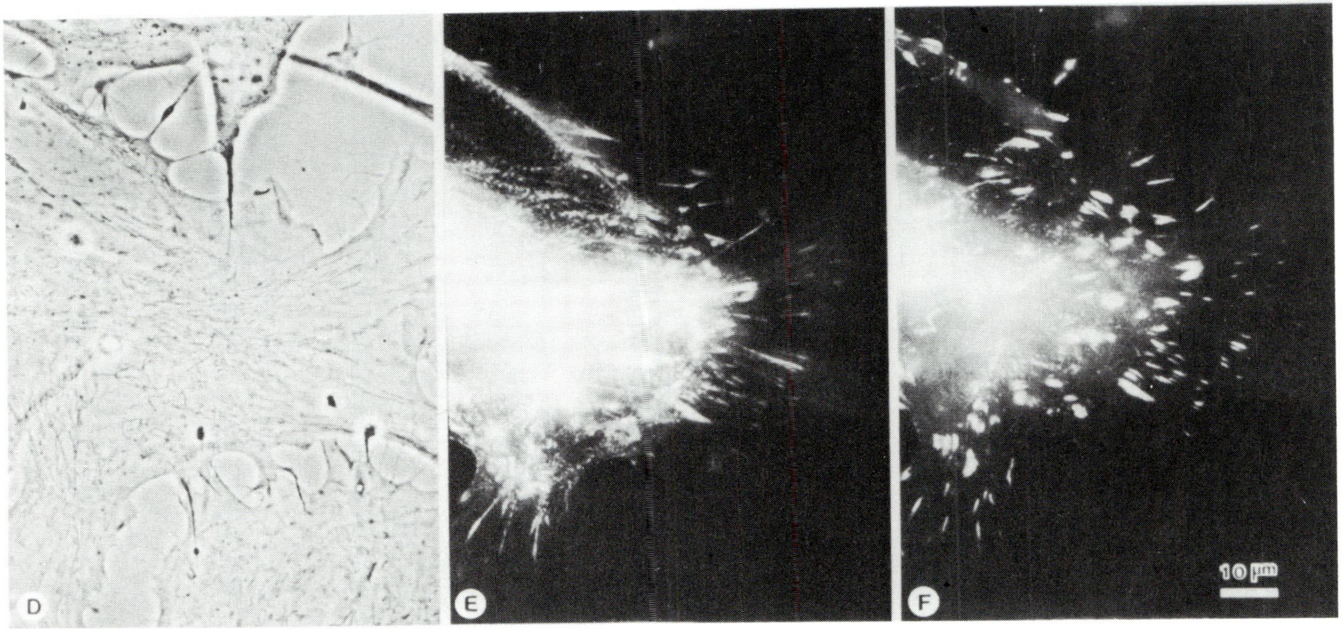

Fig. 1. Incorporation of FITC-vinculin and RITC-α-actinin simultaneously in living cell cytoskeletal systems following their microinjection. A mixture of FITC-vinculin (Burridge and Feramisco, 1980) and TMRITC-α-actinin (Feramisco, 1979) was injected into the cytoplasm of gerbil fibroma cells. Three hours later, the cells were visualized (alive) by phase-contrast (A and D) of epifluorescence photomicroscopy using filters specific for FITC-vinculin (C and F) or specific for TMRITC-α-actinin (B and E). The field shown in panels A, B, and C and the fields in panels D, E, and F are identical, respectively. Note the α-actinin-containing stress fibres terminating in the vinculin-containing adhesion plaques.

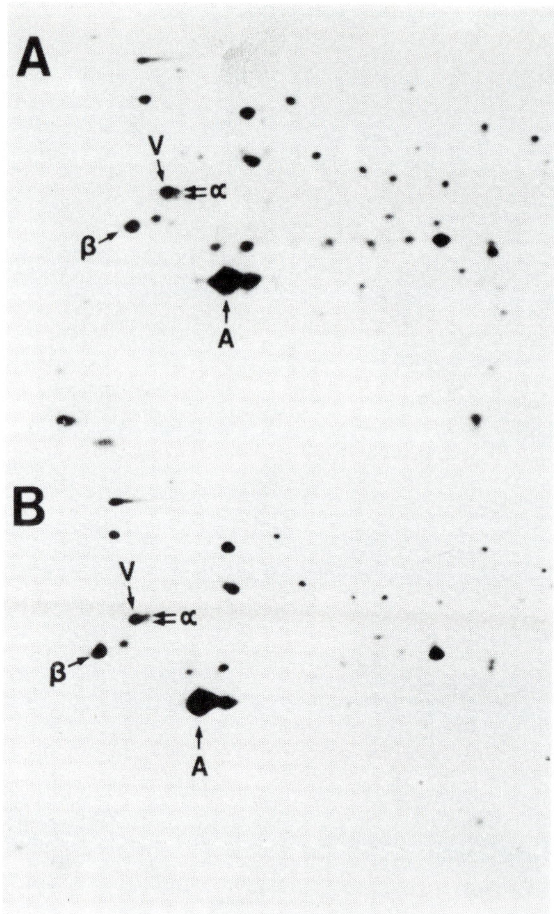

Fig. 2. Two-dimensional gel analysis of newly synthesized proteins in CHO cells following microinjection of soluble alpha- and beta-tubulin. A, Protein synthesis pattern from uninjected cells; B, pattern of protein synthesis from cells injected with the microtubule buffer lacking EGTA; *Opposite*: C, pattern from cells microinjected with hamster brain microtubule protein at an initial concentration of ~15 mg/ml in buffer lacking EGTA; D, pattern from cells microinjected with 6 mg/ml of phosphocellulose-purified porcine brain tubulin. Arrows indicate the positions of actin (A), α-tubulin (α), β-tubulin (β) and vimentin (V), respectively. Unambiguous determination of the positions of the α- and β-tubulin polypeptides was achieved by two-dimensional analysis of immunoprecipitated proteins using an antibody to α- and β-tubulin. For proteins synthesized by each aliguot of 15–20 cells during the 1 h labelling period, the fluorographs shown have been normalized by varying the exposure times over 2–4 days.

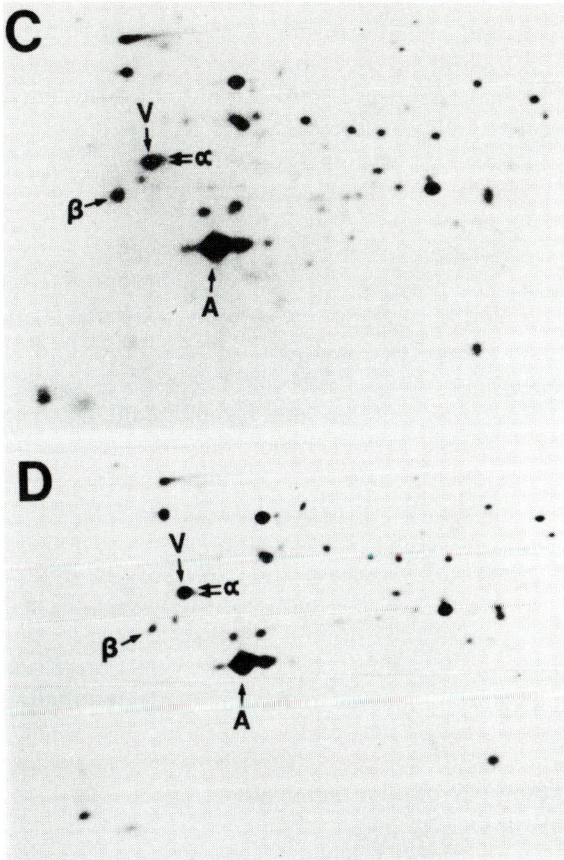

proteins purified by classical procedures in the absence of any knowledge concerning the biochemical function of the protein. This is evidenced by the fact that the gerbil fibroma cells were able to recognize the purified and infected chicken α-actinin and vinculin molecules and to incorporate these proteins into the same structures as those found for the endogenous gerbil α-actinin and vinculin proteins. Secondly, these studies illustrate the apparent dynamic state of the cytoskeleton and allow for further studies aimed at understanding events involved during the assembly of the cytoskeleton. For example, there must exist a steady state of assembly/disassembly of various cytoskeletal elements since the microinjected α-actinin and vinculin proteins became incorporated into the stress fibres and adhesion plaques, respectively, over the 3 h incubation period following their injection. (Using time-lapse video microscopy, the kinetics of such assembly/disassembly can in fact be measured.) Finally, the injection of proteins into living cells affords the possibility of studying various parameters affecting the organization of the cytoskeleton *in vivo*. For example, questions regarding the dependence, if any, of other cellular processes such as transcription, translation, or physical parameters such as temperature, confluency of the cells, etc., and the ability of the cells to incorporate and properly distribute the microinjected proteins can be addressed. This latter point will be amply illustrated in the following section.

Previous studies have shown that most eukaryotic cells regulate the synthesis of α- and β-tubulin in response to drugs which cause microtubule depolymerization and the consequent increase in the intracellular level of free α- and β-tubulin. These studies have prompted the suggestion that cells constitutively synthesize both α- and β-tubulin unless the free subunit pool rises above a specified level. Once this level is reached, a feedback mechanism operates to cease new tubulin synthesis via turn-over of the mRNA encoding the two proteins. To test this hypothesis directly and to avoid the pleitropic effect of using drugs which depolymerize the microtubules we, along with Cleveland and coworkers, investigated the effect of microinjecting purified tubulin subunits into living cells and examining the response of the cells at the protein synthesis level (Cleveland *et al.*, 1983). The hypothesis predicted that elevating the level of free tubulin subunits in the cell should be accompanied by a cessation of new tubulin synthesis. CHO cells were grown on 35 mm plastic dishes in which small wells had been constructed using silicon grease. Approximately 15–20 cells per well were injected with either tubulin buffer alone, purified 6S hamster tubulin, or with purified procine brain 6S tubulin. After 2 h, the control and injected cells were labelled for 1 h with high specific activity [^{35}S]-methionine in DMEM lacking methionine. Following the labelling period, the cells were solubilized and analysed by two-dimensional gel electrophoresis (Fig. 2). Injection of the purified hamster 6S tubulin (Fig. 2C) resulted in a slightly decreased synthesis of both α- and β-tubulin as compared to either those cells injected with the tubulin buffer alone (Fig. 2B) or the uninjected control cells (Fig. 2A). Microinjection of the purified porcine brain 6S tubulin depressed the *in vivo* synthesis of tubulin to an even greater extent (Fig. 2D). This depression of tubulin synthesis was specific for the injected 6S tubulin since microinjection of either preimmune IgG, bovine serum albumin, or a variety of purified mammalian heat-shock proteins had no effect on tubulin synthesis (data not shown). These results then strongly favour the idea that the free level of 6S tubulin in the cell can act to repress further tubulin biosynthesis and indicates that eukaryotic cells, like prokaryotes, utilize autoregulatory control mechanisms. Again, as described earlier, these results also demonstrated that the hamster cells can recognise exogenously added proteins (even when derived from other species) and utilize these proteins in a manner similar to that found for their own analogous endogenous proteins.

III. INVESTIGATION OF THE MAMMALIAN HEAT-SHOCK RESPONSE USING MICROINJECTION

Our laboratory has also been examining the response of mammalian cells to physiological stress (Welch and Feramisco, 1982; Welch *et al.*, 1983; Welch and Feramisco, 1984). Mammalian cells, when confronted with a diverse array of environmental insults (heat-shock, exposure to heavy metals, amino acid analogues, ethanol, etc.), respond by elevating the synthesis of a small number of proteins referred to as the heat-shock or stress proteins (for review see Ashburner and Bonner, 1979). Accumulation of the stress proteins appears to afford the cell protection, especially when confronted with subsequent stress situations. The most highly induced stress protein in all cells, including prokaryotes, yeast, and all higher eukaryotes, is a polypeptide of approximately 70000 daltons. This protein, referred to in our laboratory as the 72 kDa stress protein, is present in negligible amounts in normal cells but is synthesized at extremely high levels in cells undergoing the stress response. Using a polyclonal antibody specific for the protein, we had found that the 72 kDa stress protein localizes within the nucleus and more prominently the nucleolus of cells following heat-shock treatment (Welch and Feramisco, 1984). We have purified the 72 kDa protein from heat-shock treated HeLa cells, covalently coupled it with rhodamine, and re-introduced it into the cytoplasm of living cells via microinjection (Welch and Feramisco, 1985a). In the case of the injected cells maintained at normal temperatures (i.e., 37°C), the fluorescently labelled protein distributed within both the nucleus and to a lesser extent the cytoplasm (Fig. 3A and B). No nucleolar fluorescence was observed. Following heat-shock treatment of the cells for a short period of time, however, the microinjected protein relocalized within the nucleus and quite prominently the nucleolus (Fig. 3B), a location, as mentioned above, identical to that found for the endogenous protein using indirect immunofluorescence analysis. Again these results demonstrate that: (1) the protein we have purified has indeed been obtained in "native" form; (2) that the protein is apparently well conserved since the rat fibroblasts were able to both recognize and utilize the exogenous HeLa protein in a manner similar to that found for the endogenous rat 72 kDa protein; and (3) that the nucleolar distribution of the protein occurs only when the cells enter into a heat-shock response.

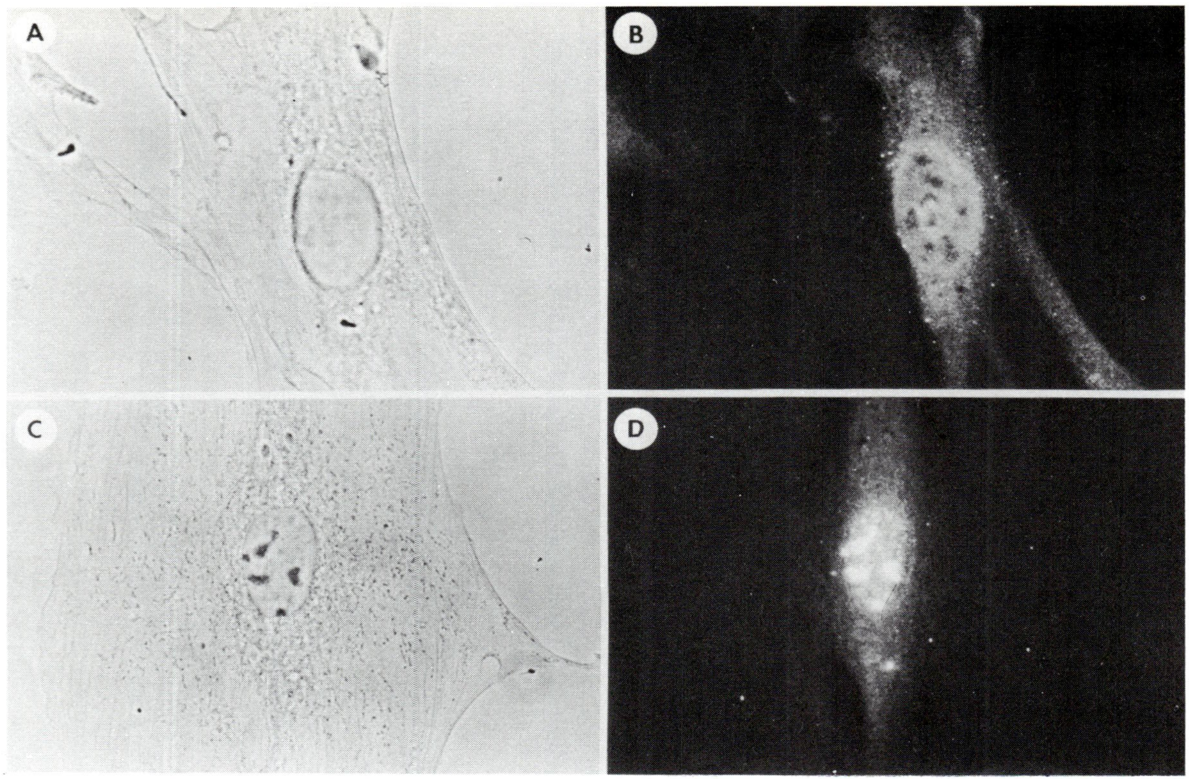

Fig. 3. Microinjection of fluorescently labelled 72 kDa and 73 kDa stress proteins. The purified 72 kDa and 73 kDa stress proteins were conjugated with the chromophore tetramethyl rhodamine isothiocyanate. The fluorescently labelled proteins were microinjected into the cytoplasm of 37°C rat embryo fibroblasts and the cells incubated at either 37°C (A and B) or at 42°C (C and D). The proteins were visualized by fluorescence microscopy using the appropriate filters. Shown in panels A and C are the phase-contrast micrographs and in panels B and D the corresponding fluorescence micrographs.

We have also used the mammalian heat-shock response to examine the dependence, if any, of new transcription, translation, and protein translocation events and the integrity of the cytoskeleton (Welch and Feramisco, 1985b). Using drugs which disrupt and/or depolymerize the cytoskeleton (e.g. colcemid and cytochalasin E), we have examined whether cells containing no integral cytoskeleton can undergo the heat-shock response as assayed by synthesis of the stress proteins and the proper translocation of the 72 kDa protein into the nucleus/nucleolus. We found that the cells could respond to the heat-shock treatment in typical fashion regardless of the state of microfilaments, intermediate filaments or microtubules. Moreover, we found that translocation of the major induced 72 kDa protein from the cytoplasm into the nucleus and nucleolus occurred irrespective of an organized cytoskeleton. For example, in Fig. 4 are shown the results of microinjecting the purified and fluorescently labelled 72 kDa protein into normal cells or cells treated with either colcemid, cytochalasin E, or a mixture of both colcemid and cytochalasin E and subsequent heat-shock treatment. As was shown previously in Fig. 3, microinjection of the protein into normal cells and subsequent heat-shock treatment resulted in a nuclear/nucleolar distribution of the protein (Fig. 4A and B). Similarly, the microinjected cells treated with colcemid (Fig. 4C and D), cytochalasin E (Fig. 4E and F) or a mixture of the two (Fig. 4G and H) all still showed a somewhat typical nuclear and nucleolar distribution of the 72 kDa protein despite the dramatic morphological alterations of the cells due to the drug treatments. A similar result was observed in cells microinjected with the adenovirus nuclear protein, ElA). Again regardless of the state of the cytoskeleton, the ElA protein, injected into the cytoplasm of rat cells, was efficiently translocated to the nucleus (data not shown). We concluded from these experiments that in fact new transcription, translation, and protein translocation events can occur in cells regardless of the state of the three major cytoskeletal networks.

IV. MICROINJECTION OF THE *ras* PROTEIN OR ANTIBODIES AGAINST THIS PROTEIN INTO LIVING CELLS

Very recent studies in our laboratory have focused on the molecular events involved in cellular transformation with a particular emphasis on the function of the *ras* proteins. In human cells the *ras* proteins actually consist of a family of proteins, each of which appear to have proto-oncogenic (wild-type) and oncogenic (activated) forms (Tabin *et al.*, 1982; Taparowsky *et al.*, 1982). In general, the oncogenic forms of the genes differ from the proto-oncogenic forms in only one codon, clustering around either codon 12 or 61.

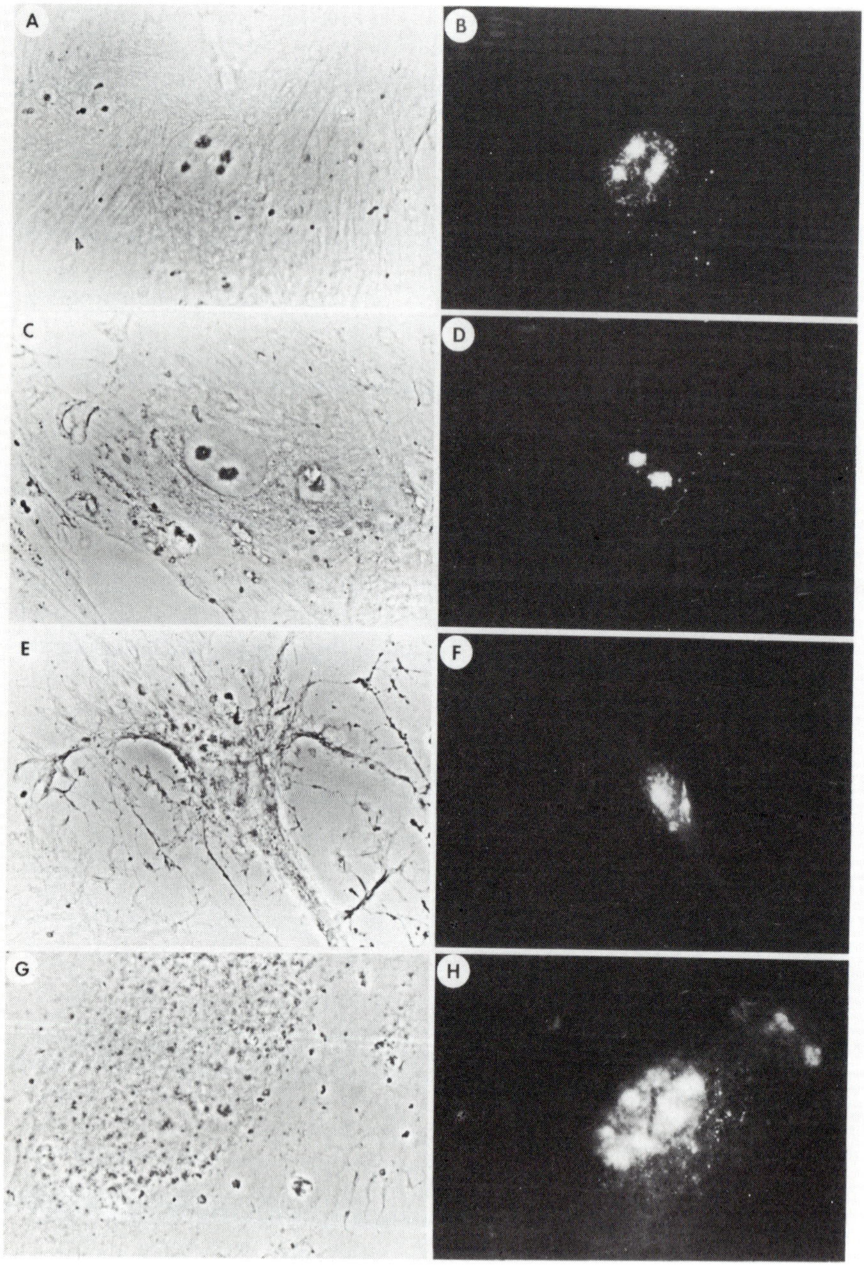
A
B
C
D
E
F
G
H

In order to study the biochemical and biological activities of the proto-oncogenic and oncogenic forms of the *ras* proteins, collaborative studies with Mike Wigler and his colleagues at Cold Spring Harbor Laboratory and Martin Rosenberg and his colleagues at Smith Kline and Beckman Laboratories were initiated which led to the production of the proto- and oncogene forms of the human H-*ras* protein (M. Gross, G. Sathe, R. Sweet, M. Rosenberg, O. Fasano, M. Goldfarb and M. Wigler, unpub. res.; Feramisco *et al.*, 1984). We have examined the effects of microinjection of the various purified *ras* proteins into living cells. An example of these studies is shown in Fig. 5. Here confluent monolayers of an established rat embryo fibroblast cell line were injected with either the wild-type, proto-oncogenic form or the oncogenic T-24 form of *ras*. Approximately 30 cells were injected in the centre of the two fields of cells and the cells further incubated for 20 h. The cells were photographed 30 min (Fig. 5A and E), 4 h (Fig. 5B and F), 12 h (Fig. 5C and G) or 20 h (Fig. 5D and H) post-injection. It can be seen that within 12 h the cells injected with the oncogenic form of the *ras* protein (Fig. 5E to H) began rounding up and dividing. Even up to 20 h the cells continued to show high levels of cell division. Note that the uninjected cells (those surrounding the injected cells) as well as the cells injected with the proto-oncogenic form of *ras* (Fig. 5A to D) showed little or no change.

The cells injected with the oncogenic form of *ras* protein were indeed committed to new growth, as evidenced by the studies examining DNA synthesis. Again, approximately 30–40 cells, in a confluent quiescent monolayer, were injected with the human oncogene *ras* protein, or with the proto-oncogenic form of *ras*, the cells incubated in the presence of [^{3}H]-thymidine for 24 h and then fixed and processed for emulsion autoradiography. Cells injected with the oncogenic *ras* protein showed high levels of DNA synthesis (Fig. 6A). In contrast, the uninjected cells (those cells shown on the border of Fig. 6A) or the cells injected with the proto-oncogenic form of *ras* (Fig. 6B) showed little or no active DNA synthesis. These studies

---

Fig. 4. Microinjected, rhodamine-labelled 72 kDa heat-shock protein is translocated to the nucleus/nucleolus of cells containing a disrupted cytoskeleton. Ref 52 cells growing on glass coverslips at 37°C were treated with either colcemide (2 μM, 5 h), cytochalasin E (2 μg/ml, 2 h) or with a mixture of colcemide/cytochalasin E (2 μM, 5 h and 2 μg/ml, 2 h, respectively). Fluorescently labelled purified HeLa 72 kDa/73 kDa were microinjected into the cytoplasm of the cells, the cells incubated for 30 min at 37°C, and then further incubated at 42°C for 2.5 h in the presence of the drugs. Following the heat-shock treatment the cells were fixed with 3.7% formaldehyde and examined by phase-contrast and fluorescence microscopy. Phase-contrast (A, C, E and G) and fluorescence micrographs (B, D, F and H) are shown.

A and B; Heat-shocked, control cells. C and D: Heat-shocked, colcemide treated cells. E and F: Heat-shocked, cytochalasin E treated cells. G and H: Heat-shocked, colcemide/cytochalasin E treated cells.

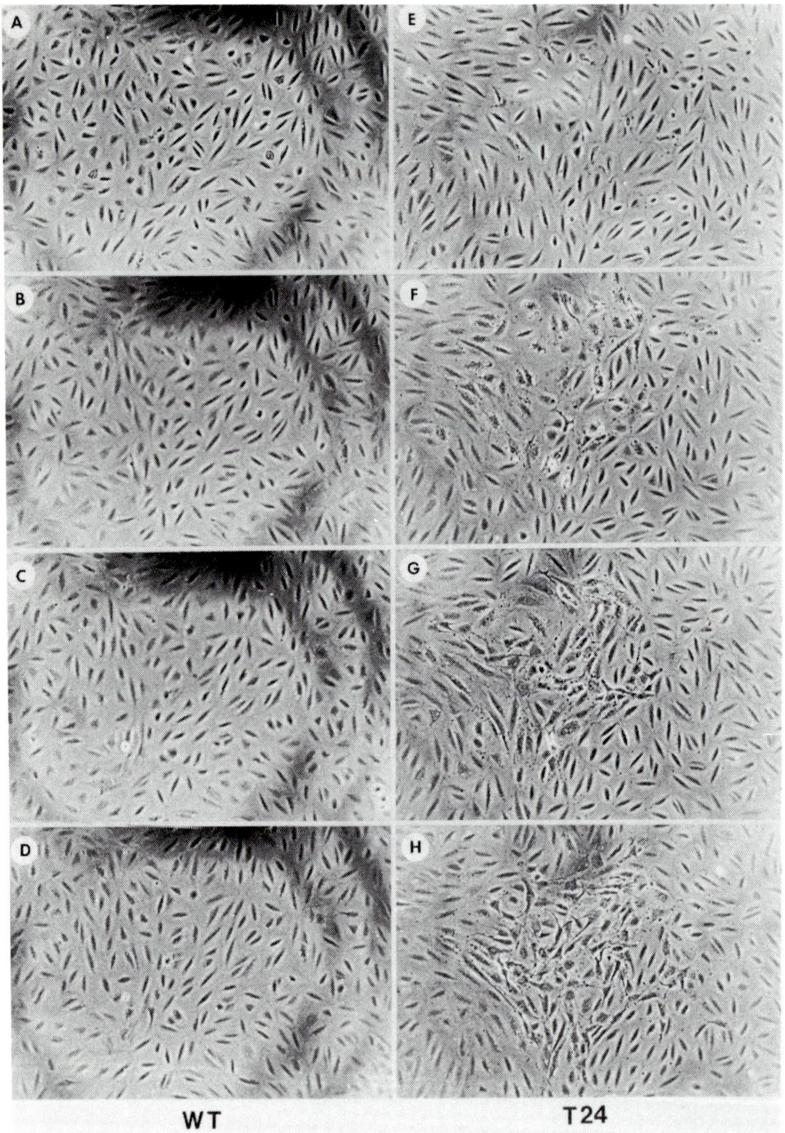

Fig. 5. Effect of microinjection of *ras* proteins into Ref 52 cells. Areas of a confluent monolayer of Ref 52 cells in DMEM containing 8% foetal bovine serum (FBS) were injected with either 5 × 10^5 molecules/cell of the proto-oncogenic form of H-*ras* (A–D) or 8 × 10^5 molecules/cell of the oncogenic form of H-*ras* (E–H). About 30 cells were injected in the centres of the two fields. The fields were photographed by phase-contrast microscopy (10× lens) at 30 min (A, E), 4 h (B, F), 12 h (C, G) and 20 h (D, H) post-injection.

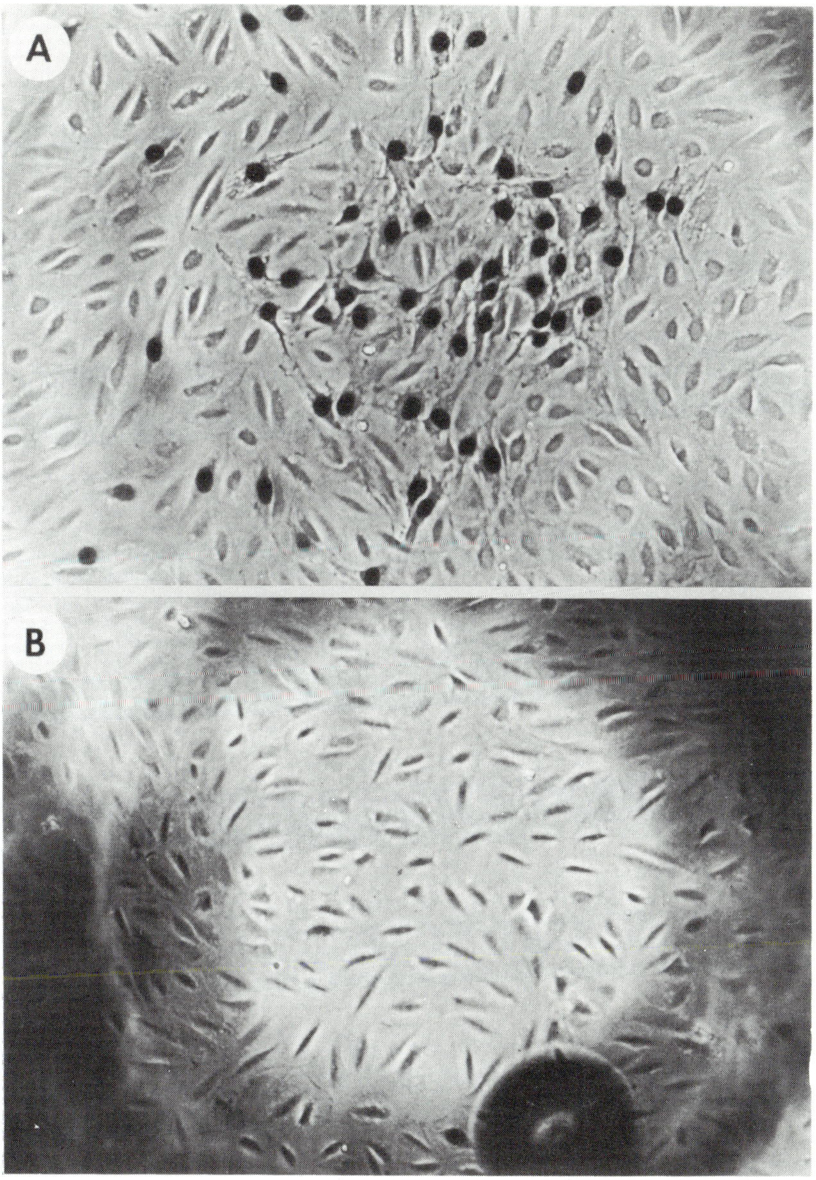

Fig. 6. Stimulation of DNA synthesis in quiescent rat embryo fibroblasts (Ref 52) after microinjection of the human H-*ras* oncogene protein. Thirty cells in the middle of each panel were injected with the human oncogene (A) or proto-oncogene (B) form of the H-*ras* protein and incubated with [^{3}H]thymidine. Twenty-four hours post-injection, the cells were fixed and processed for emulsion autoradiography. The fields were then photographed by phase-contrast microscopy with a 10× lens. Note that only the oncogene form of the H-*ras* protein stimulated DNA synthesis.

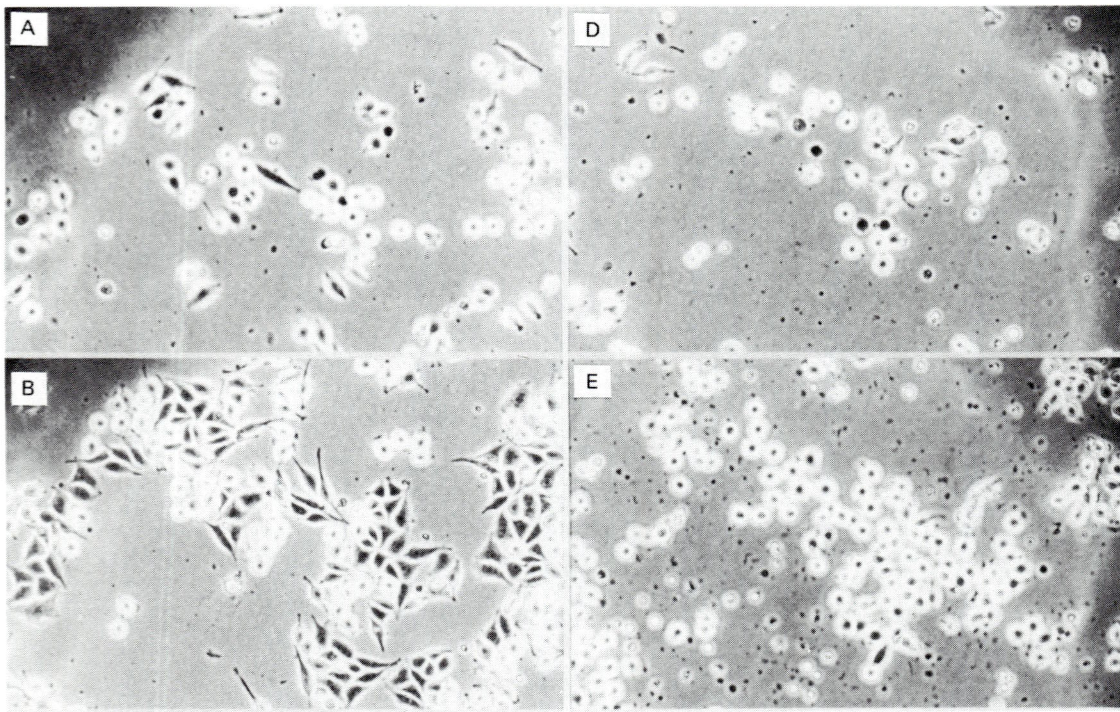
A
D
B
E

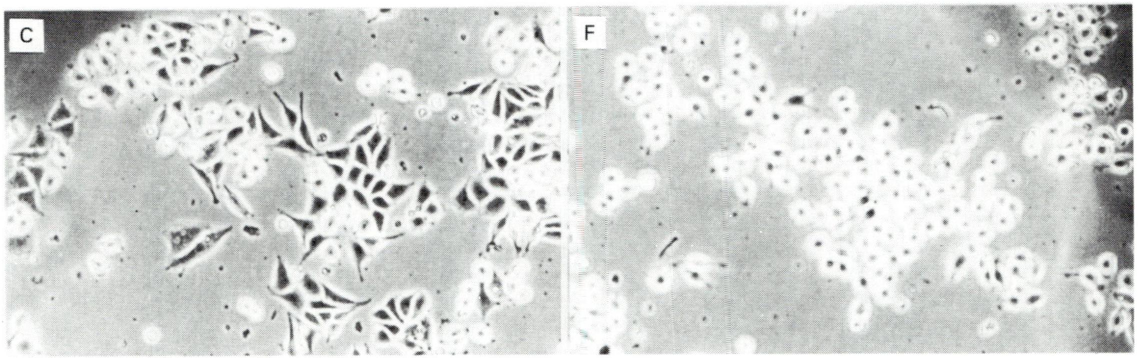

Fig. 7. Morphology of v-Ki-NRK cells after microinjection of anti-p21-ser and control IgG. Approximately 35 v-Ki-NRK cells in each of the two areas (demarcated by ink circles under the dish) were microinjected with anti-p21-ser (panels A–E) or non-immune IgG (panels D–F). Phase-contrast photomicrographs (10× lens) were taken of the two areas 30 min (A, D), 24 h (B, E), and 36 h (C, F) post-injection. Notice that the cells injected with anti-p21-ser preparation show a normal flattened morphology for some time and grow at a slower rate than the surrounding uninjected cells or the cells injected with the control IgG

demonstrated that introduction of the oncogenic, but not the proto-oncogenic, form of the *ras* protein resulted in a stimulation of cell growth as shown by both increased DNA synthesis and cell division. Using this assay, we and our collaborators are currently examining other cellular factors which either stimulate or inhibit this *ras*-induced cell proliferation. In addition, similar to the tubulin studies shown in Fig. 2, we are analysing both the pattern of protein synthesis as well as changes in the phosphorylation state of certain cellular proteins following introduction of the oncogenic *ras* protein into living cells.

Complementary to the studies examining the action of *ras* in living cells, we (in collaboration with the Human Genetics Group at Cetus Corporation) have also investigated whether antibodies against certain forms of the *ras* protein, when introduced into *ras* transformed cells, will result in a reversal of the transformed phenotype (Feramisco *et al.*, 1985). In these studies an antibody specific for only the oncogenic, v-Ki-*ras* oncogene protein, and not for the wild-type proto-oncogenic form, was produced by Frank McCormick and his colleagues (Clark *et al.*, 1985). NRK cells, transformed with the *ras* oncogene (Ki-NRK cells), were injected with this specific antibody or with non-immune IgG antibody. At 30 min, 24 h and 36 h post-injection, the cells were photographed as shown in Fig. 7. In Fig. 7A, C and E are shown the time-course of cells injected with the anti-V-*ras* antibody and in Fig. 7D, E and F the time-course of cells injected with pre-immune serum. The cells injected with the anti-V-*ras* antibody showed a normal flattened morphology and a much slower rate of cell division as compared to the surrounding uninjected cells or the cells injected with the pre-immune serum. With time, as the antibody was presumably turned-over in the cell, the injected cells returned to a more rounded and transformed phenotype and displayed an accompanying increase in the rate of cell division.

V. CONCLUSION

While it is certain that we have as yet to take full advantage of the wide range of experiments involving direct microinjection, some interesting concepts have been put forward. The work of several groups has shown that functional proteins can be directly placed inside living somatic cells, and indeed alter the biology of the recipient cells. For example, cellular DNA or protein synthesis, cell structure, or membrane potential have been altered by these microinjected proteins (e.g. Tjian *et al.*, 1978; Feramisco *et al.*, 1984; DeRiemer *et al.*, 1985). As we improve our microanalytical procedures, it will be possible to analyse many more types of biological responses using these types of microinjection studies.

A second class of microinjection experiments utilizing fluorescently labelled proteins has also begun to be exploited with considerable success. For example, individual protein components of the cell are purified and "tagged" with a visual probe, and then injected into the living cell. By using either photomicroscopy or time-lapse microscopy (Willingham and Pastan, 1978), it is possible to follow both the distribution and the fate of the protein (e.g. half-life) in the cell. While this approach has been most commonly used by those studying the cytoskeleton, a cellular macromolecular system easily visualized, this technique may prove to be useful in the studies of other cellular components. Surely as more sophisticated microscopy systems (which are less damaging than continual fluorescence microscopy) become available, this general approach will become a more useful method for examining the intracellular dynamics of individual proteins.

The third type of experiments covered in this chapter deal with the microinjection of antibodies into the cell, with the purpose being to interfere with the function of the target antigen. This approach appears extremely powerful, in that it may serve to be complementary to both biochemical studies *in vitro* as well as to the aforementioned approach of microinjection of functional proteins into the cell. Armed with a suitable antibody of the desired specificity, it is possible transiently to eliminate or diminish the activity of the target antigen, thereby allowing the investigator a time period in which to assess the biological consequence(s) of this inhibited activity. While there is no guarantee that the antigen will be accessible to the injected antibody (thereby giving a negative result), the several cases where the antigen appears accessible are striking. For example, the role of intermediate filaments (Klymkowski, 1981; Lin and Feramisco, 1981), myosin (Mabuchi and Okuno, 1977), vinculin (Kreis and Birchmeier, 1981), or actin (Scheer *et al.*, 1984) in the biology of the cell have been studied in this way. In addition, the direct role of the *ras* oncogene protein in maintaining the transformed state of the cell has also been established using this approach (Feramisco *et al.*, 1985). There is little doubt that numerous antigens will be destroyed in living cells by microinjection of specific antibodies, yielding direct information concerning the biological functions of the antigens.

All in all, these sorts of microinjection experiments are proving to be most useful in studying the structural organization and functions of cellular components and will continue to be invaluable to the investigator for the studies of the structure and function of various macromolecules.

ACKNOWLEDGEMENTS

We especially thank all our colleagues who have participated in various aspects of the studies described herein. Thanks are due to Dr J. D. Watson for his continuing encouragement and support. The technical assistance of G. Binns, N. Kronenberg, P. Renna and M. Szadkowski is gratefully acknowledged. Support for many of these studies was provided in part by N.I.H. grants GM28277 (J.R.F.), GM33551 (W.J.W.), and HL 23848 (W.J.W.).

REFERENCES

Antman, K. H. and Livingston, D. (1980). *Cell* **19**, 627–635.

Ashburner, M. and Bonner, J. J. (1979). *Cell* **17**, 241–254.

Burridge, K. and Feramisco, J. R. (1980). *Cell* **19**, 587–595.

Clark, R., Wong, G., Arnheim, N., Nitecki, D. and McCormick, F. (1985). *Proc. Natl. Acad. Sci. USA* **82**, 5280–5284.

Cleveland, D. W., Pittenger, M. F. and Feramisco, J. R. (1983). *Nature* **305**, 738–740.

DeRiemer, S. A., Strong, J. A., Albert, K. A., Greengard, P. and Kaczmarek, L. K. (1985). *Nature* **313**, 313–316.

Feramisco, J. R. (1979). *Proc. Natl. Acad. Sci. USA* **76**, 3967–3971.

Feramisco, J. R. and Blose, S. H. (1980). *J. Cell Biol.* **86**, 608–615.

Feramisco, J. R., Clark, R., Wong, G., Arnheim, N., Milley, R. and McCormick, F. (1985). *Nature* **314**, 639–642.

Feramisco, J. R., Gross, M., Kamata, T., Rosenberg, M. and Sweet, R. W. (1984). *Cell* **38**, 109–117.

Geiger, B. (1979). *Cell* **18**, 193–205.

Keith, C., Feramisco, J. R. and Shelanski, M. (1981). *J. Cell Biol.* **88**, 234–240.

Klymkowski, M. (1981). *Nature* **291**, 249–251.

Kreis, T. E. and Birchmeier, W. (1981). *Experimentia* **37**, 650a.

Kreis, T. E., Winterhalter, K. H. and Birchmeier, W. (1979). *Proc. Natl. Acad. Sci. USA* **76**, 3814–3818.

Lin, J. J. C. and Feramisco, J. R. (1981). *Cell* **24**, 185–193.

Mabuchi, I. and Okuno, M. (1977). *J. Cell. Biol.* **74**, 251–263.

Scheer, U., Hinssen, H., Franke, W. and Jockusch, B. (1984). *Cell* **39**, 111–122.

Tabin, C. J., Bradley, S. M., Bergmann, C. I., Weinberg, R. A., Papageorge, A. G., Scolnick, E. M., Dhar, R., Lowy, D. R. and Chang, E. H. (1982). *Nature* **300**, 143–149.

Taparowsky, E., Suard, Y., Fasano, O., Shimizu, K., Goldfarb, M. and Wigler, M. (1982). *Nature* **300**, 762–765.

Tjian, R., Fey, G. and Graessmann, A. (1978). *Proc. Natl. Acad. Sci. USA* **75**, 1279–1283.

Warner, A. E., Guthrie, S. C. and Gilula, N. B. (1984). *Nature* **311**, 127–131.

Wehland, J. and Weber, K. (1980). *Exp. Cell Res.* **127**, 397–408.

Welch, W. J. and Feramisco, J. R. (1982). *J. Biol. Chem.* **257**, 14949–14959.

Welch, W. J. and Feramisco, J. R. (1984). *J. Biol. Chem.* **259**, 4501–4513.

Welch, W. J. and Feramisco, J. R. (1985a). *Mol. Cell. Biol.* **5**, 1229–1237.

Welch, W. J. and Feramisco, J. R. (1985b). *Mol. Cell. Biol.* **5**, 1571–1581.

Welch, W. J., Garrels, J. I., Thomas, G. P., Lin, J. J.-C. and Feramisco, J. R. (1983). *J. Biol. Chem.* **258**, 7102–7111.

Willingham, M. C. and Pastan, I. (1978). *Cell* **13**, 501–507.

4

Studies of Retroviral Packaging

S. J. DeGudicibus, B. Gentile, R. S. Bhatt, M. S. Poonian and D. W. Stacey

I. INTRODUCTION

Viruses provide important models in biological studies because of their simplicity, both in structure and biological action. The retrovirus, for example, contains all three of its replicative genes within a single RNA genomic molecule of approximately 10 kb. The retrovirus particle contains a protein core derived from the viral *gag* gene, reverse transcriptase from the *pol* gene and envelope glycoprotein from the *env* gene. Upon infection the viral genome is reverse-transcribed to yield a double stranded cDNA which integrates into the host chromosome and serves as a template for viral mRNA synthesis. The primary viral RNA transcript contains a copy of the entire integrated proviral DNA. It is known, however, that two viral-specific RNA species are present within infected cells. A 35S transcript which is similar or identical to virion genomic RNA serves as mRNA for *gag* and for *pol* proteins. The 35S, full genomic molecule also serves as nuclear precursor to the second viral-specific mRNA present in infected cells, the subgenomic 21S *env* mRNA. When 35S genomic RNA is microinjected into the nuclei of uninfected host cells using glass capillaries, virus production results. The genomic RNA serves as precursor to subgenomic *env* mRNA only when introduced directly into the nucleus (Stacey and Hanafusa, 1978).

While approximately equal amounts of spliced and unspliced mRNA exist within an infected cell, very little spliced *env* mRNA appears in virus particles. The small amount of *env* mRNA which is found in virus particles does not appear to be packaged in a normal way. Two full genomic viral molecules are normally present within the virion. The *env* mRNA in virus particles appears to be present in addition to both full-sized molecules and may therefore be a simple contaminant (Stacey, 1979). Host cell mRNAs similarly appear to be aberrantly packaged into retroviral particles at very

Microinjection and Organelle Transplantation Techniques

ISBN: 0-12-164722-6
ISBN: 0-12-164723-4 Pbk

low frequency (Ikawa *et al.*, 1974). In this chapter we describe studies of the molecular characteristics of the genomic molecule recognized during viral packaging.

Our approach to the study of viral packaging first involved the introduction of desired nucleotide changes into a cloned viral genomic molecule. It was then necessary to determine the effect of these changes upon the viral packaging phenotype using direct microinjection (see also Chapters 1 and 2) and viral genetics.

II. RETROVIRAL PACKAGING — ASSAY

The cloned viral genome employed in this work represented a circular permutation of the linear viral genomic molecule (Fig. 1). Circular viral DNA obtained from infected cells was introduced into pBR322 after a single restriction endonuclease cleavage within the *env* gene. Subsequent expression of *env* would, therefore, require that the gene be reconstituted by ligation. To accomplish this, viral-specific sequences were freed from vector sequences by restriction enzyme cleavage.

We were pleased to find that remarkably rapid and accurate ligation was carried out by the recipient cell following microinjection of restriction endonuclease-cleaved DNA into the nucleus (Kopchick and Stacey, 1983). In addition, the properly ligated molecules served well as templates for transcription without apparent integration (as required during normal virus infection). Consequently, cloned viral DNA was freed of pBR322 sequences and injected into the nuclei of host (chick embryo) cells. Viral RNA and protein then appeared within the treated cells as directed by the injected template.

A final aspect of our packaging assay involved viral genetics. In any given culture few cells could be injected due to physical constraints. Injections were, therefore, made into cells infected and transformed by the viral mutant RSV(−). This sarcoma virus contains the *src* oncogene in place of the viral *env* gene. Viral *gag* and *pol* functions are expressed in RSV(−) cells but infectious virus production requires complementation with viral envelope glycoprotein. We selected for injection mutants we knew would provide the *env* function. In this way, regardless of the proportion of injected cells, infectious virus was released by all those receiving injections. Within these cells two types of viral genomic RNA would exist and be available for packaging. Genomic RNA of the transforming RSV(−) virus would contain the *src* gene but not *env*. Transcripts of injected DNA, on the other hand, would uniquely be *env*-positive (Pugatsch and Stacey, 1983). Genetic analysis of virus released following injection yielded a ratio of these two

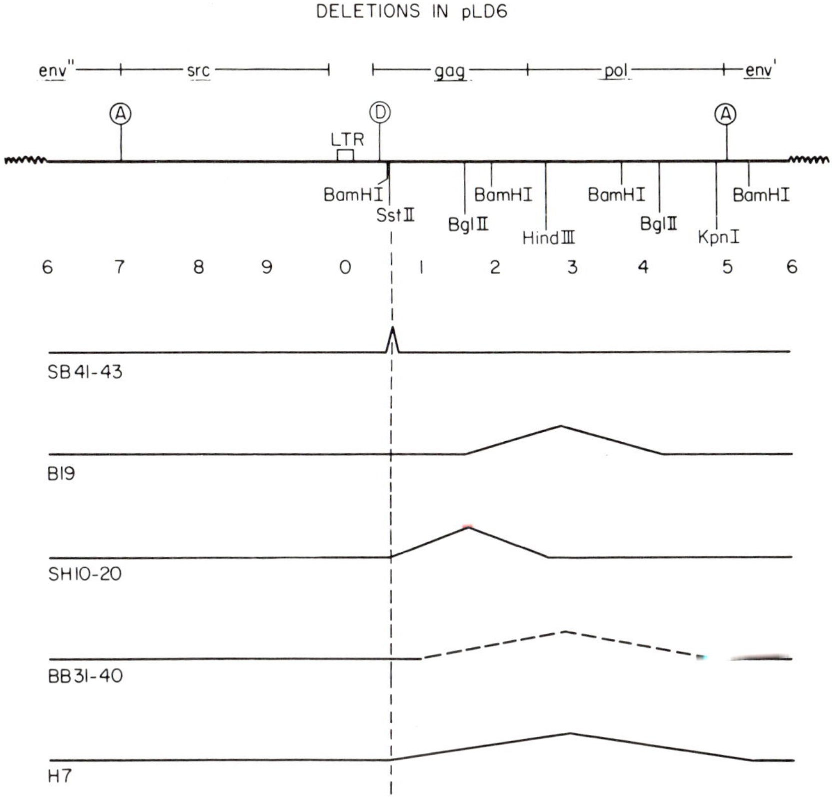

Fig. 1. Cloned viral genome and deletions. The cloned retroviral genome is diagrammed along with relevant restriction sites, the location of viral gene coding regions, and splice donor and acceptor sites (circled letters). Numbers refer to kbp. Lines below indicate the location of deletions analysed for packaging efficiency (from Pugatsch and Stacey, 1983). The dashed line (SB31-40) indicates that deletions vary significantly in length.

types of virus and, therefore, a comparison of packaging efficiency of the two genomic molecules (Fig. 2).

Initial studies identified a region of the viral genome required for proper packaging recognition. Subsequent studies to be reported here, however, reveal the complexity of the nucleotide recognition mechanism involved. T. Pugatsch reasoned that a sequence required for packaging must be removed during splicing of full genomic viral RNA to yield *env* mRNA, since the spliced mRNA is poorly packaged. This intron, however, is almost 5 kbp in length.

At first, attempts were made to identify the general location of packaging sequences. A deletion of 2.6 kbp located entirely within the *env* intron

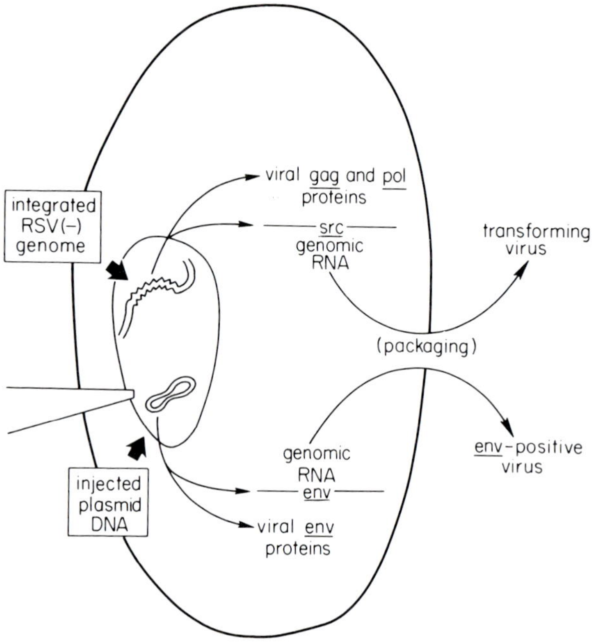

Fig. 2. Diagram of microinjection packaging assay. An RSV(−) cell is diagrammed. The integrated sarcoma viral genome is transcribed to yield genomic RNA containing *src*, along with mRNA for viral *gag* and *pol* proteins. No infectious virus are released due to viral *env* gene deficiency. Injected plasmid DNA is transcribed to yield *env*-containing genomic RNA along with *env* mRNA able to complement the cells in virus production. Upon introduction of the *env*-containing plasmid DNA, therefore, virus production begins. Infectious particles may package either genomic RNA transcribed from the RSV(−) genome or transcripts of injected DNA. The ratio between these can be determined by genetically analysing virus released. This ratio serves as an indication of relative packaging efficiency of the two viral RNAs.

(between BglII sites; B19, Fig. 1) was removed. The resulting deleted viral genomic molecule was then injected into RSV(−) cells. The proportion of *env*-positive virus released following injection was almost identical to that observed when unaltered viral genomic DNA was injected. Approximately 10 *env*-containing DNA transcripts were packaged for each RSV(−) genome RNA. Thus, no sequence contained within the 2.6 kbp BglII fragment was involved in packaging; nor was the full size of the transcript important. Further studies involved extending the size of the deletion to more than 3.0 kbp (BB31-40, Fig. 1) yet the resulting transcripts were packaged well (Pugatsch and Stacey, 1983).

The deletions described were all located in the *pol* gene and extended into the 3′ half of *gag*. Since this genomic region seemed not to be required for packaging the 5′ portion of the *gag* gene was analysed. Fortunately, a unique

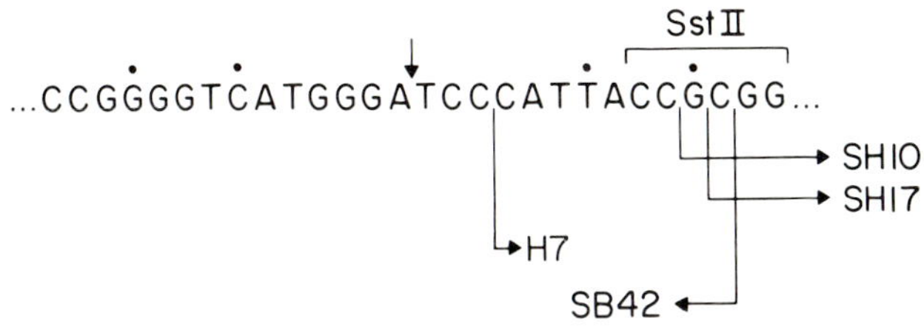

Fig. 3. Location of sequences required for virus packaging. The viral genome is diagrammed along with location of viral protein coding regions and location of a self-complementary 28 bp sequence believed to be required in packaging. The sequence is presented along with the position at which deletions begin or terminate within the sequence. (Note, A at position 9 from left is actually C.) Of the deletion mutants listed only SH17 was packaged normally (from Pugatsch and Stacey, 1983).

SstII restriction site was located in this area. Four deletions of 40–70 bp were introduced into the viral plasmid at this site (SB41-43, Fig. 1). When DNAs of the resulting plasmids were microinjected into RSV(−) cells a 10-fold excess of RSV(−) genomic molecules compared to transcripts of the injected DNA was packaged. Previously, the transcripts had always been packaged in a 10-fold excess. Thus, the short deletions near the SstII site (approximately 100 bp downstream of the splice donor site) had resulted in a 100-fold reduction in packaging efficiency (Pugatsch and Stacey, 1983). This region was obviously very important in packaging and attempts were made to analyse the region even more critically.

Deletions were introduced beginning at the SstII site and extending into the *pol* gene. Several were generated and all but one had a normal packaging phenotype. Sequence studies of the one deletion whose packaging was also reduced by 100-fold (SH10, Fig. 3) showed that it lacked only two base pairs more than a deletion which was packaged normally (SH17, Fig. 3: one base was derived from each terminus of the deletion). The two base pairs identified appeared, therefore, to be critical in packaging. These happened to be located at the 3′ terminus of a sequence of 28 bp, 22 of which form a self-complementary structure believed to be involved in binding the two genomic molecules together within the virion (Pugatsch and Stacey, 1983). At this point it seemed apparent that the palindrome was necessary for packaging.

To assess directly the involvement in packaging of the 28 bp region described, site-specific mutagenesis was employed as follows. The 28 bp region was bounded at one terminus by a unique SstII restriction site and at the other by a SmaI site. Deletions introduced into the viral plasmid removed all SmaI sites except the one described. This required generating deletions of a 4 kbp EcoRI restriction fragment containing the *src* gene along with a BglII fragment from *gag* and *pol*. Synthetic oligonucleotides were

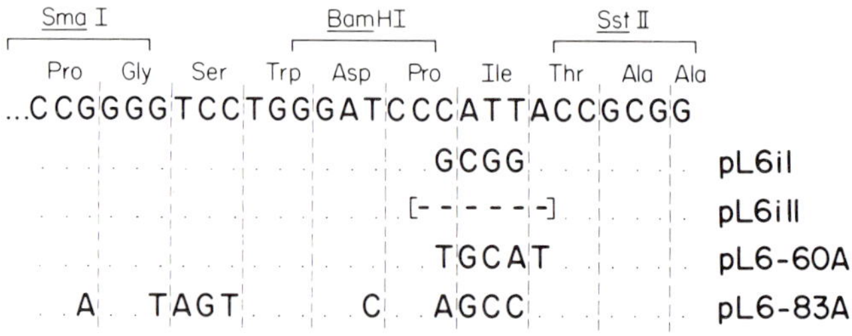

Fig. 4. Site-specific sequence alterations analysed for packaging efficiency. The sequence of the self-complementary 28 bp region described in Fig. 3 is diagrammed along with restriction sites and amino acid codons. The sequence of 4 mutants analysed is presented. Only those bases altered from wild-type are listed.

then constructed and inserted between the SstII and the SmaI sites. Recipient clones were identified by hybridization with the labelled oligonucleotides. The previously deleted genomic regions were then reintroduced to generate the full virus and sequences were verified by DNA sequence analysis. A 4 bp region was first altered to yield clone pL6i1. In addition, an exact 6 bp deletion was generated at this same location to yield pL6ill. In the first an Ile was changed to an Arg, while in the second Ile and Thr were deleted (Fig. 4). When pL6il was injected into uninfected chick cells a productive infection resulting in virus production at high titre resulted, indicating that neither the base change nor the amino acid alteration had significantly affected any viral function.

The phenotype of pL6ill, on the other hand, was dramatically altered. Little virus production was observed after injection into chick cells. In addition, injection into RSV(−) cells yielded little virus, indicating that the production of *env* mRNA was greatly reduced. It is not known why such a dramatic alteration resulted, especially since large deletions in the same area did not affect *env* mRNA synthesis. It was not possible to make any conclusion regarding packaging due to the low levels of *env* mRNA produced with pL6ill.

It was clear from results with pL6il that minor alterations in the palindrome were tolerated in packaging. Consequently, two more dramatic alterations were constructed. In pL6-60A a 5 bp alteration was introduced resulting in the substitution of an Ile for an Ala and Thr for Ser. Where 22 of 28 bp were self-complementary in the original virus now only 16 of 28 were complementary (Fig. 4). This virus was injected into RSV(−) cells and the packaging phenotype analysed. Surprisingly, the packaging phenotype was unaltered from wild-type (data not shown). The final construct involved alteration of 10 bp resulting in a single amino acid change from Ile to Ala and only 12 of 28 bp were self-complementary (Fig. 4). Again packaging phenotype was unaltered in this mutant pL6-83A.

III. DISCUSSION

Previous work clearly demonstrated that a self-complementary region of the Rous sarcoma viral genome near the SstII restriction site is required for packaging. While deletion of 3 kbp elsewhere in the viral genome did not affect packaging, deletion of 40 to 70 bp at this region consistently resulted in a 100-fold decrease in packaging efficiency.

Unpublished data are reported here to extend these studies. Unexpectedly, alteration of from 4 to 10 bp within the self-complementary region did not affect the packaging phenotype. A deletion of 6 bp in this region had a generally depressing effect upon a variety of viral functions. Clearly the molecular restraints in identification of viral genomic molecules during viral packaging is not simple. It appears that the ability to form a stable base-paired structure near the SstII site is not required since packaging occurs when 10 of 22 bp are disrupted (see Norton and Coffin, 1985). Furthermore, it is known that base-pairing probably does not occur until the virus has budded, which further suggests that base-pairing is not involved in packaging (Canaani *et al.*, 1973).

The previous results with deleted viral genomic DNA clearly indicate that the genomic region described is important in packaging. Deletions disrupt not only base composition but secondary structure of the RNA as well. Others have reported regions in the untranslated leader or near the 3′ terminus of the viral genome to be required (Shank and Linial, 1980; Sorge *et al.*, 1983; Kawai and Koyama, 1984; Norton and Coffin, 1985). Our results are consistent with the observation that packaging recognition is complicated and may involve multiple genomic regions. These may be important in the actual recognition or in the formation of the RNA secondary structure necessary to expose the sequences which are directly recognized during viral packaging.

REFERENCES

Canaani, E., von der Helm, K. and Duesberg, P. (1973). *Proc. Natl. Acad. Sci. USA* **70**, 401–405.

Ikawa, Y., Ross, J. and Leder, P. (1974). *Proc. Natl. Acad. Sci. USA* **71**, 1154–1158.

Kawai, S. and Koyama, T. (1984). *J. Virol.* **51**, 147–153.

Kopchick, J. J. and Stacey, D. W. (1983). *J. Biol. Chem.* **258**, 11 528–11 536.

Norton, P. A. and Coffin, J. M. (1985). *Mol. Cell. Biol.* **5**, 281–290.

Pugatsch, T. and Stacey, D. W. (1983). *Virology* **128**, 505–511.

Shank, P. R. and Linial, M. (1980). *J. Virol.* **36**, 450–456.

Sorge, J., Ricci, W. and Hughes, S. H. (1983). *J. Virol.* **48**, 667–675.

Stacey, D. W. (1979). *J. Virol.* **29**, 949–956.

Stacey, D. W. and Hanafusa, H. (1978). *Nature* **273**, 779–782.

5

Erythrocyte-Mediated Transfer: Methods

R. A. Schlegel and M. C. Rechsteiner

I. INTRODUCTION

Mammalian erythrocytes offer several advantages as carriers for introducing materials into living, nucleated cells. Because erythrocytes are non-nucleated and contain only vestiges of other organelles, they are genetically and nearly metabolically inert. Because they are small, their contents do not unduly perturb recipient cells. A mammalian erythrocyte fused to a typical culture cell increases its volume by only about 6% and its plasma membrane by 20%. Because their membranes are simple and the most well-studied of eukaryotic cells, they are amenable to manipulations which can exchange their contents, making them carriers of specific materials. For these reasons, it is not surprising that several systems have been devised to exploit erythrocytes as carriers of materials into eukaryotic culture cells (see also Chapters 6 and 12).

In 1974 Okada and colleagues detected the transfer of endogenous haemoglobin from erythrocytes to culture cells with which they had been fused. The percentage of culture cells which were positive for haemoglobin was 36%. However, when fluorescein isothiocyanate was substituted for haemoglobin in the erythrocytes, fewer than one in a hundred culture cells fused with a loaded erythrocyte (Furusawa *et al.*, 1974). Apparently, the hypotonic procedure used to load the erythrocytes had reduced their capacity to fuse. This problem was rapidly remedied with the description of protocols for loading and fusion which resulted in the transfer of loaded materials from erythrocyte carriers into a large fraction (up to 90%) of as many as 10^7 culture cell recipients (Schlegel and Rechsteiner, 1975; Loyter *et al.*, 1975; Nishimura *et al.*, 1976).

Microinjection and Organelle Transplantation Techniques

ISBN: 0-12-164722-6
ISBN: 0-12-164723-4 Pbk

II. ERYTHROCYTE LOADING

When erythrocytes are placed in a sufficiently hypotonic solution, they swell from osmotic pressure, and pores appear in their plasma membranes. Substances dissolved or suspended in the solution are thus allowed access to the erythrocytes' interior. Equilibration of internal and external pressure through release of haemoglobin leads to cell shrinking and closure of the pores, which can be most effectively sealed by incubation at 37°C, thus trapping exogenous substances inside the cell.

Available information leads to a generalization concerning the ability of erythrocytes loaded by hypotonic haemolysis to be fused with culture cells using Sendai virus: as the tonicity of the environment to which the erythrocytes are exposed during loading decreases and as the length of exposure to these conditions increases, the capacity to be fused decreases. For instance, the addition of large volumes of hypotonic lysing buffer to erythrocytes exposes them to very hypotonic conditions as the salts liberated from the cells are diluted. Conversely, lysis by reduced volumes maintains more physiological conditions. The following loading protocols have been designed with these precepts in mind. However, as discussed below, such restrictions do not necessarily apply when polyethylene glycol (PEG) is used as fusogen.

Human erythrocytes are most often used for erythrocyte-mediated injection. Not only are they usually the easiest to obtain, but they are also the most readily fused by Sendai virus. Yamaizumi *et al.* (1978a) have reported that guinea pig, dog and cow erythrocytes fuse with efficiencies of 90%, 50% and 40% of human erythrocytes, respectively. Rabbit (Kaltoft *et al.*, 1976), guinea pig (Heumann *et al.*, 1981) and commercially available sheep erythrocytes (Kriegler *et al.*, 1978) have also been successfully used, the latter two in fusions using PEG where relative fusion efficiencies of erythrocytes from different species have not been examined. The fusion efficiencies of different human ABO blood types are similar using Sendai as fusogen (Yamaizumi *et al.*, 1978a). Outdated as well as fresh blood can be used (Wasserman *et al.*, 1976), although use of the latter may necessitate special precautions to stabilize loaded erythrocytes as mentioned below. Furusawa *et al.* (1976) report that washed erythrocyte suspensions can be stored at 4°C for several days before they are loaded, but others advise that they should be used as soon as possible after washing, since loading is significantly reduced following overnight storage (Rechsteiner, 1975). This discrepancy may be a reflection of the differing procedures which these investigators employ to load erythrocytes.

The most popular procedures for loading erythrocytes are the dialysis method and the pre-swell method. Two standard dialysis protocols and a pre-swell protocol are described, followed by variations on these themes and a description of alternate procedures.

A. Dialysis loading

In the dialysis protocol of Yamaizumi *et al.* (1978a), two ml of an isotonic 10% suspension of washed erythrocytes are placed in a dialysis bag containing a solution of the molecule to be loaded. This mixture is dialysed against 500 ml of isotonic buffer diluted 1:6 with H_2O. After 30 min at 4°C, at which time there is no further entry of molecules into the reversibly lysed erythrocytes, the suspension is dialysed against 500 ml of isotonic buffer for 30 min at room temperature to afford resealing of the erythrocyte membrane. The percentage of the initial concentration of the molecule which is trapped inside the erythrocytes is dependent upon molecular weight, as discussed below. However, using a fluorescence-activated cell sorter (FACS) to analyse erythrocytes loaded with fluoresceinated bovine serum albumin (fl-BSA), Mekada *et al.* (1978b) found a linear increase in the average fluorescence of erythrocytes with increasing concentration of fl-BSA in the dialysis bag up to at least 15 mg/ml. Under these conditions all cells were loaded and the coefficient of variation in the FACS pattern was small, indicating that nearly equivalent amounts of fl-BSA were contained in each cell.

This linear uptake applies as long as the concentration of erythrocytes in the dialysis bag is lower than 30%. At this point, the concentration loaded begins to plateau, probably as a result of inhibition of haemolysis caused by release of large amounts of haemoglobin. Indeed, at a 40% concentration of erythrocytes many intact, unlysed erythrocytes are found (Yamaizumi *et al.*, 1978a). Therefore, if a small amount of a precious material is to be loaded, one should employ no more than one part erythrocytes to two parts of a solution of the molecule to be loaded. Furusawa (1980) also recommends that under these circumstances a specially devised microdialyser be used and that dialysis be against H_2O for 15 min at 0°C followed sequentially by dialysis against isotonic buffer for 15 min at 0°C and incubation at 37°C for 90 min to afford resealing. Smaller ratios of buffer to erythrocytes, down to 1:1, can be handled using the pre-swell method described below.

The dialysis protocol of Wasserman *et al.* (1976) is similar to the general one just described except that erythrocytes are dialysed for a longer period of time against less dilute buffer (2 h against 40 mM NaCl, 10 mM Tricine-NaOH). Tonicity is restored by addition of a small volume of a concentrated salt solution, and resealing is performed by incubation for 30 min at 37°C. A significant difference is that cytochrome C is included at 0.5 mg/ml in the erythrocyte suspension during dialysis. This measure is required for efficient subsequent fusion of erythrocytes to culture cells and may be necessary only when using aged blood, as these investigators do, since the Japanese group apparently found no such requirement. Loading characteristics are the same as reported by the Japanese group: trapping is a linear function of the concentration of the macromolecule to be loaded, from 1–30 mg/ml in the case of BSA, for erythrocyte concentrations from 2.5 to 35%. Again, at concentrations higher than 35%, the efficiency of loading falls off, probably because not all cells lyse due to a high osmotic pressure in the haemolysate (Kulka and Loyter, 1979).

B. Pre-swell loading

The pre-swell method of loading was devised by Rechsteiner (1975) to permit efficient loading of erythrocytes at low ratios of lysing buffer to erythrocytes, which preserves precious materials. In addition, very small quantities of erythrocytes and consequently small volumes of materials can be easily handled. Briefly, erythrocytes are placed in a hypotonic solution which is dilute enough that the cells swell, but not so dilute that any haemoglobin is released. These "pre-swollen" cells are primed so that addition of a volume of lysing buffer only equivalent to the volume of a pre-swollen cell pellet will lyse and load nearly every erythrocyte. Two minutes after lysis is initiated by addition of buffer, a small volume of concentrated saline is added to restore isotonicity and cells are resealed by incubation at 37°C for 30–60 min. Detailed descriptions of the protocol can be found in Schlegel and Rechsteiner (1978), Rechsteiner (1982), and Schlegel and McEvoy (1985).

C. Characteristics of loading and of loaded erythrocytes

The ultimate haemolytic event appears to be the same whether the dialysis of pre-swell method is used. With each method there is a linear increase in material loaded with increasing concentration during lysis, and each method is characterized by a progressive exclusion or sieving of larger materials by the membrane. After dialysis, 100% of the initial concentration of a protein of 22000 Da (fragment A of diphtheria toxin) can be loaded, 50% of a 68000 Da protein (BSA) and 30% of a 160000 Da protein (IgG) (cited in Mekada *et al.*, 1978b). A similar size dependence is seen with the pre-swell method (Rechsteiner, 1982). Although loading of RNA molecules has not been systematically examined with respect to such factors as size and folding, some information is available. Small RNA molecules such as tRNA (Kaltoft *et al.*, 1976; Schlegel *et al.*, 1976) and small nuclear RNAs (Rechsteiner, 1982) can be efficiently loaded, as apparently can small mRNA molecules such as those coding for globin (Anderson *et al.*, 1978; Furusawa, 1980) and protamine (Boogaard and Dixon, 1983a). Information on loading of larger messages has not yet appeared. With respect to ribosomal RNAs, extensive degradation during loading by the pre-swell method has been reported (Rechsteiner, 1982), although Celis (1977) recorded success using a large-dilution method of loading. Therefore, the jury is still out on whether it is possible to efficiently load larger RNA molecules.

Loading of DNA into erythrocytes has also met with mixed success. To determine the size limitation on entry of double-stranded DNA into erythrocytes, Rechsteiner *et al.* (1984b) hypotonically lysed cells in the presence of a mixture of DNA fragments which were multiples of 200 bp in length. Only the fragments of 200–800 bp were found to be loaded in greater than trace amounts. Loading was quantified using single radioactively labelled fragments of defined lengths. Approximately 4% of 140-bp fragments and 2% of 400-bp fragments could be loaded. In an attempt to increase the size and quantity of fragments loaded, liquid crystal ψ forms of DNA were used in loadings, reasoning that these collapsed, compact structures of DNA might more readily penetrate the membrane pores than their extended, long and linear counterparts. However, loading did not occur (Rechsteiner *et al.*, 1984b). Nevertheless, Straus and Raskas (1980) have reported that enough adenovirus DNA can be loaded by the dialysis method to subsequently infect culture cells to which the loaded erythrocytes are fused.

The foregoing information can be translated into copies of molecules loaded into each erythrocyte. By either the dialysis or pre-swell method, nearly 10^7 copies of proteins with molecular weights around 25000 Da can be loaded per cell. Proteins with molecular weights roughly equivalent to BSA at 68000 Da can be loaded at from 2–5 × 10^6 copies. This number decreases to about 10^6 for proteins with a molecular weight near that of IgG molecules (180000 Da) and 10^5 for proteins of roughly 500000 Da. When small RNA molecules are considered, each erythrocyte can be loaded with from 5 × 10^6 to 10^7 molecules of tRNA. Loading of 140 and 400 bp of DNA translates to 3 × 10^5 and 5 × 10^4 molecules per cell, respectively, and the number of copies of adenovirus DNA per erythrocyte protected from DNAase digestion following loading was calculated to be 180. Another, reportedly more successful, method of loading DNA is described in the next section.

Once loaded, erythrocytes can be stored for reasonably long periods before they are used in fusions. Furusawa (1980) reports that cells loaded by the dialysis procedure leak only 10% of their contents over a 4-day period when kept at 4°C. At 37°C, however, 90% of loaded material is lost in a day. Similarly, pre-swell loaded erythrocytes lose only a trace of loaded material after overnight storage on ice, and even exhibit only a small amount of lysis after 24 h at 37°C if they are in culture medium (Rechsteiner, 1982).

Although the ability of loaded erythrocytes and even erythrocytes to fuse with culture cells has been reported to decrease dramatically beyond one day of storage at 4°C (Neff *et al.*, 1981), successful injections have been performed with loaded erythrocytes stored on ice for eight days (Rechsteiner, 1982). In the latter case $MnCl_2$ was added to the buffer in which the cells were stored to stabilize their membranes. Perhaps also of note is that the fusogens used in these two instances were not the same, PEG being employed in the first case and Sendai virus in the second. Once loaded, macromolecules are generally quite stable inside the erythrocyte due to a paucity of proteases and nucleases. A brief summary of the information available concerning stability is presented in Rechsteiner (1982).

D. Freeze–thaw loading

Recently, a pair of loading procedures which do not utilize hypotonic haemolysis or use it only as an adjunct have been developed for the expressed purpose of loading high molecular weight DNA. Both use freeze–thaw cycles to lyse cells, but they differ significantly in simplicity and somewhat in efficiency of loading.

In the procedure of Iino *et al.* (1983), one volume of erythrocytes is simply added to six volumes of a DNA solution, the suspension is frozen at −80°C for 30 s and then thawed at 37°C. Of the input DNA, roughly 2–3% is found associated with the cells, either within them or firmly attached to their membranes; most is resistant to DNase I. The upper size limit of DNA which can be loaded is around 10 kb. Loading of a pBR322 plasmid of 6.4 kb containing a thymidine kinase gene resulted in the association of 30 copies per erythrocyte when DNA at 50 μg/ml was used for loading, and the transformation of thymidine kinase-negative cells when fused with erythrocytes. Apparently proteins can also be loaded by this procedure since BSA was trapped at 40% of its initial concentration up to a concentration of 10 mg/ml.

The freeze–thaw method of Wiberg *et al.* (1983) begins with haemoglobin-free, unsealed erythrocytes prepared according to the procedure of Kaltoft and Celis (1978), described below under Alternative Procedures. To a 50-μl pellet of these cells is added 5 μg of DNA in a volume of 15 μl. Three freeze–thaw cycles performed at −70°C and 37°C are followed by the addition of concentrated saline to restore isotonicity, 5 min on ice and incubation at 37°C for 45 min for resealing. Six to 14% of plasmid DNA ranging in size from 3740 to 15 000 bp was found stably associated with cells, as judged by resistance to release by 1% NP-40. The amount associated was linearly related to the amount of DNA used for loading between 0.1 and

10 μg so that from 8–800 genome equivalents of polyoma form I DNA could be loaded per erythrocyte and used to transfect recipient cells to which they were fused.

E. Alternative procedures

Circumstances may arise where it is necessary to clear the erythrocyte of some endogenous molecule before loading. For instance, Capecchi *et al.* (1977) were interested in measuring the expression of HGPRT in mutant cells following injection of suppressor tRNA and therefore needed to reduce the level of the enzyme endogenous to erythrocytes. They did so by adapting the pre-swell method. Pre-swollen erythrocytes were treated with 6 vol of hyptonic buffer and then resealed as usual. The cells in which HGPRT activity had thus been reduced by seven-fold were then loaded normally by the pre-swell method using an equal volume of lysing buffer in which the tRNA was dissolved.

This approach has been taken several steps further by Boogaard and Dixon (1983a) in their "multiple lysis technique". Again, the pre-swell technique was used, this time at a dilution ratio of five, carrying the cells through 3–4 successive cycles in order drastically to reduce their endogenous contents. Finally, cells were loaded by the pre-swell method using an equal volume of lysing buffer containing the molecules to be loaded. Although the majority of tRNA loaded by either the simple pre-swell method or the multiple lysis method was still found to be full-sized when recovered from the cells, fewer molecules loaded by the latter technique were degraded. There is, however, a trade-off, since the amount of material which is trapped progressively decreases with each succeeding cycle such that at the fourth cycle nearly a factor of 10 less tRNA is loaded compared to the first cycle. In addition, cells were reported to lose their shape progressively with each cycle and to become increasingly smaller and more fragile.

Kaltoft and Celis (1978) have taken even more drastic measures to remove any possible interfering substances from erythrocytes prior to loading. Erythrocytes are lysed by 50 vol of hypotonic buffer and washed 3–4 times with the same buffer to remove haemoglobin. Molecules to be loaded are then added to these still unsealed cells (followed by freeze–thaw in the DNA-loading procedure described in the preceding section), isotonicity is restored and cells are resealed by incubation at 37°C.

As noted in the beginning of this section, exposure of erythrocytes to prolonged and drastic hypotonic conditions greatly reduces their ability to be fused by Sendai virus, whether they are fused with each other (Peretz *et al.*, 1974) or with culture cells (Furusawa *et al.*, 1974). In the latter case, erythrocytes were lysed by 5 vol of distilled water and washed in their unsealed state three times before being loaded and resealed, resulting in fusion with fewer than 1% of culture cells. Simply omitting the washing step appears to increase fusion to 10% (Wille and Willecke, 1976), whereas the dialysis or pre-swell method results in up to 90–95% of culture cells fusing with erythrocytes. If harsh conditions during loading result in such low fusion frequencies, how can the erythrocytes loaded after extensive washing as described in the preceding paragraph and those additionally frozen and thawed, or the distorted erythrocytes produced by the multiple-lysis technique, fuse perfectly well to culture cells? The answer is that in each of these cases PEG, not Sendai virus, was used as fusogen. Apparently, harsh treatments perturb the membrane such that Sendai virus can either no longer recognize its receptors or is unable to induce the membrane perturbations necessary to initiate fusion. These membrane alterations are of no consequence in fusion induced by chemicals such as PEG, the only factor of importance being that the erythrocytes are resealed so that their membranes neither leak erythrocyte contents prior to fusion nor cellular contents following it. Therefore, taking care in preparing erythrocytes which retain their capacity to fuse applies primarily to fusions where Sendai virus is used.

As a final note on loading, adaptation of any of the above standard procedures to satisfy particular experimental requirements may result in some erythrocytes which do not lyse or some which lyse but do not reseal. Should this occur, Kruse and Popjak (1981) have described a Percoll density gradient method for separating successfully loaded cells from intact erythrocytes or empty ghosts.

III. IDENTIFICATION AND ENUMERATION OF INJECTED CULTURE CELLS

Efficiency of microinjection refers to the fraction of culture cells in a population which have fused with one or more erythrocytes. To determine this value, a means of identifying injected cells is required. Both the transfer of endogenous erythrocyte components and of exogenous tracer molecules which are readily detectable at the level of single cells have been successfully used. Endogenous components can be either membrane or cytoplasmic erythrocyte constituents. Immunofluorescent staining using antibodies directed against erythrocytes has been used to detect erythrocyte membrane components incorporated into culture cell membranes upon fusion (Wasserman *et al.*, 1976; Yamaizumi *et al.*, 1978a). Transfer of haemoglobin from erythrocytes to the cytoplasm of culture cells upon fusion can be detected by benzidine staining (Furusawa *et al.*, 1974; Yamaizumi *et al.*, 1978a; Rechsteiner, 1982). Finally, Jonak and Mora (1980) identified cells which had been injected by fusion with loaded hen erythrocytes based on the presence of the distinctive, small and temporarily inert hen erythrocyte nuclei within injected heterokaryons.

Detection by transfer of the cytoplasmic marker haemoglobin suffers from lack of sensitivity if haemoglobin becomes sufficiently diluted during loading. One solution is to stain for the presence of injected haemoglobin using anti-haemoglobin antibodies and a second fluoresceinated antibody (Hendil, 1980). Alternatively, cytoplasmic tracers can be introduced into the erythrocytes upon loading. Fluoresceinated BSA, which becomes uniformly distributed within the cytoplasm of culture cell recipients within 5 min of its injection (Yamaizumi *et al.*, 1978a; Wojcieszyn *et al.*, 1981), has quite often been used, as has fluoresceinated IgG (Yamaizumi *et al.*, 1979; Ohara and Watanabe, 1982). Because these molecules are excluded from the nucleus of healthy cells, fluorescence microscopy of live or fixed cells also permits healthy injected cells to be distinguished from those which are dead or damaged. Finally, not only can these fluoresceinated cytoplasmic tracers be used to identify and enumerate injected cells, but they can also be used to separate injected cells from uninjected ones, and even to separate cells according to the number of erythrocytes to which they have fused, using FACS as described below under methods for isolating injected cells.

Almost any molecule which can be loaded and for which an antibody is available can also be used to identify injected cells. For instance, loading and injection of IgG molecules and detection by fluoresceinated anti-IgG has often been used (Antman and Livingston, 1980; Petrie *et al.*, 1982; Schlegel, 1984). Although radioactively labelled molecules can also be loaded, and injected cells identified by autoradiography (see, for example, Rechsteiner and Kuehl, 1979; Neff *et al.*, 1981), delays of usually at least several days are required for proper exposure of emulsions.

Many of the foregoing methods require a fluorescence microscope for detection. If one is not available, alternative cytological detection systems can be used. For instance, second antibodies conjugated with horseradish peroxidase (HRP) can be substituted for fluoresceinated antibodies and their presence detected by sequential application of H_2O_2 and a benzidine reagent. In fact, HRP itself can be loaded into erythrocytes as a cytoplasmic marker and detected histochemically in injected cells (Heumann *et al.*, 1981) with perhaps a ten-fold greater sensitivity than fluoresceinated cytoplasmic markers (Rechsteiner, 1982).

IV. FUSION

Each of the originators of erythrocyte-mediated microinjection used Sendai virus as fusogen. Because the initial description of the technique coincided with the advent of the use of PEG as a fusogen in the production of somatic cell hybrids, it was not long thereafter that several procedures were devised for its use in erythrocyte-mediated microinjection. Protocols employing each type of fusogen are described.

A. Sendai virus

Fusion employing Sendai virus can be performed either in suspension or in monolayer. Fusions in suspension offer logistical advantages when large numbers of cells are to be injected. On the other hand, when numerous variables or time-points are to be examined in a single experiment, as few as 10^3–10^4 cells plated on a coverslip are sufficient for each experimental point when cells are injected in monolayer. In addition, spread cells can be examined microscopically almost immediately after fusion.

(1) Suspension

The experimental conditions used for fusions in suspension vary little among investigators (Schlegel and Rechsteiner, 1978; Kulka and Loyter, 1979; Furusawa, 1980). From 10^6 to 10^7 culture cells, a 100-fold excess of loaded erythrocytes and from 400 to 1000 HAU of UV-inactivated Sendai virus (depending on number and type of culture cells and on the virus preparation) are combined in a small volume. After 10–15 min at 0°C to allow agglutination, the mixture is incubated at 37°C with gentle shaking for 20 min. Fusion is then terminated by placing cultures at 0°C and/or diluting with buffer. This simple procedure routinely results in a microinjection efficiency of 60–70%. There is general agreement that most injected cells result from fusion with 1–3 erythrocytes under these conditions. If culture cells remain viable after fusion with more than three erythrocytes, they may still be unrecoverable if attachment to a surface is required, since their surface has been considerably altered by the incorporation of large amounts of non-adherent erythrocyte membrane.

The only real variable in the above procedure is the divalent (or trivalent) cation which is included during fusion. Although Furusawa (1980) makes no specific mention of divalent cation requirements, Ca^{2+} is present during fusion at 1 mM in his protocol. Rechsteiner (1982) recommends that loaded erythrocytes be stored in buffer containing 2 mM Mn^{2+} to stabilize the cells against leakage and that it also be present at the same concentration during fusion to counteract some of the lysis induced by the virus. On the other hand, Wasserman *et al.* (1976, 1977) found Mn^{2+} to be inhibitory to protein synthesis by recipient cells following fusion. They recommend Ca^{2+} at 10 mM be used to reduce lysis of erythrocytes during fusion and yet maintain the health and viability of injected cells. However, not all types of cells can be efficiently fused in the presence of Ca^{2+}. In such cases they recommend the use of La^{3+} which prevents lysis of erythrocytes and stimulates fusion, but is somewhat toxic to recipient cells, although not as much so as Mn^{2+}. Therefore, unless the cell lines used are ones that have previously been tested, optimal choice of kind and concentration of cation may require some experimentation.

Cloning efficiency of a population of injected cells is a valid test of the viability of injected cells as long as they represent a very high fraction of the population. Under such conditions cloning efficiency has been found by most investigators to be 85–100% of uninjected controls. In several instances the fate of only the injected cells has been followed, identifying them by the presence of injected protein. Indicative of nearly normal cell division, the proportion of injected cells in a population was found to decrease only slightly over 4 days (Schlegel and Rechsteiner, 1978), the decrease possibly being attributed to a reported 1-day lag in the resumption of division (Yamaizumi *et al.*, 1978a). In the very best test of viability, injected cells were separated from uninjected cells by FACS, as described in a later section, and their cloning efficiencies compared. Injected cells were found to have a cloning efficiency of 90–100% of uninjected controls (Mekada *et al.*, 1978a, b).

Because erythrocytes are used in 100-fold excess over culture cells, the vast majority of them do not fuse to culture cells and must somehow be removed. Although some of the schemes described here for their removal were devised for fusions other than those induced by Sendai in suspension, all are nonetheless applicable. The simplest method is to plate the fusion mixture and wash out the non-adherent erythrocytes after the culture cells have adhered. Because erythrocytes settle and adhere to culture cells upon prolonged incubation, presumably due to residual Sendai particles adsorbed to both types of cells, it is best to wash out the erythrocytes as soon as possible. Residual erythrocytes of this type can be removed by a brief trypsin treatment which does not detach the culture cells (Rechsteiner, 1982), by two 10-min treatments with 0.83% NH_4Cl (Kaltoft *et al.*, 1976) or by a 10-s treatment with 10 mM buffer (Kruse *et al.*, 1981), the latter two of which preferentially lyse the erythrocytes. If time-points earlier than the time required for plating are desired, other steps can be taken.

Differential centrifugation is an effective way to remove a large fraction of unfused erythrocytes. Rechsteiner (1982) dilutes fusion mixtures to 10 ml with culture media and centrifuges for a short period at low *g* forces, which produces a tight pellet of culture cells overlaid with a fluffy coat of erythrocytes. After the latter is removed by decanting or pipetting and the operation repeated several times, erythrocytes outnumber culture cells by only 2:1, and less than 10% of the culture cells have been lost. Using a very similar procedure, Yamaizumi *et al.* (1978d) are able by repeated centrifugations to reduce erythrocyte levels to less than 0.5%, though loss of culture cells, which also increases with each centrifugation, was not reported.

Another commonly used tactic for erythrocyte removal is sedimentation of cells through a shelf of calf serum. Fusion mixtures are layered over serum and centrifuged at low speed for a short period, the majority of the erythrocytes which do not readily penetrate the shelf being removed by aspiration (Wasserman *et al.*, 1976; Yamaizumi *et al.*, 1979; Bennett *et al.*, 1983). Although contamination by erythrocytes has been reported to be reduced to levels from 0.5 to 0.04%, loss of culture cells can also be considerable.

Ohara and Watanabe (1982) have used a "panning" system specific for B lymphocyte recipients but probably applicable for other cell types as well. After injection of mouse splenic lymphocytes, fusion mixtures were incubated in dishes coated with rabbit-antimouse $F(ab')_2$ fragments, thus resulting in selective attachment of B lymphocytes through their surface immunoglobulins. After contaminating erythrocytes (and also T lymphocytes) were washed away, the adherent cells, removed by a rubber policeman, were found to contain <0.1% erythrocytes. Although recipients in this example were non-adherent, presumably if non-tissue culture dishes were used, any cell for which an antibody to a surface component not found on erythrocytes was available could be freed of erythrocytes by this method.

(2) Monolayer

Most investigators have found fusion of erythrocytes to culture cells in monolayer to be much less efficient than fusion in suspension. However, the Japanese workers have used this approach with success and employ it routinely.

Mercer (1980) found that only 5–10% of culture cells in monolayer fused with erythrocytes. Attempts to increase this efficiency by exposing the cultures to a brief treatment with trypsin prior to fusion met with no success. Kulka and Loyter (1979) reported that repeated attempts to inject a variety of cell lines in monolayer failed. However, cells treated with vinblastine or colcemid to dissociate microtubules could be injected, and fusion was further enhanced by supplementation with cytochalasin B.

The procedure which the Japanese workers have adopted is the following. Virus is added to monolayers at 4°C and removed 4 min later; after a further 20 min at 4°C, erythrocytes are added and cultures are incubated at 37°C for 20 min. When this protocol is followed, microinjection efficiencies are quite variable ranging from about 15–20% (Yamaizumi *et al.*, 1978c; Iino *et al.*, 1983) all the way up to 84% (Yamaizumi *et al.*, 1978a). At a microinjection efficiency of about 60%, 30% of recipients fused with one erythrocyte, 30% with two and 40% with three or more (Yamaizumi *et al.*, 1979), perhaps indicating that culture cells in monolayer fuse more readily with multiple erythrocytes than in suspension, or at least that the products of such multiple fusions are more recoverable in monolayer, although the efficiency of microinjection is usually lower than in suspension (Furusawa, 1980).

As a final note, Kruse *et al.* (1981) have isolated the HN (haemagglutinin) and F (fusion) glycoproteins from Sendai virus particles and have used these components in place of the whole virus to induce fusions in monolayer. They report that microinjection efficiency is comparable to that achieved with whole virus: depending on the experiment, usually an average of from 4–10 (but up to 14) erythrocytes fuse with each recipient, calculated from the total amount of arginase transferred from loaded erythrocytes to populations of culture cells.

B. PEG

As was the case with Sendai virus, both suspension and monolayer procedures have been developed for the use of PEG as fusogen. Although some general guidelines have been provided for the selection of the most fusogenic and least toxic PEG (Schlegel and McEvoy, 1985), the articles referenced below should be consulted with respect to the brand and molecular weight of the PEG used, since these considerations may be of importance if a particular procedure is selected.

(1) Suspension

Several investigators (Boogaard and Dixon, 1983b; Wiberg *et al.*, 1983) have directly adopted procedures originally designed to fuse culture cells to produce hybrid cells. Culture cells and erythrocytes (again in considerable excess) are combined in a very small volume or in a pellet, and 1 ml of 50–55% PEG is added. After 1 min at 37°C, the fusion mixture is slowly diluted with buffer or media and the products are washed. Unfused erythrocytes can be removed by the methods described in the preceding section.

Some investigators have found it necessary to adapt this basic procedure in order to increase microinjection efficiencies to acceptable levels. In particular, bringing erythrocytes into closer apposition with culture cells has been found to greatly enhance fusion (see also monolayer procedures below). Closer approach of cells was achieved by Ohara and Watanabe (1982) by incorporating poly-L-arginine at 5 μg/ml in their PEG solution. They reported a microinjection efficiency of 80% using this tactic.

Enhancement of fusion has also been accomplished by immunospecific targeting of erythrocytes to recipients (Godfrey *et al.*, 1983). In this method, culture cells are treated with antibodies directed against their surface antigens, to which biotin has been conjugated. Loaded erythrocytes whose surfaces have been derivatized with avidin then home to and become tenaciously attached to recipients. Microinjection efficiencies are thereby increased from 1–2% in the absence of targeting to 20–66%, depending on the cell line, and viabilities determined by dye exclusion are in the 70–85% range. The greatest advantage of this immunospecific method over the non-specific method of attachment, however, is that selected cells within a mixed population can be targeted for injection. For instance, by treating spleen cells with biotinylated polyclonal or monoclonal antibodies specific for B lymphocytes, only those types of cells formed rosettes upon addition of avidin-derivatized erythrocytes. Microinjection efficiencies of targeted cells were 30% and viability was 60–90%. In the absence of targeting <1% of recipients were injected.

(2) Monolayer

As was the case with fusions performed in suspension, some investigators find it unnecessary to add agents which enhance erythrocyte–culture cell contacts. Dice and coworkers (Neff *et al.*, 1981; Dice, 1982; Backer *et al.*, 1983) simply add a 100-fold excess of loaded erythrocytes in a small volume to a confluent culture of fibroblasts and swirl to distribute the erythrocytes evenly. Only a small volume of PEG is used to induce fusion in order to increase the frequency of interactions between erythrocytes and fibroblasts. After it is added, the PEG is also evenly distributed by swirling, and after 1 min at room temperature 4–5 volumes of medium is added with minimal disturbance of the PEG layer. After 30 min at 37°C, the medium is removed and the monolayer washed. Using this protocol, microinjection efficiencies of 50–60% are reported with an average of 0.5–1.0 erythrocytes fusing with each recipient. Importantly, rates of protein synthesis, net protein accumulation, and rates of protein degradation were not disturbed by the procedure when assayed at 2, 6 and 24 h after fusion.

The monolayer procedure of Kriegler and Livingston (1977) is similar to that just described, except that the loaded erythrocytes are suspended in the PEG prior to its addition to confluent monolayers, again presumably to enhance contact between erythrocytes and culture cells. Microinjection efficiencies of 90% are reported, although the cloning efficiency of injected populations is reduced to 12–20% of controls, perhaps due to the formation of syncytia which remain viable for only short periods of time and are unable to divide.

Enhancement of cell contact is promoted mechanically in a procedure devised by Kaltoft and Celis (1978). Culture cells plated onto coverslips are grown to 80% confluency. Coverslips are then placed in flat-bottomed centrifuge tubes, a suspension of erythrocytes is added, followed by media, and the tubes are centrifuged at 6000 × *g* for 5 min. After removal of the media, PEG is added to the culture to induce fusion. Using this protocol, microinjection efficiencies of 80% are possible, and recipient cells fuse with an average of 5–10 erythrocytes, the latter number considerably higher than that attained with the basic procedure, probably as a result of increased cell–cell contact. Viability at 22 h after fusion is about 85% as assessed by dye exclusion and at least 90% of mononucleated cells divide during the first 30 h after fusion. Certain cell lines must be grown and fused on plastic rather than glass coverslips if viability is to be preserved following fusion (Celis *et al.*, 1980). This procedure can be adapted to microinject non-adherent cells by centrifuging a mixture of culture cells and erythrocytes onto a coverslip (Celis *et al.*, 1980), and has been successfully used to fuse loaded hen erythrocytes with monolayers of culture cells (Jonak and Mora, 1980).

Another tack taken to enhance fusion by bringing cells into close apposition is the use of an agglutinin. Schlegel and colleagues (Mercer *et al.*, 1979; Schlegel and Mercer, 1980; Schlegel and McEvoy, 1985) have used the lectin phytohaemagglutinin (PHA) which recognizes the carbohydrate portion of glycoproteins on the surfaces of both erythrocytes and culture cells and thereby brings them into contact. PHA is added to a suspension of loaded erythrocytes just prior to addition of the mixture to monolayers of culture cells. After a brief incubation period to allow the erythrocytes to attach, those which did not attach are removed by aspiration, and PEG is added to induce fusion. Using this protocol, from 60–90% microinjection frequencies have been attained with a wide variety of culture cell lines. Several advantages accrue from the use of this procedure. First, sparsely plated culture cells are quite easily microinjected, thereby reducing the possibility of generating non-viable multikaryons during fusion. Second, use of the lectin allows fusion to be induced by concentrations of PEG as low as 44%, rather than the normal 50–55%. Because the toxicity of PEG to culture cells increases at higher concentrations, the viability of microinjected cultures remains high, usually in the 80–95% range. Even fragile, quiescent fibroblasts maintained in low serum for several days prior to fusion remain viable after fusion and retain their capacity to proliferate following stimulation by serum (Schlegel and Mercer, 1980). An additional precaution found helpful by Heumann *et al.* (1981) to reduce cell damage in this protocol is a 5-min exposure to ice-cold PEG, rather than a 1-min exposure at room temperature. Finally, selectivity can be introduced into this protocol by substitution of specific antibody targeting for non-specific agglutination. Using the biotin–antibody, avidin–erythrocyte system described in the preceding section, microinjection efficiencies and viabilities equivalent to those with PHA were obtained (Godfrey *et al.*, 1983).

One problem encountered with the use of PHA as agglutinin is the extreme difficulty in removing non-fused erythrocytes from cultures. Substitution of agglutinating agents whose binding is readily reversible circumvents this problem (Schlegel and McEvoy, 1985). When the lectin concanavalin A (con A) is used in place of PHA, erythrocytes can be easily removed from fused cultures by chelation of Ca^{2+} and Mg^{2+} with EDTA, since these divalent cations are required for con A binding, augmented by exposure to sugars which compete for con A binding sites. Alternatively, polylysine can be used as the agglutinin. Because this polycation binds electrostatically, it and its agglutinating capacity can be simply removed by thorough washing of cultures after fusion. Both of these alternative agglutinating agents yield microinjection efficiencies and viabilities comparable to those obtained with PHA.

A final cautionary note concerns the presence of divalent cations during and immediately after fusion. Several groups of investigators have found that the toxicity of PEG to cells fused in monolayer is reduced by specifically excluding Ca^{2+} from fusion and post-fusion buffers for at least 15 min following fusion (Schneiderman *et al.*, 1979; Schlegel and Mercer, 1980). How many cell lines are covered by this caveat is not known, but for those which display this sensitivity to Ca^{2+}, the con A method just described would best not be used since Ca^{2+} is required for the lectin to bind. This effect is apparently restricted to fusions where PEG is used as fusogen since, as described in a previous section, Ca^{2+} can be used to enhance fusions induced by Sendai virus, and in fact the extent of toxicity produced by Ca^{2+} is dependent on the brand of PEG used (Mercer and Baserga, 1982).

C. Other fusogens

The haemagglutinin (HA) of Influenza induces fusion of virus particles with the membrane of endocytic vesicles, inside of which they are brought into the cell, upon acidification of the vesicle interior. Doxsey *et al.* (1985) have taken advantage of a fibroblast cell line stably transformed by the cloned HA gene to facilitate erythrocyte-mediated injection. When loaded erythrocytes are added to cells of the line, they tightly bind to the HA that is constitutively synthesized by the cells and efficiently expressed on their surface. A brief drop in pH to 5.0 triggers the fusogenic activity of the protein resulting in the fusion of erythrocytes with culture cells. At present the efficiency of microinjection is 50%. This elegant method eliminates the necessity of exogenous agglutinins or fusogens and will no doubt find great popularity in studies of both general cellular processes and cell type-specific processes, should HA-expressing lines derived from more specialized cells become available.

D. Stability of injected molecules

The usefulness of erythrocyte-mediated transfer is highly dependent upon whether the molecules, once introduced into the milieu of the recipient, assume the identity of endogenous constituents, or in the case of molecules not normally in the cytoplasm, such as antibodies, persist for periods long enough to be of value. With regard to nucleic acids, molecules of tRNA introduced by this technique are broken down at rates similar to those of endogenous tRNAs (Schlegel *et al.*, 1978); an extensive literature, reviewed in Rechsteiner *et al.* (1984a), is available concerning the half-lives of injected proteins. The ultimate test of usefulness is, however, whether injected molecules function normally within injected recipients. That consideration is one of the primary topics of the companion article on applications of erythrocyte-mediated injection.

V. SEPARATION OF INJECTED FROM UNINJECTED CELLS

Actual sorting of injected from uninjected cells following fusion requires a means of distinguishing the two. Several of the methods described in Section III for identifying injected cells have been applied to just this task. Mekada *et al.* (1978a) set themselves the goal of isolating only mononuclear, injected cells using FACS. Erythrocytes and multinucleated cells could be distinguished from mononuclear cells and eliminated from further consideration by light scattering. Injected cells could be distinguished from uninjected cells by their fluorescence intensity following sequential application of antierythrocyte antiserum and fluoresceinated anti-IgG antibody. Therefore, a two-parameter sort yielded a mononuclear population which contained 95% injected cells (confirmed by benzidine staining) from a starting population which was only 50% pure. Importantly, the sorted cells had a cloning efficiency of 90%, just the same as unfused, unstained and unsorted cells. A much less expensive method, using erythrocyte-specific antibodies might be panning (as described at the end of Section IV.A.1) for injected cells using antibody-coated dishes, once unfused erythrocytes had been removed by any of the several methods described in the preceding sections.

Another dimension is added to sorting by using fl-BSA to identify injected cells. In contrast to the use of the fluoresceinated surface marker, the distribution of fluorescence intensity within a population injected with the cytoplasmic marker is sharp enough that peaks corresponding to cells fused with one, two or three erythrocytes are resolved (Mekada *et al.*, 1978b). Therefore, mononuclear cells have been sorted by FACS on the basis of the amount of material with which they were injected. The cloning efficiency of cells injected by two erythrocytes was found to be equivalent to cells injected by only one (and to sorted, uninjected cells and the unsorted population as well, 60%), indicating that, at least within these bounds, dosage does not affect viability. More than a mere exercise, the method has been successfully employed to separate cells injected with different quantities of an experimental protein by including fl-BSA as a tracer during loading (Yamaizumi *et al.*, 1978b). When it is crucial to know the amounts of material injected or when dosage effects are under investigation, this separation method can be extremely valuable.

Another approach for obtaining only those cells which are injected does not require sorting at all. This method relies on the ability of an injected substance to rescue a cell. Yamaizumi *et al.* (1978c, 1979) injected cells with antibody to fragment A of diphtheria toxin, the fragment which when liberated into the cytoplasm kills cells by its ability to modify soluble polypeptide elongation factor 2 and thus inhibit protein synthesis. Injected cells were found to be protected from the effects of a subsequent challenge of toxin. Therefore, if anti-fragment A is included during loading of the primary molecule of interest, only injected cells will survive exposure to toxin. One problem with this method is that several days are required for uninjected cells to be eliminated from culture. By this time the coloaded and coinjected primary molecule may have undergone considerable degradation within the cell. This problem can be circumvented by using ricin instead of diphtheria toxin (Rogers and Rechsteiner, unpub. ob.), because ricin kills cells within 24 h. Because ricin and its antibody are commercially available, this approach is both feasible and practical.

VI. CONCLUSION

Clearly, a range of procedures is available for introducing molecules into cells by erythrocyte-mediated microinjection. Experimental requisites will often dictate whether a monolayer or suspension procedure is selected. If fusions are performed in suspension, a large body of literature recommends the use of Sendai virus as fusogen. If fusions are performed in monolayer, the most reproducibly efficient injections employ PEG as fusogen. Beyond these general guidelines, the procedure chosen can be tailored to meet individual needs and demands. What can be ultimately expected is that as few as 10^3 or as many as 10^7 culture cells can be microinjected with efficiencies up to 90%; as many as 10^6–10^7 protein molecules or 10^8 small RNA molecules can be transferred into each cell; loading requires several and injection only one, with most of the time occupied by washing; viabilities and cloning efficiencies approach those of uninjected controls.

By its nature, erythrocyte-mediated microinjection precludes direct injection of molecules into the nucleus. If, however, proteins of nuclear origin are injected into the cytoplasm by this procedure, they rapidly accumulate in the nucleus (Yamaizumi *et al.*, 1978d; Rechsteiner and Kuehl, 1979; Rechsteiner *et al.*, 1984b). Yet the situation remains that most non-nuclear proteins when injected into the cytoplasm remain there. This problem becomes acute if the function of nuclear proteins is to be studied by injection of their specific antibodies, since these molecules are excluded from the nucleus. Antibodies and other molecules can, however, gain access to the nucleus if recipients are synchronized in mitosis when injected. As the cells leave mitosis following injection, the nuclear membrane reforms around injected molecules, enclosing even those normally excluded (Schlegel, 1984). Therefore, erythrocyte-mediated microinjection can be used to indirectly introduce molecules into the nucleus as well as directly into the cytoplasm, as needed.

REFERENCES

Anderson, W. F., Deisseroth, A., Nienhuis, A. W., Gopalakrishnan, T. V., Huang, A. and Kreuger, L. (1978). *Natl. Cancer Inst. Monogram* **48**, 65–73.

Antman, K. H. and Livingston, D. M. (1980). *Cell* **19**, 627–635.

Backer, J. M., Bourret, L. and Dice, J. F. (1983). *Proc. Natl. Acad. Sci USA* **80**, 2166–2170.

Bennett, F., Busch, H., Lischwe, M. A. and Yeoman, L. C. (1983). *J. Cell Biol.* **97**, 1556–1572.

Boogaard, C. and Dixon, G. H. (1983a). *Exp. Cell Res.* **143**, 175–190.

Boogaard, C. and Dixon, G. H. (1983b). *Exp. Cell Res.* **143**, 191–205.

Capecchi, M. R., Von der Haar, R. A., Capecchi, N. E. and Sveda, M. M. (1977). *Cell* **12**, 371–381.

Celis, J. E. (1977). *Brookhaven Symp. Biol.* **29**, 178–196.

Celis, J. E., Kaltoft, K. and Bravo, R. (1980). *In* "Introduction of Macromolecules into Viable Mammalian Cells", (R. Baserga, C. Croce and G. Rovera, eds) pp. 99–123. Alan Liss, New York.

Dice, J. F. (1982). *J. Biol. Chem.* **257**, 14624–14627.

Doxsey, S., Helenius, A. and White, J. (1985). *J. Cell Biol.* **101**, 19–27.

Furusawa, M. (1980). *Int. Rev. Cytol.* **62**, 29–67.

Furusawa, M., Nishimura, T., Yamaizumi, M. and Okada, Y. (1974). *Nature* **249**, 449–450.

Furusawa, M., Yamaizumi, M., Nishimura, T., Uchida, T. and Okada, Y. (1976). *Meth. Cell Biol.* **14**, 73–80.

Godfrey, W., Doe, B. and Wofsy, L. (1983). *Proc. Natl. Acad. Sci. USA* **80**, 2267–2271.

Hendil, K. B. (1980). *J. Cell Physiol.* **105**, 449–460.

Heumann, R., Schwab, M. and Theonen, H. (1981). *Nature* **292**, 838–840.

Iino, T., Furusawa, M., Furusawa, I. and Obinata, M. (1983). *Exp. Cell Res.* **148**, 475–480.

Jonak, G. J. and Mora, M. (1980). *In* "Introduction of Macromolecules into Viable Mammalian Cells", (R. Baserga, C. Croce and G. Rovera, eds) pp. 157–167. Alan Liss, New York.

Kaltoft, K. and Celis, J. E. (1978). *Exp. Cell Res.* **115**, 423–428.

Kaltoft, K., Zeuthen, J., Engberg, F., Piper, P. W. and Celis, J. E. (1976). *Proc. Natl. Acad. Sci. USA* **73**, 2793–2797.

Kriegler, M. P. and Livingston, D. M. (1977). *Somatic Cell Genet.* **3**, 603–610.

Kriegler, M. P., Griffin, J. D. and Livingston, D. M. (1978). *Cell* **14**, 983–994.

Kruse, C. A. and Popjak, G. (1981). *Biochem. Biophys. Res. Commun.* **102**, 258–264.

Kruse, C. A., Spector, E. B., Cederbaum, S. D., Wisnieski, B. J. and Popjak, G. (1981). *Biochim. Biophys. Acta* **645**, 339–345.

Kulka, R. G. and Loyter, A. (1979). *Curr. Topics Memb. Transport* **12**, 365–430.

Loyter, A., Zakai, N. and Kulka, R. G. (1975). *J. Cell Biol.* **66**, 292–304.

Mekada, E., Yamaizumi, M. and Okada, Y. (1978a). *J. Histochem. Cytochem.* **26**, 62–67.

Mekada, E., Yamaizumi, M., Uchida, T. and Okada, Y. (1978b). *J. Histochem. Cytochem.* **26**, 1067–1073.

Mercer, W. E. (1980). Ph.D. Dissertation, The Pennsylvania State University.

Mercer, W. E. and Baserga, R. (1982). *In* "Techniques in Somatic Cell Genetics", (J. W. Shay, ed.) pp. 22–34. Plenum Press, New York.

Mercer, W. E., Terefinko, D. J. and Schlegel, R. A. (1979). *Cell Biol. Int. Rep.* **3**, 265–271.

Neff, N. J., Bourret, L., Maio, P. and Dice, J. F. (1981). *J. Cell Biol.* **91**, 184–194.

Nishimura, T., Furusawa, M., Yamaizumi, M. and Okada, Y. (1976). *Cell Struct. Funct.* **1**, 197–200.

Ohara, J. and Watanabe, T. (1982). *J. Immunol.* **128**, 1090–1096.

Peretz, H., Toister, Z., Laster, Y. and Loyter, A. (1974). *J. Cell Biol.* **63**, 1–11.

Petrie, H. T., McDonel, J. L. and Schlegel, R. A. (1982). *Cell Biol. Int. Rep.* **6**, 705–711.

Rechsteiner, M. (1975). *Exp. Cell Res.* **93**, 487–492.

Rechsteiner, M. (1982). *In* "Techniques in Somatic Cell Genetics", (J. W. Shay, ed.) pp. 385–398. Plenum Press, New York.

Rechsteiner, M. and Kuehl, L. (1979). *Cell* **16**, 901–908.

Rechsteiner, M., Chin, D., Hough, R., McGarry, T., Rogers, S., Rote, K. and Wu, L. (1984a). *In* "Cell Fusion", (D. Evered and J. Whelan, eds) Ciba Foundation Symposium 103, pp. 181–195. Pitman, London.

Rechsteiner, M., Wu, L. H. and Miller, A. O. A. (1984b). *In* "Red Blood Cells as Carriers for Drugs" (J. R. DeLoach and U. Sprandel, eds). pp. 142–149. S. Karger, Basel.

Schlegel, R. A. (1984). *In* "Red Blood Cells as Carriers for Drugs", (J. R. DeLoach and U. Sprandel, eds). pp. 134–141. S. Karger, Basel.

Schlegel, R. A. and McEvoy, L. (1985). *Methods Enzymol.* (in press).

Schlegel, R. A. and Mercer, W. E. (1980). *In* "Introduction of Macromolecules into Viable Mammalian Cells", (R. Baserga, C. Croce and G. Rovera, eds) pp. 145–155. Alan Liss, New York.

Schlegel, R. A. and Rechsteiner, M. C. (1975). *Cell* **5**, 371–379.
Schlegel, R. A. and Rechsteiner, M. C. (1978). *Methods Cell Biol.* **20**, 341–354.
Schlegel, R. A., Darrah, L. B. and Rechsteiner, M. C. (1976). *In* "Molecular Mechanisms in the Control of Gene Expression", (D. Nierlich, W. Rutter and C. F. Fox, eds), pp. 465–470, Academic Press, New York and London.
Schlegel, R. A., Iverson, P. and Rechsteiner, M. C. (1978). *Nucl. Acids Res.* **5**, 3715–3729.
Schneiderman, S., Farber, J. L. and Baserga, R. (1979). *Somatic Cell Genet.* **5**, 263–269.
Straus, S. E. and Raskas, H. J. (1980). *J. Gen. Virol.* **48**, 241–245.
Wasserman, M., Zakai, N., Loyter, A. and Kulka, R. G. (1976). *Cell* **7**, 551–556.
Wasserman, M., Loyter, A. and Kulka, R. G. (1977). *J. Cell Sci.* **27**, 157–165.
Wiberg, F. C., Sunnerhagen, P., Kaltoft, K., Zeuthen, J. and Bjursell, G. (1983). *Nucl. Acids Res.* **11**, 7287–7302.
Wille, W. and Willecke, K. (1976). *FEBS Lett.* **65**, 59–62.
Wojcieszyn, J. W., Schlegel, R. A., Wu, E.-S. and Jacobson, K. A. (1981). *Proc. Natl. Acad. Sci. USA* **78**, 4407–4410.
Yamaizumi, M., Furusawa, M., Uchida, T., Nishimura, T. and Okada, Y. (1978a). *Cell Struct. Funct.* **3**, 293–304.
Yamaizumi, M., Mekada, E., Uchida, T. and Okada, Y. (1978b). *Cell* **15**, 245–250.
Yamaizumi, M., Uchida, T., Okada, Y. and Furusawa, M. (1978c). *Cell* **13**, 227–232.
Yamaizumi, M., Uchida, T., Okada, Y., Furusawa, M. and Mitsui, H. (1978d). *Nature* **273**, 782–784.
Yamaizumi, M., Uchida, T., Mekada, E. and Okada, Y. (1979). *Cell* **18**, 1009–1014.

6

Erythrocyte-Mediated Transfer: Applications

M. C. Rechsteiner and R. A. Schlegel

I. INTRODUCTION

In the preceding chapter, we presented a number of ways for loading macromolecules into RBCs and fusing the loaded RBCs to mammalian cells. Here we review applications of RBC-mediated microinjection to specific biological problems. Although the technique has been used to transfer DNA and RNA as well as proteins, by far the most applications have involved proteins. In fact, the majority of published studies relate to the injection of antibodies or to intracellular proteolysis. Consequently, a considerable portion of this review is devoted to these two topics. The remainder of the chapter presents other types of studies to which the injection methodology has been applied.

Although the merits of the various techniques available for introducing macromolecules into cells have recently been considered (Celis, 1984; see also Chapter 12), certain comparisons which illustrate the particular advantages of each are worth repeating. For example, either direct microinjection or RBC-injection could be used to determine whether fluoresceinated G-actin forms filaments after introduction into cultured fibroblasts. Since more protein can be injected per cell using glass capillaries, this method might be preferred. On the other hand, if it were important to know whether fluoresceinated actin underwent modification within the recipient cell, RBC-mediated injection would clearly be the method of choice. Because such small numbers of cells can be injected by glass capillaries, it would be virtually impossible to recover enough fluorescent actin for biochemical analysis. Thus, RBC-mediated injection, where large recoveries are possible, is best suited for studies in which the injected molecule must be re-examined biochemically or where the introduced molecule generates a

Microinjection and Organelle Transplantation Techniques

ISBN: 0-12-164722-6
ISBN: 0-12-164723-4 Pbk

response only measurable with large numbers of injected cells. RBC-mediated injection is also preferred for cytological experiments that require an abundance of injected cells such as the studies on internuclear migration of proteins discussed below. It is less useful for the transfer of large macromolecules, which are progressively excluded during loading (see previous chapter). Moreover, the technique is severely limited when compared to glass capillaries since it does not permit the direct transfer of molecules into the nuclei of interphase cells.

II. INTRACELLULAR PROTEOLYSIS

The extensive use of RBC-mediated injection for studies on intracellular protein degradation is due in part to an interest in this subject among the developers of RBC-injection and in part to the unique suitability of the technique for studying the complex, multicomponent reactions involved in proteolysis. It has long been known that intracellular proteolysis requires ATP (Simpson, 1953) and exhibits remarkable substrate specificity (Schimke and Doyle, 1970). However, an *in vitro* proteolytic system with these properties was developed only recently (Etlinger and Goldberg, 1977). For this reason, several investigators adopted the alternative strategy of introducing protein substrates into cells. This approach offered a number of technical advantages. Studies on protein turn-over using biosynthetic labelling are complicated by the vast array of proteins that become labelled and because these newly labelled proteins can enter diverse cellular compartments, such as mitochondria, rough endoplasmic reticulum, etc. The ability to introduce individually labelled proteins into cells permits accurate measurement of the degradation rate, location, and modifications of these injected proteins. Moreover, almost all injected proteins are confined to the cytosol-nuclear compartments so that proteases within the secretory pathway or mitochondria contribute little, if anything, to their degradation.

Early papers describing RBC-mediated injection commented on the stability of the injected molecules, but Wasserman *et al.* (1977) were the first to apply this technique specifically for studies on intracellular proteolysis. They reported that injected IgG molecules were degraded in two phases, and they noted the absence of intracellular degradation products. There soon appeared two papers which underscored the usefulness of microinjection for measuring the intracellular stability of proteins. Zavortink *et al.* (1979) injected several iodinated proteins into HeLa cells and found that the proteins were degraded at first-order rates with half-lives varying from 3 h to 60 h, depending upon the protein. A year later Hendil (1980) elegantly demonstrated the selective degradation of an injected protein. He showed that the degradation rate of haemoglobin could be increased more than ten-fold by exposing injected BHK fibroblasts to low levels of phenylhydrazine, which oxidized the haeme iron and thereby denatured the injected haemoglobin. Two subsequent studies provided evidence that the selective degradation of injected proteins is a faithful representation of normal intracellular processes. Freikopf-Cassel and Kulka (1981) found that the degradation of microinjected glutamine synthetase was responsive to the concentration of glutamine in the medium, an observation in accord with the behaviour of endogenous glutamine synthetase. And Neff *et al.* (1981) reported that a mixture of cytosolic proteins injected into IMR-90 human fibroblasts were degraded as expected for endogenous cytosolic proteins. That is, larger proteins were degraded faster than smaller, and negatively charged proteins were degraded faster than positively charged species.

Recent studies on intracellular proteolysis using RBC-injection have focused on three major questions. Are lysosomes involved in the degradation of injected proteins? What structural features of proteins correlate with their intracellular stability? And does covalent modification precede proteolysis of injected proteins?

A. Lysosomes and the degradation of microinjected proteins

There seems to be little doubt that proteins entering cells by endocytosis are subsequently degraded within lysosomes (Fambrough and Devreotes, 1976; Wall *et al.*, 1980). Similarly, there is an impressive body of evidence that lysosomal proteases play a major role in enhanced protein degradation resulting from nutritional deprivation of animal cells (Mortimore, 1982). However, the extent to which lysosomes are involved in the degradation of endogenous, cytosolic proteins in cells maintained under normal physiological conditions (basal proteolysis) has been a controversial issue for more than 10 years. It is well established that cytosolic patterns exhibit a wide range of half-lives (Schimke and Doyle, 1970; Goldberg and St. John, 1976), so one must invoke a mechanism either for the selective transfer of proteins into lysosomes or selective degradation within the cytosol. In this regard, Dean (1975) proposed that soluble proteins could be selectively adsorbed onto membranes which then form autophagic vacuoles and fuse with lysosomes. Other models involving selective uptake of proteins directly by lysosomes (Lloyd, 1978) or bulk uptake of proteins followed by selective release of resistant proteins have also been advanced (Haider and Segal, 1972).

During the past four years, RBC-mediated injection has been used to determine the degree of lysosomal involvement in basal proteolysis. In the first studies, Bigelow *et al.* (1981) coupled ^{14}C-sucrose-labelled bovine serum albumin (^{14}C-sucBSA) to polylysine and exposed monolayers of L929 cells to the conjugates. The ^{14}C-sucBSA polylysine conjugates were taken up by pinocytosis, and the ^{14}C-sucrose-labelled peptides that arose upon degradation accumulated exclusively within lysosomes. In contrast, when ^{14}C-sucRSA or ^{14}C-sucrose-labelled pyruvate kinase (^{14}C-sucPK) were microinjected into L929 cells, over half of the ^{14}C-sucrose-labelled peptides derived from the injected proteins were present in the post-lysosomal supernatant. Control experiments demonstrated that the microinjection procedure itself did not cause ^{14}C-sucrose peptides to leak from lysosomes. The presence of substantial amounts of the degradation products from injected ^{14}C-sucBSA and ^{14}C-sucPK in the cytosol led the authors to conclude that a major proteolytic system exists within this compartment of animal cells. These results were apparently confirmed (Dice *et al.*, 1981), but more recent observations suggest that a predominance of non-lysosomal degradation of injected proteins may not hold for all proteins. J. F. Dice (pers. commun.) has found that although 70% of the TCA-soluble ^{3}H-rhaffinose-labelled products arising upon degradation of injected ^{3}H-rhaffinose-labelled BSA is found in the cytosol, virtually all TCA-soluble ^{3}H-rhaffinose-labelled products arising from injected ^{3}H-rhaffinose-RNaseA are present in lysosomes.

The tertiary amines, ammonia and chloroquine, accumulate within lysosomes resulting in a marked increase in intralysosomal pH and inhibition of proteolysis within these organelles (Ohkuma and Poole, 1978). From the results obtained with sucrose-labelled proteins, one would expect the degradation of microinjected proteins to be generally insensitive to lysosomotropic agents. These predictions were tested by Rote and Rechsteiner (1983) who injected radioiodinated proteins into HeLa cells and then exposed the injected cells to inhibitors of lysosomal proteolysis. The degradation of injected BSA was unaffected by chloroquine, NH_3Cl, or a variety of agents such as colcemid that inhibit autophagy. Although degradation of lactate dehydrogenase (LDH) and pyruvate kinase (PK) was inhibited one-third by chloroquine or ammonia, compounds inhibiting autophagy had no effect. In contrast, enhanced degradation of PK as a result of depriving injected HeLa cells of amino acids and serum was inhibited 70% by colcemid and abolished by chloroquine or ammonia. Similarly, degradation of ^{14}C-sucrose-labelled BSA–polylysine conjugates taken up by HeLa cells was inhibited as much as 80% by chloroquine and ammonia. The sensitivity of both enhanced proteolysis and degradation of exogenous proteins to ammonia or chloroquine demonstrates that these compounds are effective inhibitors of lysosomal proteolysis in HeLa cells. Consequently, their failure to inhibit degradation of injected BSA and the modest inhibition of the degradation of injected LDH or PK indicate that virtually all BSA molecules and most PK or LDH molecules are degraded by a non-lysosomal proteolytic system.

Similar results were obtained by Katznelson and Kulka (1983). ^{125}I-BSA and ^{125}I-lysozyme were degraded rapidly with pseudo first-order kinetics after microinjection into HTC cells. When HTC cells were depleted of ATP degradation of both proteins was inhibited, thereby implicating an ATP-dependent pathway. Proteolysis was not, however, inhibited by ammonia, methylamine or chloroquine, indicating that the injected proteins were not degraded by lysosomal proteases.

In a significant extension of the inhibitor approach, Rogers and Rechsteiner (1985) measured the effects of ammonia or chloroquine on the degradation of 35 different proteins following their injection into HeLa cells. These authors plotted the half-lives for the thirty-five proteins (16–214 h) against the percentage of each protein degraded within lysosomes, assuming that the extent to which ammonia and chloroquine inhibited the degradation of an injected protein was directly proportional to the fraction of that protein degraded within lysosomes. Ammonia and chloroquine had no effect on the degradation rates of proteins with half-lives less than 45 h, and the data for longer-lived proteins formed a reasonable line ($r = 0.76$) that extrapolated to a half-life of 310 h for the hypothetical protein totally impervious to cytosolic proteolysis, i.e. a protein whose degradation was totally inhibited by ammonia or chloroquine. These data imply that all proteins are transferred by lysosomes at comparable rates so that the fraction degraded in lysosomes depends upon the rate of degradation within the cytosol; thus short-lived proteins whose degradation is inhibited by lysosomotropic agents are simply not observed. These results are in good agreement with those of Hendil (1981) who used RBC-mediated injection to introduce ^{3}H-dextran, a compound resistant to degradation, into BHK fibroblasts. He then found that ^{3}H-dextran accumulated in lysosomes at rates estimated between 0.19 and 0.036%/hr, values that imply that a protein completely resistant to cytosolic proteolysis should still exhibit a half-life of between 200 and 350 h due to basal autophagy.

Temperature was employed in a third approach to the question of lysosome involvement in the degradation of injected proteins. If the selective degradation of injected proteins requires their transfer into lysosomes, then the proteins must somehow traverse the lysosomal membrane. Many membrane processes exhibit curved or "broken" Arrhenius plots attributed to progressive immobilization of phospholipids upon cooling. To determine the shape of Arrhenius plots for intracellular proteolysis, Hough and Rechsteiner (1984) injected a number of proteins into HeLa cells and measured the degradation of these proteins at temperatures between 6°C and 37°C. There were no "breaks" in the Arrhenius plots obtained, and this result was taken as evidence that membranes are not involved in the degradation of microinjected proteins, a conclusion strengthened by examining the degradation of injected proteins in HeLa cells grown in nutrient-poor medium. Under those conditions, curved Arrhenius plots were observed since enhanced degradation occurred only above 20°C. It has been shown that fusion of lysosomes with phagocytic or pinocytic vesicles ceases below 20°C (Kielian and Cohn, 1980; Dunn *et al.*, 1980), so Hough and Rechsteiner suggested that either the formation of autophagic vacuoles or the fusion of autophagic vacuoles with lysosomes was similarly inhibited below 20°C.

B. Protein structure and intracellular stability

The structure of a protein must certainly influence its intracellular stability because there is good evidence for the rapid degradation of mutant proteins (Capecchi *et al.*, 1974; Goldberg and St. John, 1976) and proteins containing amino acid analogues (Rabinowitz and Fisher, 1964; Etlinger and Goldberg, 1977). Over the past decade there have been a number of attempts to correlate protein structure with intracellular degradation rates. It has been suggested that larger proteins are degraded faster than smaller (Dice *et al.*, 1973; Dice and Goldberg, 1975; Hendil, 1977) and that negatively charged proteins are degraded faster than those which are positively charged (Acton and Gupta, 1979; Dice and Goldberg, 1975). However, other investigators do not observe such correlations (Brinster *et al.*, 1979; Mosteller *et al.*, 1980; Russell *et al.*, 1980), and this question has become controversial.

Previous attempts to correlate protein structure and stability have been restricted by the absence of data on *both* stability and structure. Those key metabolic enzymes for which half-life measurements are available have rarely been sequenced or crystallized. Conversely, those proteins for which we have the most detailed structural information are either extracellular or they have been obtained from diverse species. Hence, their intracellular stabilities have not been measured. RBC-mediated injection permits measurement of the half-lives of this latter set of proteins, and this technique is sure to provide a wealth of information on the relationship between structure and stability.

The use of natural proteins, as opposed to synthetic polypeptide substrates, offers two approaches for discovering this relationship. One could take a single protein, systematically modify it either by mutation or chemical means, and then measure the half-life of each modified form after microinjection into culture cells. If one obtained a sufficient spectrum of half-lives and knew the structure of each form, then eventually it should be possible to deduce key aspects of protein structure promoting intracellular breakdown. Alternatively, one could take a collection of different proteins of known structure and measure their half-lives after microinjection. One would then hope to discover those features of protein structure often present in the rapidly degraded proteins and scarce among the stable proteins. Both approaches are being tried.

J. F. Dice and his colleagues have adopted the former approach, focusing on RNase A and several of its derivatives. They have shown that following iodination RNase A retains enzymatic activity and that its *in vitro* susceptibility to proteases does not increase. It is therefore a reasonable candidate for probing intracellular proteolysis by injection studies (Neff *et al.*, 1981). Early passage human fibroblasts have been found to degrade RNase A with a half-life of approximately 90 h, but in late-passage (senescent) fibroblasts its half-life increases to between 125 and 250 h (Dice, 1982). Reduced capacity to degrade microinjected RNase S protein, RNase B, aldolase and lysozyme was also observed in senescent IMR-90 fibroblasts. Thus, it appears that intracellular proteolysis becomes impaired in ageing fibroblasts.

Neff *et al.* (1981) also showed that the degradation of injected RNase A increases about 2-fold upon serum withdrawal. Backer *et al.* (1983) have recently reported that the enhanced degradation of RNase A requires the presence of the amino terminal 20 amino acids. RNase A is cleaved between alanine 20 and serine 21 by subtilisin to produce RNase S. The nicked protein can, in turn, be separated into S protein (residues 21–124) and S-peptide (1–20). Although S protein was degraded with a half-life similar to RNase A, its catabolism did not increase upon serum deprivation. In surprising and interesting contrast, S peptide alone showed the 2-fold increase in degradation upon serum withdrawal. Moreover, reconstituted RNase S also showed the 2-fold enhancement. Backer *et al.* (1983) conclude that recognition of RNase A for enhanced breakdown during serum deprivation is based on some feature of its N terminal 20 amino acids, and they are now trying to identify the key residues (J. F. Dice, pers. commun.).

Immunoglobulin G molecules have also been used to probe the selectivity properties of the intracellular degradation pathway(s). These molecules offer a unique opportunity to study the proposed isoelectric correlation because sequence diversity in the variable regions of heavy and light chains produces immunoglobulins with differing isoelectric points even though they have equivalent conformations. McGarry *et al.* (1983) undertook a fairly extensive study on the degradation of IgGs injected into HeLa cells and found no correlation between isoelectric point and degradation rate. They also reported that whereas heavy and light chains were degraded at the same rate when whole IgG molecules were injected, Fab fragments produced by papain cleavage were more stable than intact IgGs or Fc fragments. These results suggest that the Fc portion of IgG molecules contains the primary site(s) recognized by the intracellular degradation system and that once degradation of IgG is initiated, the whole molecule is degraded. Support for the idea that intracellular proteolysis is all-or-none has been obtained in preliminary studies using rapidly degraded proteins cross-linked to the hinge sulphhydryls of IgGs. When such conjugates were microinjected into HeLa cells, their degradation rate closely matched that of the protein added at the hinge. Moreover, for at least 80% of molecules, all chains disappeared at the same rate (Hough and Rechsteiner, unpub. obs.).

Using the latter survey approach to the structure–stability problem, Rogers and Rechsteiner (1985) have obtained more than 35 proteins of known sequence and whose X-ray structure has been resolved to less than 0.35 nm. Each protein was labelled by at least two methods, injected into HeLa cells, and its half-life measured. As mentioned above, ammonia or chloroquine was used to correct for the contribution of lysosomes to the overall degradation rate. Half-lives obtained for a few proteins differed significantly depending upon the labelling protocol and will therefore require verification by a third labelling technique. Nevertheless, the search for correlations between structural features of proteins and their intracellular stability has begun, but so far no significant correlations have been detected between half-life and subunit molecular weight, reported isoelectric point, proportion of α-helix, or β-sheet. However, these data are in the early stages of analysis, and other features of protein structure, such as density of β-turns, types of β-turns, etc. have not yet been considered.

C. Intracellular protein modification

It is becoming increasingly clear that ubiquitin plays a key role in the intracellular degradation of proteins in animal cells (Hershko and Ciechanover, 1982). Significant progress has been made in this area by traditional biochemical fractionation techniques, methods which should continue to prove successful since a major goal is to isolate the components of the degradation pathway. However, there have also been several microinjection studies directed at elucidating the role of ubiquitin in intracellular proteolysis. Atidia and Kulka (1982) injected radioiodinated ubiquitin into HTC cells and observed its covalent attachment to a variety of intracellular proteins. Chin *et al.* (1982) injected radioiodinated ubiquitin into HeLa cells and then analysed various cell fractions using SDS-acrylamide gel electrophoresis. They found that HeLa nuclei contained two major labelled proteins: ubiquitin and the histone H2A–ubiquitin conjugate, protein A24. HeLa cytosol contained ubiquitin and a series of ubiquitin–protein conjugates of diverse relative molecular masses. When the injected HeLa cells were treated with phenylhydrazine to denature the cotransferred haemoglobin, a series of prominent ubiquitin–globin conjugates appeared. The identity of these conjugates was established by microinjection experiments in which either protein was labelled. At low doses of phenylhydrazine, the intracellular concentration of globin–ubiquitin conjugates was proportional to the rate of haemoglobin degradation. This result, together with the observation that ubiquitin conjugation to globin is markedly enhanced by phenylhydrazine-induced denaturation of haemoglobin, provides support of the hypothesis that the covalent attachment of ubiquitin to proteins plays an important role in intracellular proteolysis.

Ubiquitin is known to attach to the ε-amino group on lysine, and several investigators (Chin *et al.*, 1982; Katznelson and Kulka, 1983; Tanaka *et al.*, 1983) have examined the degradation of proteins with blocked lysine residues on the assumption that if ubiquitin conjugation were mandatory for proteolysis and lysines were the exclusive conjugatable residues, such modified proteins would be stable. Katznelson and Kulka (1983) showed that exhaustive methylation of BSA or lysozyme almost completely inhibited their degradation in rabbit reticulocyte lysates, but methylation had virtually no effect on the degradation of the same molecules within HTC cells. They concluded that HTC cells degrade BSA and lysozyme by a non-lysosomal pathway different from the ubiquitin-dependent pathway in reticulocytes.

Rechsteiner *et al.* (1984a) treated five proteins with *O*-methylisourea to convert lysine residues to homoarginine, a process termed guanidination. They then compared the intracellular stabilities of the five proteins in their guanidinated (G) versus non-guanidinated forms. The results were quite variable. Guanidinated bovine serum albumin was degraded four times faster, there was little change in the degradation of carbonic anhydrase or IgG, and lysozyme and cytochrome C were 2–3 times more stable in their guanidinated forms. They also examined the degradation of guanidinated proteins in reticulocyte lysates observing that G-lysozyme was degraded by an ATP-dependent, haemin-sensitive process, but failing to detect ubiquitin conjugates of G-lysozyme on SDS-PAGE. Although their studies suggest that ubiquitin conjugation is not required for the degradation of G-lysozyme, they recognized that such an interpretation was not conclusive. Haemin, added to prevent proteolysis, might also have inhibited conjugation to residues on G-lysozyme other than lysine, or possibly to other proteins in the proteolytic pathway. Alternatively, ubiquitin may have formed very labile bonds to G-lysozyme.

D. Cell type variation

RBC-mediated injection has also shown that intracellular proteolysis does not vary significantly among cell types. Zavortink *et al.* (1979) found that the half-life of radioiodinated bovine serum albumin varied less than 2-fold among eight mammalian cell lines. Consistent with these data are observations that the half-life of RNase A is 75 h in IMR-90 human fibroblasts and 40 h in chick myotubes (Neff *et al.*, 1981; McElligott and Dice, 1983). In a recent survey (Rechsteiner *et al.*, 1984b), the half-lives of aldolase, pyruvate kinase, lactate dehydrogenase, lysozyme, bovine serum albumin and mouse IgG were measured following their injection into 5 mammalian cell lines. Only the half-life of lactate dehydrogenase varied more than 2-fold among the 5 cell lines, which included a differentiated hepatoma, a melanoma and a glioma.

III. INJECTION OF ANTIBODIES

As mentioned above, injected IgG molecules have been used to probe the selective properties of the intracellular proteolytic system. Specific antibodies have also been used in a number of injection experiments to inactivate intracellular proteins or to complex with intracellular metabolites. This application of RBC-mediated injection has tremendous potential since the ability to inactivate a specific intracellular protein is equivalent to having a temperature sensitive mutation in the same protein.

A. Intracellular inactivation of antigens

Yamaizumi *et al.* (1978a) first showed that antibody–antigen reactions could occur in the cytoplasm of living cells and were able to prevent biochemical reactions catalysed by the antigen. They injected antibodies to the A fragment of diphtheria toxin into toxin-sensitive human FL cells and found that the cells were resistant to diphtheria toxin 4 h after injection. In an extension of these experiments (Yamaizumi *et al.*, 1979), they demonstrated that the functional activity of anti-fragment A antibodies was relatively stable within FL cells ($t_{1/2}$ about 24 h) and that reaction of antibody and antigen occurred as efficiently within the cytoplasm of living cells as in the test tube.

Intracellular toxin neutralization is not restricted to diptheria toxin. Okada and Rechsteiner (1982) found that RBC-mediated injection of anti-ricin antibodies into L929 cells conferred resistance to subsequent toxin challenge. In contrast, Petrie *et al.* (1982) found that antibody to *Clostridium perfringens* enterotoxin did not protect against toxin killing after injection into Vero cells. Since neutralizing antibody was shown to be present in cytoplasmic extracts from injected cells, their results supported the suspicion that *C. perfringens* toxin acted at the plasma membrane rather than at an intracellular site.

There are a number of other examples of the use of antibody injection to inactivate intracellular processes. Antman and Livingston (1980) prepared IgG fractions that reacted with SV40 T antigen from the sera of hamsters injected with SV40 tumours. Microinjection of immune IgG into SV40-infected green monkey cells correlated with inhibition of viral DNA synthesis in this permissive cell line, whereas pre-immune hamster IgG was inactive in this assay. Microinjection of immune antibody also inhibited SV40-induced abortive transformation in two non-permissive cell lines. The inhibition of abortive transformation depended upon the intracellular delivery of the appropriate antibody molecules, since no inhibition was observed when uninjected cells were exposed to immune IgG in the medium. As with the inhibition of viral DNA synthesis, the blockage of abortive transformation depended upon a stoichiometric interaction of antibody and antigens, since graded inhibition of abortive transformation was observed when the concentration of immune IgG presented to an infected cell was varied.

Smith *et al.* (1983) have injected antibodies against ribonucleoprotein particles containing the small nuclear RNA, U1, in an attempt to determine whether (U1)-RNPs were responsible for the suppression of protein synthesis observed at mitosis. They found the injected antibodies did not prevent the mitotic suppression of protein synthesis and concluded that U1 and U2 small nuclear RNPs probably do not play a role in translational control.

In most studies, it has been found that intact IgG molecules are excluded from the nuclei of injected cells (see below). To circumvent this limitation, Schlegel (1984) and Schlegel, Miller and Rose (submitted) injected antibodies into metaphase cells since the nuclear membrane is absent at mitosis. They found that when the injected mitotic cells were allowed to enter G1 phase, antibodies were present in the nucleoplasm as well as the cytoplasm. In contrast, antibodies were excluded from the nucleus of cells injected during interphase. To determine whether antibody molecules introduced into the nuclear compartment by this manoeuvre retained their specificity, they microinjected antibodies prepared against RNA polymerase I, the enzyme responsible for transcription of rDNA sequences. When injected cells were examined after entry into G1 using immunofluorescence, nuclear fluorescence was localized primarily to nucleoli, the sites of rRNA synthesis. Following injection with anti-polymerase the cells were pulsed with ^{3}H-uridine at various times to measure their ability to synthesize RNA. Relative to cells injected with non-specific antibodies or not antibodies at all, total RNA synthesis was reduced by 30–40% in cells injected with anti-polymerase molecules. Based on considerations of mitotic index, micro-injection efficiency and the proportion of total RNA synthesis catalysed by RNA polymerase I, their results were consistent with total suppression of rRNA synthesis within injected cells.

Microneedles have been used for most injection studies relating to the cytoskeleton. However, in one study, designed to assess the effects of antibodies on intermediate filaments, Eckert and Daley (1981) introduced antibodies to vimentin via RBC ghosts. Microinjection of anti-keratin antibodies resulted in formation of a perinuclear cap of keratin within 20 minutes and a loss of keratin filament bundles from the cytoplasm within one hour. The authors suggest that cap formation results from antibody interference with normal interactions between cytokeratin and other cytoskeletal structures. In a similar approach Vogt *et al.* (1983) injected metaphase ptk_1 cells with both polyclonal and monoclonal antibodies to tubulin. In most treated cells microtubule number was reduced, with the remaining microtubules usually associated with the centrosome, kinetochore or both. In approximately a third of the treated cells the spindle elongated without associated chromosomal motion. Microinjection of metaphase cells with monoclonal antibodies to α-tubulin produced changes in spindle structure different from that observed with the polyclonal antibodies. Electron microscopy showed that fragmentation of spindle microtubules, which occurred without a major loss of spindle microtubule polymer, was so complete that there was no continuity of microtubules in either half spindle.

An unusual and surprisingly successful use of antibody injection has been reported by Ohara and Watanabe (1982), who injected antibodies to cyclic AMP into murine lymphocytes. They found that in non-stimulated lymphocytes antigen binding activity of anti-cyclic AMP antibodies was stable and intact even 24 h after microinjection, whereas the activity rapidly decreased in mitogen-stimulated lymphocytes, suggesting that some immunologic or enzymatic mechanisms for inactivating antibodies were induced in mitogen-stimulated cells. Furthermore, microinjection of anti-cyclic AMP markedly enhanced the proliferative responses of lymphocytes to mitogens such as concanavalin A or lipopolysaccharide (LPS) and reversed the effect of a known elevator of intracellular cyclic AMP.

In a subsequent paper using mouse monoclonal antibodies to cAMP rather than rabbit polyclonal antibodies, Ohara *et al.* (1982) reported that microinjection of monoclonal antibody molecules into lymphocytes at a very early stage of LPS stimulation resulted in a marked enhancement of DNA synthetic responses as well as increased numbers of plaque-forming cells. Intracellular cyclic AMP levels were found to be markedly decreased suggesting that lowering the intracellular cyclic-AMP level in the B lymphocytes at an early stage of stimulation might have induced the enhanced proliferative as well as differentiative responses to LPS. Similar enhancing effects on cell proliferation were obtained when antibodies were injected 18 h after stimulation. Microinjection of anti-cyclic AMP at 12 h after culture, however, inhibited the DNA synthetic responses, and induction of plaque-forming cells was suppressed when anti-cyclic AMP was injected 6 h after

LPS stimulation. The authors suggest biphasic regulatory roles for cyclic AMP at the early stage of B lymphocyte activation. They also emphasize the usefulness of this approach for identifying regulatory molecules in B lymphocytes induced by mitogenic or antigenic stimulation.

B. Antibodies as probes of nuclear entry

Antibody injection has also been used to measure the permeability properties of the nuclear envelope. There is abundant evidence that certain features of a protein's structure (for example, leader or transit peptides, phosphomannose residues) can determine the intracellular compartment in which the protein accumulates (Kaplan *et al.*, 1977; Sando and Neufeld, 1977; Chua and Schmidt, 1978; Highfield and Ellis, 1978; Blobel, 1980). Whether there are specific signals which direct proteins to the nucleus remains unresolved. DeRobertis *et al.* (1978) injected a mixture of ^{125}I-labelled non-histone chromosomal proteins into *Xenopus* oocytes and found a striking accumulation of the injected proteins within the germinal vesicle. They suggested that nuclear proteins possess a common feature responsible for entry into the nucleus. Supporting this idea are several recent studies which show that nucleoplasmin entry into *Xenopus* nuclei depends upon the presence of a distinct portion of the protein chain (Dingwall *et al.*, 1982), that the nuclear entry of SV40 T antigen is abolished by mutations in a specific peptide sequence (Kalderon *et al.*, 1984; Lanford and Butel, 1984), and that the 116 kDa subunit of β-galactosidase can be targeted to yeast nuclei by fusion to the N terminus of yeast nuclear proteins (Hall *et al.*, 1984; Silver *et al.*, 1984).

On the other hand, there are studies which suggest that size primarily determines whether proteins enter the nucleus (Bonner, 1975; Paine *et al.*, 1975). Results obtained after RBC-mediated injection of immunoglobin G molecules support both hypotheses. McGarry *et al.* (1983) found that Fab and Fc fragments distributed evenly between nucleus and cytoplasm, whereas intact non-immune IgG molecules were excluded from the nucleus. The apparent distribution did not change during a 17 h period following fusion, indicating that exclusion was probably complete. These results, obtained by autoradiography on thin sections, are in accord with the immunofluorescence studies of Schlegel (1984) mentioned above. Moreover, several microneedle injection studies suggest that intact IgG molecules do not readily cross the nuclear membrane. Capecchi (1980) found that ^{125}I-IgG molecules remained within L929 nuclei after microneedle injection into that compartment, and Stacey and Allfrey (1984) observed that rhodamine-labelled IgGs remained in the cytoplasm of HeLa cells for at least 8 h after microneedle injection.

Different results were obtained by Bennett *et al.* (1983) who used RBC-fusion to introduce antibodies against the nucleolar antigen, C23, into rat Walker 256 cells. Affinity purified antibodies were found in the cytoplasm and nucleolus 3 h after injection, and by 17 h the antibodies were almost exclusively within the nucleolus. In contrast to the behaviour of anti-C23 antibodies, pre-immune immunoglobulins remained in the cytoplasm 36 h after injection. The authors consider several possibilities for the divergent results including fixation artifacts or entry during mitosis, and with good justification they discount them. They also observe that anti-C23 antibodies enter the nucleolus even when protein synthesis is inhibited, suggesting that anti-C23 antibodies do not enter the nucleus after complexing with *newly synthesized* C23 antigen in the cytoplasm. The apparent exclusion of pre-immune IgGs and the entry of anti-C23 IgGs into Walker 256 nucleoli are not easily reconciled. However, if C23 antigen normally shuttles between nucleus and cytoplasm, the possibility remains that anti-C23 antibodies do, in fact, enter the nucleolus after complex formation with endogenous C23 antigen.

Whatever the eventual explanation for this seeming paradox, RBC-mediated injection should continue to be a valuable tool for studying the mechanism of nuclear localization of proteins. For example, it would not be difficult to determine whether antibodies covalently coupled to specific nuclear antigens thereby gain entry to the nucleus. In a similar fashion, it would be easy enough to inject large proteins chemically coupled with specific peptide sequences identified by site-specific mutagenesis or gene fusion as possible signals for directing proteins to the nucleus. Subsequent localization of these proteins and their unmodified counterparts could provide a powerful assay for nuclear entry signals.

C. Antibody injection for cell and mutant selection

As mentioned in the previous chapter, introduction of antitoxin antibodies permits selection of injected cells. Yoshimori *et al.* (1984) have recently proposed that monoclonals to diphtheria toxin CRM176 be used for such a selective procedure. Antibody injection can also be used to select for hybrid cells. Wright (1984) has introduced anti-ricin antibodies into one set of human cells and anti-diphtheria antibodies into another. The two populations were then fused, exposed to both toxins, and only heterokaryons were resistant to both toxins. Although Wright introduced the antitoxin antibodies by osmotic lysis of pinosomes (Okada and Rechsteiner, 1982), RBC-mediated injection should prove equally successful for such selections.

One of us (MCR) is using antibody injection in an attempt to select for temperature-sensitive mutants in intracellular proteolytic pathways. Since antibodies against ricin and diphtheria toxin protect cells from the lethal activity of these toxins, all injected cells should survive low levels of toxin immediately after fusion. However, cells which degrade the injected antibody should become increasingly sensitive to the toxins, while cells with temperature-sensitive defects in proteolysis are expected to remain resistant at the non-permissive temperature.

Success of the antibody injection studies reported above was by no means assured. The cytoplasm of living cells is a reducing environment and disulphide bonds play an important role in antibody structure. Accordingly, the injected IgG molecules might have easily lost activity upon reduction of disulphide bridges. Fortunately, this does not appear to occur. Or if it does, complex formation between antibodies and antigens is not prevented.

We do not know with certainty the ultimate fate of intracellular antibody–antigen complexes. Stacey and Allfrey (1977), using microneedles, injected haemoglobin into HeLa cells followed by antihaemoglobin antibodies, and observed cytoplasmic precipitation and perinuclear aggregation of the haemoglobin–antihaemoglobin complexes. They suggested that these complexes were degraded within lysosomes, but they also report that some precipitates were extruded from the cells.

Yamaizumi *et al.* (1982) have measured the half-lives of wild-type and CRM mutants of diphtheria toxin fragment A injected into Ehrlich ascites cells. The wild-type fragment A was relatively stable in mouse cytoplasm at 37°C and at least 80% was recovered from cells after 24 h of incubation. In contrast, fragment A molecules from CRM176 and CRM1975 were unstable and were degraded with half-lives of about 2.5 h under similar conditions. When a rabbit anti-fragment A IgG fraction was introduced with wild-type A, the rate of degradation of A was accelerated, whereas the rates of degradation for mutant fragment As were retarded by the same antibody. In every instance the degradation rate appeared to be that of the IgG fraction itself ($t_{1/2}$ = 7.5 h). This rate seems too rapid for the autophagy–lysosomal pathway so it is not clear where antibody–antigen complexes are degraded.

IV. INJECTION OF NUCLEAR PROTEINS

RBC-mediated injection has been used to study the intracellular behaviour of nuclear proteins. Yamaizumi *et al.* (1978b) isolated non-histone chromosomal proteins from rat liver, radiolabelled them with ^{125}I and reintroduced them into Ehrlich ascites tumour cells. They fractionated the injected cells at various times and found that about 20% of the injected proteins were associated with nuclei immediately following injection. The absolute amount of injected protein within nuclei did not change appreciably over the next 24 h whereas there was a 5-fold decrease in the amount of injected proteins that remained in the cytoplasm. They concluded that non-histone chromosomal proteins are rapidly transferred to nuclei and suggested that there is some machinery in the cytoplasm for such selective transfer.

Rechsteiner and Kuehl (1979) studied the intracellular behaviour of a specific chromosomal protein, the high mobility group protein, HMG1. Following its injection into HeLa cells and bovine fibroblasts, HMG1 was found to associate rapidly with nuclei although a number of non-nuclear proteins did not. Autoradiography of thin sections showed that ^{125}I-labelled HMG1 was within the nuclei and that it remained associated with metaphase chromosomes at mitosis. When uninjected HeLa cells were fused with ^{125}I-HMG1-injected HeLa cells, the labelled molecules equilibrated between nuclei within 12 h. Similar results were obtained with bovine fibroblasts, indicating that a dynamic equilibrium exists between HMG1 and chromatin. Electrophoresis of ^{125}I-HMG1 retrieved from HeLa cells or bovine fibroblasts showed that more than 80% of the molecules were intact, and autoradiographic analysis produced apparent half-lives for ^{125}I-HMG1 of 80 h in HeLa cells and 100 h in bovine fibroblasts.

Wu *et al.* (1981) extended these studies by comparing the intracellular behaviour of microinjected HMG1 and HMG2 molecules following the report by Seyadin and Kistler (1979) that the levels of HMG2, but not HMG1, correlated with the proliferative activity of various rat tissues. Coinjection of ^{125}I-HMG1 and ^{131}I-HMG2 into HeLa cells revealed that the two molecules display virtually equivalent distributions upon cell fractionation, identical stability, identical intracellular distributions, and equal rates of equilibration between nuclei. Importantly, HMG1 and HMG2 did not differ in their partitioning upon fractionation nor in their stability between growing and non-growing 3T3 cells. This similarity in the intracellular behaviour of HMG1 and HMG2 was observed in human, bovine, and murine cells.

Recently, Wu, Kuehl and Rechsteiner (in prep.) have injected histone H1 into HeLa cells to determine whether H1 remains stably associated with nucleosome core particles. The molecule was purified from bovine thymus and labelled with ^{3}H by reductive methylation. ^{3}H-labelled H1 was found to associate rapidly with HeLa chromatin following its injection into S phase HeLa cells, and a number of tests indicate that this association faithfully mimics the behaviour of endogenous H1. Injected ^{3}H-H1 copurified with HeLa nuclei and remained associated with chromatin unless the NaCl concentration exceeded 0.5 M. ^{3}H-H1 exhibited a half-life of 110 h, in good agreement with several *in vivo* labelling studies (Gurley and Hardin, 1969; Sakagami *et al.*, 1982). Also, microinjected ^{3}H-H1 molecules were phosphorylated at mitosis like endogenous histone H1 molecules (Gurley *et al.*, 1978). When ^{3}H-H1 injected HeLa cells were fused with 3T3-4E mouse cells to form heterokaryons, autoradiography showed that there was virtually no exchange of H1 between HeLa and mouse nuclei. However, immediately following mitosis ^{3}H-H1 molecules were distributed evenly between human and mouse chromosomes, suggesting that H1 molecules are either in dynamic equilibrium within nuclei but cannot leave the nucleus or that there is extensive redistribution of H1 molecules at mitosis.

V. INJECTION OF MISCELLANEOUS PROTEINS

There are a number of reports in which other specific proteins have been introduced into cells using RBC mediated injection. We cover these here briefly because much more space would be required to describe the process under study in sufficient detail for full comprehension.

Prior to their work on antibody injections described above, Yamaizumi *et al.* (1978c) had injected purified fragment A of diphtheria toxin into toxin-resistant mouse L cells. They varied the number of toxin molcules per RBC and obtained convincing evidence that a single molecule of the A fragment was sufficient to kill an injected cell. Similarly, several years before they used antibodies to inhibit T antigen function, Livingston and his colleagues (Kriegler *et al.*, 1978) had shown that microinjected T antigen would function within recipient cells. African green monkey cells were injected with purified SV40 T antigen and infected with a temperature-sensitive mutant of SV40 (tsA209) defective in the initiation of viral DNA synthesis. Using *in situ* hybridization as an assay method, they found that microinjection of purified T antigen resulted in an increase in the amount of viral DNA sequences in the monolayer. Thus injection of SV40 T antigen led to phenotypic complementation of the tsA defect.

RBC-mediated injection has been used in two studies relating to the action of growth factors. Wille and Willecke (1980) introduced macrophage growth factor into cultivated mouse peritoneal macrophages and found that macrophage DNA synthesis was induced within 40 h. In contrast, Heumann *et* al. (1981) found no effect on neurite outgrowth from PC12 phaeochromacytoma cells by RBC-mediated injection of nerve growth factor. In addition, they injected anti-NGF antibodies into PC12 cells and also failed to inhibit fibre outgrowth, concluding that binding of NGF to its receptor generated a second messenger responsible for neurite development.

Kishimoto *et al.* (1982) provided some evidence for a second messenger from studies on lymphocyte receptors. B lymphocytes are able to differentiate into immunoglobulin-(Ig) producing cells through several activation processes, i.e., activation by signals provided through Ig receptors by antigens or anti-Ig, proliferation by B cell growth factor(s), and final differentiation by B cell differentiation factor(s), such as T cell replacing factor (TRF). Injection of the cytoplasm from a TRF-stimulated B lymphoblastoid cell line into non-stimulated cells induced an increase in IgG-producing cells whereas injection of TRF itself did not. Active substance(s) in the cytoplasm were generated 2 h after TRF stimulation, and IgG-producing cells reached their maximum level at 40 h after injection of the factor(s). The authors suggested that binding of TRF with its receptor generated cytoplasmic factor(s) involved in the transmission of TRF-mediated signals from membrane to nuclei. Since there is a 50- to 100-fold dilution of cytoplasmic contents upon RBC-mediated injection, the TRF second messenger must either be present in very high concentration or be a stably activated enzyme.

Boney *et al.* (1983) used RBC-mediated injection of purified beef heart cAMP-dependent protein kinase catalytic subunit to test its effects on tyrosine aminotransferase activity in cultured rat H35 hepatoma cells. Although the microinjection procedure itself produced temporary fluctuations in protein synthesis and in tyrosine aminotransferase activity in H35 cells, after a recovery period of 8–12 h these parameters returned to normal. No significant change in the activity of the aminotransferase was detected 8 to 16 h after fusion of H35 cells with unloaded ghosts, ghosts loaded with bovine serum albumin or mock-loaded with the partially purified protein kinase catalytic subunit. In contrast, fusion with ghosts loaded with the catalytic subunit at concentrations between 0.1–2 mg/ml produced 2- to 3-fold increases in enzyme activity. Homogeneous preparations of the catalytic subunit exhibited even greater potency as an inducer. The effect was both time and concentration dependent and was abolished by inactivation of the catalytic subunit with *N*-ethylmaleimide prior to loading.

In a recent application, Osawa *et al.* (1984) have injected pancreatic DNase I into mouse Y1 adrenal tumour cells to complex actin and test whether this would inhibit the steroidogenic responses of Y1 cells to ACTH and cAMP. They found that microinjection of DNase I, but not albumin, ovalbumin, boiled DNase I, or DNase I with excess G-actin, inhibited the increase in production of 20 α-dihydroprogesterone produced by ACTH and dibutyryl cyclic AMP. Inhibition, shown to be concentration dependent, was exerted at the step in the steroidogenic pathway at which cholesterol is transported to mitochondria, the site at which steroidogenesis begins. Since DNase I is known to form a one to one complex with G-actin, they suggested that at least some of the G-actin in the cells is necessary for the steroidogenic responses to ACTH and cyclic AMP.

VI. DIFFUSIBILITY OF INJECTED PROTEINS

Our knowledge of the physical properties of the cytosol is at present limited, but this aspect of cell biology is attracting increasing interest (Porter, 1984), and two fundamental questions in this area have been approached using RBC-mediated injection. Wojcieszyn *et al.* (1981a,b) have measured the diffusion of proteins in the cytoplasm of human fibroblasts. Bovine serum albumin and immunoglobulin G were labelled with fluroscein and introduced into human diploid fibroblasts by RBC fusion. The authors then bleached a portion of the cytoplasm and recorded fluorescence recovery in the bleached spot. The apparent diffusion coefficients of the two molecules were $\sim 10^{-8}$ cm^2/sec at 22°C, consistent with the kinetics of spreading of the fluorescent probe following microinjection and ~1/70 the values in aqueous buffer. The diffusion of labelled bovine serum albumin was shown to be strongly dependent on temperature and, in fact, similar to that expected in a 61% aqueous sucrose solution. However, the marked reduction in diffusion at 5°C could be fully reversed by incubation with 1.0 mM colchicine. Jacobsen and Wojcieszyn (1984) have recently extended these studies by showing that in fibroblast cytoplasm, diffusion coefficients (D) of test macromolecules ranging in relative molecular mass from 12000 to 440000 exhibited almost no dependence on molecular weight or cellular energy metabolism. However, hypotonic treatment increased D for bovine serum albumin nearly two-fold and hypertonic treatment halved it. Withdrawing the free waster from the cell by exposure to 44% polyethylene glycol abolished the translational mobility of the test molecules. They concluded that diffusion in the cytomatrix is dominated by binding of the diffusing species to elements of the cytomatrix rather than by steric hindrance through it.

The second question relates to the extent to which "soluble" cytoplasmic proteins are actually soluble within living cells. Masters (1977) has proposed that a number of soluble glycolytic enzymes are, in fact, associated with actin filaments *in vivo*. Rogers and Rechsteiner (1985), in a preliminary report on their survey of the degradation rates for 35 structurally characterized proteins, observed that only a small portion of most injected kinases and dehydrogenases were extracted in buffers containing Triton X-100. The physiological significance of these results is uncertain, since this extraction technique is controversial. Some argue that the Triton X-100 "cytoskeleton" is a manifestation of *in vivo* protein associations between various cellular proteins and the major cytoplasmic fibre systems (Fulton *et al.*, 1980). Others urge caution in this interpretation believing that proteins may bind structures other than cytoplasmic fibres (Dang *et al.*, 1983) or that associations and insolubility may arise during the extraction procedures. In fact, a large number of proteins are found in the Triton X-100 insoluble fraction, and the relevance of protein association in such a poorly defined fraction is a very difficult question. Nevertheless, the observed retention of inject enzymes within the Triton X-100 insoluble cell fraction may be of real physiological significance. Thus, even though there is presently insufficient evidence to arrive at a clear solution to this problem, future injection experiments followed by careful measurements on rates of association, factors influencing association, etc., offer a unique approach for resolving the status of enzyme "solubility" within living cells.

VII. INJECTION OF TRANSFER RNAs

Although RBC-mediated injection has been used mainly for the introduction of proteins into cells, there have been a number of successful applications with RNA molecules. Soon after the technique was first presented, Kaltoft *et al.* (1976) injected tRNAs from yeast and *Escherichia coli* into mouse cells. They showed that at least 50% of the yeast tRNAs and somewhat less *E. coli* tRNA could be recovered intact from the injected cells. They pointed out in this paper and elsewhere (Celis, 1977) the potential of RBC-mediated injection of tRNAs for identifying nonsense mutants in cultured mammalian cells.

This potential was realized in an elegant study by Capecchi *et al.* (1977). From among a large collection of HGPRT negative cell lines derived from L929 cells, these authors identified one CRM$^+$ mutant with an altered carboxyterminal peptide. Cells of this mutant line regained HGPRT activity when ochre suppressor tRNA was injected into them, but not when amber-suppressor or wild-type tRNAs were transferred. They concluded that the CRM$^+$ mutant under study contained an ochre nonsense mutation (UAA) in the C-terminal region of HGPRT.

Schlegel *et al.* (1976, 1978) also demonstrated that tRNA molecules remain intact after RBC-mediated injection into culture cells. In the second of these studies, they examined in detail the turn-over of tRNA molecules injected into SV3T3 mouse cells or TC7 cells, an African green monkey kidney line. The turn-over of endogenous tRNA, measured by labelling with ^{3}H-methionine, was first-order with half-lives of approximately one day in SV3T3 and two days in TC7 cells; injected ^{32}P-tRNA, whether isolated from *E. coli* or TC7 cells, was degraded at the same rate as the endogenous tRNAs. This demonstrated that cellular processes, not properties inherent to tRNAs, are responsible for the different rates of turn-over observed between SV3T3 and TC7 cells, and that the mechanism of tRNA turn-over in mammalian cells does not distinguish between prokaryotic and eukaryotic tRNAs. In contrast to unmodified tRNAs, glyoxalated tRNA was rapidly degraded after injection. Thus altered tRNAs, like altered proteins, turn over more rapidly in animal cells. The original intent of the tRNA injections of Schlegel *et al.* (1978) was to determine whether specific tRNA molecules play a role in permissiveness to SV40 lytic infection. From the failure of TC7 tRNA molecules to produced infective SV40 virus upon injection into SV3T3 cells, they concluded that tRNA molecules, by themselves, were not the permissive factor present in African green monkey cells.

VIII. INJECTION OF MESSENGER RNAs

There are two reports of the successful transfer of mRNA molecules using RBC-mediated injection. Anderson and Krueger (1976) describe the injection of rabbit globin mRNA into CHO cells. After injection of either mRNA or buffer only, CHO cells were incubated in medium containing 300 μCi ^{3}H-leucine. The injected cells were then harvested by trypsinization, lysed by repeated freeze–thaw, and the lysate was analysed by electrophoresis on SDS-polyacrylamide gels or by chromatography on carboxymethyl cellulose in two buffer systems with ^{14}C-uniformly labelled rabbit globin as marker. In each case, ^{3}H-material comigrating with the rabbit globin marker occurred in the cells injected with rabbit globin mRNA, but not in the cells fused with buffer-loaded RBC.

In 1983 Boogaard and Dixon published two papers (1983a,b) on the loading and transfer of messenger RNA molecules using RBC ghosts. In the first of these papers they compared pre-swell loading and multiple lysis loading of tRNA and protamine mRNA molecules. As described in the previous chapter, using the pre-swell procedure, they observed greater degradation of the loaded RNAs using the pre-swell procedure which they suggest may be due to nuclease activity or oxidative damage.

The second paper describes the successful transfer of a functional protamine mRNA into HeLa cells. Boogaard and Dixon (1983b) found that recipient HeLa cells were capable of translating the messenger RNA into the three protamine polypeptides (C_{1}, C_{11}, and C_{111}). The HeLa cells also phosphorylated C_{11} after synthesis, but this phosphorylation did not occur with C_{111}. In addition, C_{11} accumulated in HeLa nuclei after synthesis whereas C_{111} did not. Thus, a correlation between post-translational modification and nuclear localization was observed. Nuclear entry of C_{11} was not followed by the same tight binding of protamine to chromatin as is seen in the homologous trout testis spermatid cells. In spermatids protamine elutes from chromatin at a salt concentration of 1.2 M NaCl; in HeLa cells the chromatin-associated C_{11} could be eluted with 0.6 M NaCl. The authors suggest that the tight binding of protamine to chromatin in trout testis may require a series of concomitant developmental events, such as core histone hyperacetylation, lacking in HeLa cells.

IX. INJECTION OF DNA

There are several reasons that the successful use of RBC-mediated injection for transfer of DNA into cells was not reported until 1980. First, two relatively easy methods for DNA transfer using $CaPO_4$ precipitation (Graham and van der Eb, 1973) and DEAE-Dextran (Vaheri and Pagano, 1965) were already available. Second, a major goal of early DNA injections was transformation of the recipient cells, and injection directly into nuclei using microneedles proved to be very efficient (Graessmann and Graessmann, 1976). Third, the pores that form in the RBC-membrane upon osmotic lysis are small and transient so that entry of large, slowly diffusing DNA molecules is restricted.

Despite the apparent shortcomings of the RBC procedure when applied to DNA molecules, it was used by Straus and Raskas (1980) to transfect KB cells with adenovirus type 2 DNA. Following fusion, radioisotope equivalent to 25 molecules of labelled DNA was injected and transported to each KB cell nucleus. A direct immunofluorescent assay demonstrated virus replication in some cells following their fusion with DNA-containing RBCs. The efficiency of transfection was considerably lower than that expected from the large number of microinjected DNA molecules, suggesting that most of the transferred DNA molecules were degraded before a successful injection could be completed.

Recently, there have been two reports of DNA transfer using RBCs loaded by freeze–thaw lysis rather than osmotic lysis (see Chapter 5 for details). With this apparently improved loading procedure Iino *et al.* (1983) report that transformation of tk-defective L cells can be achieved using ghosts loaded with a plasmid containing a Herpes simplex viral thymidine kinase (tk) gene. The efficiency of transformation ranged from 10^{-4} to 10^{-5}.

Using a similar procedure Wiberg *et al.* (1983) report that Polyoma virus DNA can be transferred into large numbers of mammalian cells. The overall recovery permitted analysis of transferred DNA immediately after fusion by Southern blot hybridization and electron microscopy. In general, more than 20% of the cells contain the transfected Polyoma DNA in their nuclei within 4 h post-fusion, however, expression of Polyoma T antigen was delayed in comparison to a normal virus infection. During the first few days an increase in polyoma DNA could be detected which the authors suggest is due to limited replication. To analyse the replication of hybrid DNA molecules consisting of Polyoma and prokaryotic plasmid DNA sequences, fusion was followed by a normal Polyoma virus infection. The resulting induction of cells to enter the S phase made possible the analysis of the replication of transfected hybrid DNA. Replicating molecules of both the θ form and rolling-circle type were observed.

Finally, Rechsteiner *et al.* (1984c) have transferred small, 100–400 bp, DNA fragments into HTC and HeLa cells using RBC-mediated injection. Although the injection of such short DNA molecules will not permit transformation of recipient cells by most genes, it might allow integration of smaller genes such as those for tRNAs, 5S RNA, or small nuclear RNAs. Moreover, if transformation is frequent, it should be possible to study the integration reactions themselves since so many cells can be injected. Perhaps the most exciting application of RBC-mediated DNA fragment injection would result if the injected DNAs will interact with endogenous DNA binding proteins. If this were to occur, then injection of specific sequence fragments could provide a genetic interference test. For example, 10^5 copies of a 100 bp fragment can be injected into each HeLa cell. If this 100 bp fragment contained the binding site of a normal, diffusible regulatory protein (either positive or negative regulating), then these fragments should disrupt normal genetic control. That is, silent genes could be activated or transcription might cease in normally active genes.

X. SUMMARY

Throughout the chapter we have indicated those areas where future applications of RBC-mediated microinjection are likely to be successful. Rather than recapitulating we would like to close with two considerations.

Many applications of RBC-mediated injection involve the introduction of *unmodified* proteins such as SV40 T antigen, enzymes or antibodies into cells. An equally large number of studies require exogenously-labelled proteins in order to follow the protein within the recipient cells. One might question the validity of the latter approach on the grounds that derivatized proteins are not valid probes of the behaviour of their unmodified counterparts. In the discussion on nuclear proteins, we cited several examples of indistinguishable behaviour between exogenously-labelled, injected proteins and their endogenous equivalents. We believe that injection of proteins modified by gentle procedures will generally produce valid results.

Support for this assumption also comes from microneedle injection studies on cytoskeleton behaviour. For example, Keith *et al.* (1981) found that fluorescein-labelled tubulin was incorporated into microtubules within 15 min of injection. Similarly, Glacy (1983) found that microinjection of rhodamine-labelled skeletal actin into cultured cardiac myocytes was followed by rapid incorporation into myofibrils within the cells. Myocytes examined as soon as 5 min post-injection displayed fluorescent bands corresponding to the sarcomeres, and this pattern of fluorescence remained essentially unchanged for at least 15 h post-injection. Glacy also showed that the myofibrils were able to contract after rhodamine-actin incorporation. Yet another example is reported by Schlessinger and Geiger (1983) who found that rhodamine-labelled actin and α-actinin were detected in stress fibres, focal contacts and leading lamella after injection into chick gizzard myoblasts. Rhodamine-labelled vinculin, on the other hand, was localized only in focal contacts and the interfibrillary space. The observed distributions of the injected proteins were fully expected on the basis of antibody localization studies of the endogenous proteins in fixed cells. Since it seems reasonable to assume that rhodaminated actin or fluoresceinated tubulin must closely match the native conformation of their unmodified counterparts to assemble into filaments and microtubules, these results support our contention that proteins derivatized at a few residues retain a high degree of native structure.

Our second consideration deals with the historical perspective. In the 1950s and 1960s, radioisotopes, microscopes and centrifuges were the major analytical tools of cell biologists. The 1970s witnessed the introduction of increased popularity of four additional methods of analysis. First, polyacrylamide electrophoresis allowed the identification of thousands of cellular proteins. Second, fluorescence microscopy and photo-bleaching became routine procedures following the development of epifluorescence lens systems and light intensification cameras. Third, the use of specific antibodies, both polyclonal and monoclonal, to localize cellular proteins became a widespread and powerful approach. Fourth, a number of techniques were developed for introducing molecules into living cells. Thus, it became possible not only to locate cellular proteins with antibodies but to interfere with the normal function of these proteins. The late 1970s and early 1980s have witnessed the emergence of another exceedingly powerful tool, recombinant DNA technology. Already this approach is being used to vary protein sequences and thereby discover the important determinants for cellular localization and function of the modified proteins.

None of the newer techniques has supplanted a previous approach. After all, electron microscopy, cell fractionation and radioisotopic studies are still widely employed in modern cell research. Rather, the newer techniques permit experiments that were not possible prior to their development. So it is our conviction that the introduction of macromolecules into living cells will become widespread as more cell biologists phrase their questions in terms of the functioning of molecules within the cytoplasmic milieu. Whether molecules will be introduced by RBC-mediated injection, osmotic lysis of pinosomes, glass capillaries, or some procedure not yet invented will depend upon specific circumstances. There can be little doubt, however, that the microinjection approach will gain increasing acceptance as a valuable tool in modern cell research.

REFERENCES

Acton, G. J. and Gupta, S. (1979). *Biochem. J.* **184**, 367–377.

Anderson, W. F. and Krueger, L. J. (1976). *J. Cell Biol.* **70**, 185a.

Antman, K. H. and Livingston, D. M. (1980). *Cell* **19**, 627–635.

Atidia, J. and Kulka, R. G. (1982). *FEBS Lett.* **142**, 72–76.

Backer, J. M., Bourret, L. and Dice, J. F. (1983). *Proc. Natl. Acad. Sci. USA* **80**, 2166–2170.

Bennett, F., Busch, H., Lischwe, M. A. and Yeoman, L. C. (1983). *J. Cell Biol.* **97**, 1556–1572.

Bigelow, S., Hough, R. and Rechsteiner, M. (1981). *Cell* **25**, 83–93.

Blobel, G. (1980). *Proc. Natl. Acad. Sci. USA* **77**, 1496–1500.

Boney, C., Fink, D., Schlichter, D., Carr, K. and Wicks, W. D. (1983). *J. Biol. Chem.* **258**, 4911–4918.

Bonner, W. (1975). *J. Cell Biol.* **64**, 431–437.

Boogaard, C. and Dixon, G. H. (1983a). *Exp. Cell Res.* **143**, 175–190.

Boogaard, C. and Dixon, G. H. (1983b). *Exp. Cell Res.* **143**, 191–205.

Brinster, R. L., Brunner, S., Joseph, X. and Levey, I. L. (1979). *J. Biol. Chem.* **254**, 1927–1931.

Capecchi, M. (1980). *Cell* **22**, 479–488.

Capecchi, M., Capecchi, N., Hughes, S. and Wahl, G. (1974). *Proc. Natl. Acad. Sci. USA* **71**, 4732–4736.

Capecchi, M. R., Von der Haar, R. A., Capecchi, N. E. and Sveda, M. M. (1977). *Cell* **12**, 371–381.

Celis, J. E. (1977). *Brookhaven Symp. Biol.* **29**, 178–196.

Celis, J. E. (1984). *Biochem. J.* **223**, 281–291.

Chin, D. T., Kuehl, L. and Rechsteiner, M. (1982). *Proc. Natl. Acad. Sci. USA* **79**, 5857–5861.

Chua, N.-H. and Schmidt, G. W. (1978). *Proc. Natl. Acad. Sci. USA* **75**, 6110–6114.

Dang, C. V., Yang, D. C. H. and Pollard, T. D. (1983). *J. Cell Biol.* **96**, 1138–1147.

Dean, R. T. (1975). *Biochem. Biophys. Res. Commun.* **67**, 604–609.

DeRobertis, E. M., Longthorne, R. F. and Gurdon, J. B. (1978). *Nature* **272**, 254–256.

Dice, J. F. (1982). *J. Biol. Chem.* **257**, 14624–14627.

Dice, J. F. and Goldberg, A. L. (1975). *Proc. Natl. Acad. Sci. USA* **72**, 3893–3897.

Dice, J. F., Dehlinger, P. J. and Schimke, R. T. (1973). *J. Biol. Chem.* **248**, 4220–4228.

Dice, J. F., Bourret, L. and Maio, P. (1981). *J. Cell Biol.* **91**, 241a.

Dingwall, C., Sharnick, S. V. and Laskey, R. A. (1982). *Cell* **30**, 449–458.

Dunn, W. A., Hubbard, A. L. and Aronson, N. N., Jr. (1980). *J. Biol. Chem.* **255**, 5971–5978.

Eckert, B. S. and Daley, R. A. (1981). *Biol. Cell* **41**, 227–230.

Etlinger, J. D. and Goldberg, A. L. (1977). *Proc. Natl. Acad. Sci. USA* **74**, 54–58.

Fambrough, D. and Devreotes, P. N. (1976). *In* "Biogenesis and Turnover of Membrane Macromolecules" (J. S. Cook, ed.) pp. 121–144. Raven Press, New York.

Freikopf-Cassel, A. and Kulka, R. (1981). *FEBS Lett.* **128**, 63–66.

Fulton, A. B., Wan, K. M. and Penman, S. (1980). *Cell* **20**, 849–857.

Glacy, S. D. (1983). *J. Cell Biol.* **96**, 1164–1167.

Goldberg, A. L. and St. John, A. C. (1976), *Ann. Rev. Biochem.* **45**, 747–803.

Graessmann, M. and Graessmann, A. (1976). *Proc. Natl. Acad. Sci. USA* **73**, 366–370.

Graham, F. and van der Eb, A. (1973). *Virol.* **52**, 456.

Gurley, L. R. and Hardin, J. A. (1969). *Arch. Biochem. Biophys.* **130**, 6.

Gurley, L. R., D'Anna, J. A., Barham, S. S., Deaven, L. L. and Tobey, R. A. (1978). *Eur. J. Biochem.* **84**, 1–15.

Haider, M. and Segal, H. L. (1972). *Arch. Biochem. Biophys.* **148**, 228–237.

Hall, M. N., Hereford, L. and Herskowitz, I. (1984). *Cell* **36**, 1057–1065.

Hendil, K. B. (1977). *J. Cell. Physiol.* **92**, 353–364.

Hendil, K. B. (1980). *J. Cell. Physiol.* **105**, 449–460.

Hendil, K. B. (1981). *Exp. Cell Res.* **135**, 157–166.

Hershko, A. and Ciechanover, A. (1982). *Ann. Rev. Biochem.* **51**, 335–364.

Heumann, R., Schwab, M. and Thoenen, H. (1981). *Nature* **292**, 838–840.

Highfield, P. E. and Ellis, R. J. (1978). *Nature* **271**, 420–424.

Hough, R. and Rechsteiner, M. (1984). *Proc. Natl. Acad. Sci. USA* **81**, 90–94.

Iino, T., Furusawa, M., Furusawa, I. and Obinata, M. (1983). *Exp. Cell. Res.* **148**, 475–480.

Jacobsen, K. and Wojcieszyn, J. (1984). *Proc. Natl. Acad. Sci. USA* **81**, 6747–6751.

Kalderon, D., Richardson, W. D., Markham, A. F. and Smith, A. E. (1984). *Nature* **311**, 33–38.

Kaltoft, K., Zeuthen, J., Engberg, F., Piper, P. W. and Celis, J. E. (1976). *Proc. Natl. Acad. Sci. USA* **73**, 2793–2797.

Kaplan, A., Achord, D. and Sly, W. S. (1977). *Proc. Natl. Acad. Sci. USA* **74**, 2026–2030.

Katznelson, R. and Kulka, R. G. (1983). *J. Biol. Chem.* **258**, 9597–9600.

Keith, C. H., Feramisco, J. R. and Shelanski, M. (1981). *J. Cell. Biol.* **88**, 234–240.

Kielian, M. C. and Cohn, Z. A. (1980). *J. Cell. Biol.* **85**, 754–765.

Kishimoto, T., Miki, Y., Kishi, H., Muraguchi, A., Kishimoto, S. and Yamamura, Y. (1982). *J. Immunol.* **129**, 1367–1371.

Kriegler, M. P., Griffin, J. D. and Livingston, D. M. (1978). *Cell* **14**, 983–994.

Lanford, R. and Butel, J. S. (1984). *Cell* **37**, 801–813.

Lloyd, J. B. (1978). *J. Biochem. Soc. Trans.* **6**, 500.

Masters, C. (1977). *Curr. Top. Cell Regul.* **12**, 75–105.

McElligott, M. A. and Dice, J. F. (1983). *Biochem. J.* **216**, 559–566.

McGarry, T., Hough, R., Rogers, S. and Rechsteiner, M. (1983). *J. Cell. Biol.* **96**, 338–346.

Mortimore, G. H. (1982). *Nutr. Rev.* **40**, 1–12.

Mosteller, R. D., Goldstein, R. V. and Nishimoto, K. R. (1980). *J. Biol. Chem.* **255**, 2524–2532.

Neff, N. T., Bourret, L., Miao, P. and Dice, J. F. (1981). *J. Cell. Biol.* **91**, 184–194.

Ohara, J. and Watanabe, T. (1982). *J. Immunol.* **128**, 1090–1096.

Ohara, J., Sugi, M., Fujimoto, M. and Watanabe, T. (1982). *J. Immunol.* **129**, 1227–1232.

Ohkuma, S. and Poole, B. (1978). *Proc. Natl. Acad. Sci. USA* **75**, 3327–3331.
Okada, C. Y. and Rechsteiner, M. (1982). *Cell* **29**, 33–41.
Osawa, S., Betz, G. and Hall, P. F. (1984). *J. Cell. Biol.* **99**, 1335–1342.
Paine, P. L., Moore, L. C. and Horowitz, S. B. (1975). *Nature* **254**, 109–114.
Petrie, H. T., McDonel, J. L. and Schlegel, R. A. (1982). *Cell Biol. Int. Rep.* **6**, 705–711.
Porter, K. (1984). *J. Cell. Biol.* **99**, 3a–12s.
Rabinowitz, M. and Fisher, J. M. (1964). *Biochem. Biophys. Acta* **91**, 313–326.
Rechsteiner, M. and Kuehl, L. (1979). *Cell* **16**, 901–908.
Rechsteiner, M., Carlson, N., Chin, D., Hough, R., Rogers, S., Roof, D. and Rote, K. (1984a). *In* "Protein Processing and Secretion" (D. Oxender, ed.) pp. 396–407. Alan Liss, New York.
Rechsteiner, M., Chin, D., Hough, R., McGarry, T., Rogers, S., Rote, K. and Wu, L. (1984b). *CIBA Found. Symp.* **103**, 181–201.
Rechsteiner, M., Wu, L. H. and Miller, A. O. A. (1984c). *In* "Red Blood Cell Carriers" (J. R. DeLoach and U. Sprandel, eds) pp. 142–149. S. Karger, Basel.
Rogers, S. W. and Rechsteiner, M. C. (1985). *In* "The Fifth International Symposium on Intracellular Protein Catabolism" (J. S. Bond, ed.). Alan Liss, New York.
Rote, K. V. and Rechsteiner, M. (1983). *J. Cell. Physiol.* **116**, 103–110
Russell, S. M., Burgess, R. J. and Mayer, R. J. (1980). *Biochem. J.* **192**, 321–330.
Sakagami, H., Mitsui, Y., Murota, S.-L. and Yamada, M.-A. (1982). *J. Cell. Physiol.* **110**, 213–218.
Sando, G. N. and Neufeld, E. F. (1977). *Cell* **12**, 619–627.
Schimke, R. T. and Doyle, D. (1970). *Ann. Rev. Biochem.* **39**, 929–964.
Schlegel, R. A. (1981). *In* "Red Blood Cell Carriers" (J. R. DeLoach and U. Sprandel, eds). S. Karger, Basel.
Schlegel, R. A. and McEvoy, L. (1985). *Methods Enzymol.* (in press).
Schlegel, R. A. and Rechsteiner, M. C. (1978). *Methods Cell. Biol.* **20**, 341–354.
Schlegel, R. A., Darrah, L. B. and Rechsteiner, M. C. (1976). *In* "Molecular Mechanisms in the Control of Gene Expression" (D. Nierlich, W. Rutter and C. F. Fox, eds) pp. 465–470. Academic Press, New York and London.
Schlegel, R. A., Iverson, P. and Rechsteiner, M. C. (1978). *Nucl. Acid Res.* **5**, 3715–3729.
Schlessinger, J. and Geiger, B. (1983). *Cell Motil.* **3**, 399–403.
Seyadin, S. M. and Kistler, W. S. (1979). *J. Biol. Chem.* **254**, 11264–11271.
Silver, P. A., Keegan, L. P. and Ptashne, M. (1984). *Proc. Natl. Acad. Sci. USA* **81**, 5951–5955.
Simpson, M. V. (1953). *J. Biol. Chem.* **201**, 143–154.
Smith, J. H., Subbarao, M. N. and Eliceiri, G. L. (1983). *J. Cell. Physiol.* **114**, 1–6.
Stacey, D. W. and Allfrey, V. G. (1977). *J. Cell. Biol.* **75**, 807–817.
Stacey, D. W. and Allfrey, V. G. (1984). *Exp. Cell Res.* **154**, 283–292.
Straus, S. E. and Raskas, H. J. (1980). *J. Gen. Virol.* **48**, 241–245.
Tanaka, K., Waxman, L. and Goldberg, A. L. (1983). *J. Cell Biol.* **96**, 1580–1585.
Vaheri, A. and Pagano, J. S. (1965). *Virology* **27**, 435–436.
Vogt, S. I., Snyder, J. A. and Mullins, J. M. (1983). *J. Cell Biol.* **97**, 191a.
Wall, D. A., Wilson, G. and Hubbard, A. L. (1980). *Cell* **21**, 79–93.
Wasserman, M., Kulka, R. G. and Loyter, A. (1977). *FEBS Lett.* **83**, 48–52.
Wiberg, F. C., Sunnerhagen, P., Kaltoft, K., Zeuthen, J. and Bjursell, G. (1983). *Nucl. Acid Res.* **11**, 7287–7302.

Wille, W. and Willecke, K. (1980). *Exp. Cell Res.* **130**, 95–99.
Wojcieszyn, J. W., Schlegel, R. A. and Jacobson, K. A. (1981a). *Cold Spring Harbor Symp. Quant. Biol.* **46**, 39–43.
Wojcieszyn, J. W., Schlegel, R. A., Wu, E.-S. and Jacobson, K. A. (1981b). *Proc. Natl. Acad. Sci. USA* **78**, 4407–4410.
Wright, W. (1984), *Proc. Natl. Acad. Sci. USA* **81**, 7822–7826.
Wu, L., Kuehl, L. and Rechsteiner, M. (1981). *J. Cell Biol.* **91**, 488–496.
Yamaizumi, M., Mekada, E., Uchida, T. and Okada, Y. (1978a). *Cell* **15**, 245–250.
Yamaizumi, M., Uchida, T., Okada, Y., Furusawa, M. and Mitsui, H. (1978b). *Nature* **273**, 782–784.
Yamaizumi, M., Uchida, T., Okada, Y. and Furusawa, M. (1978c). *Cell* **13**, 227–232.
Yamaizumi, M., Uchida, T., Mekada, E. and Okada, Y. (1979). *Cell* **18**, 1009–1014.
Yamaizumi, M., Uchida, T., Takamatsu, K. and Okada, Y. (1982). *Proc. Natl. Acad. Sci. USA* **79**, 461–465.
Yoshimori, T., Yamada, M., Sugawa, H., Mekada, E., Uchida, T. and Okada, Y. (1984). *Exp. Cell Res.* **151**, 344–353.
Zavortink, M., Thacher, T. and Rechsteiner, M. (1979). *J. Cell. Physiol.* **100**, 175–186.

7

Liposomes for Microinjection of Molecules into Cells

R. M. Straubinger and D. Papahadjopoulos

I. INTRODUCTION

Liposomes (phospholipid vesicles) are spheroidal particles, usually cell-sized or smaller, that form spontaneously when a variety of dried phospholipids are suspended in aqueous media (Bangham and Horne, 1964). Since their initial description (reviewed in Bangham, 1983), liposomes have been the subject of intense study, first as models with which to study numerous functions of biological membranes, and later as carriers of molecules of biological interest *in vivo* and *in vitro*. Investigators have produced many methods for creating liposomes with specific characteristics, such as surface charge, permeability, size, shape, and proteins incorporated in the membrane, and there exist several detailed reviews on the subject (cf. Deamer and Uster, 1980; Szoka and Papahadjopoulos, 1980).

One major area in which the carrier function of liposomes may be important *in vivo* is that of chemotherapy of tumours and of infection; liposomes can protect encapsulated material from degradation, provide for sustained release of their contents, alter the anatomic distribution of encapsulated agents (Kimelberg and Mayhew, 1978), and possibly allow targeting of specific cells by means of ligands bound to the liposome surface (Heath *et al.*, 1980; Huang *et al.*, 1980; Leserman *et al.*, 1980; Martin *et al.*, 1981; Matthay *et al.*, 1984). Another use of the carrier properties of liposomes, mostly pursued *in vitro*, is to promote the intracellular delivery of molecules. A wide variety of molecules can be encapsulated at high concentration within the aqueous interior of liposomes, and some fraction of the captured material can be delivered to the interior of cells and exert a biological effect. Several types of molecules, such as nucleic acids, proteins, or drugs have been encapsulated in

Microinjection and Organelle Transplantation Techniques

ISBN: 0-12-164722-6
ISBN: 0-12-164723-4 Pbk

liposomes for delivery to cells (see reviews by Kimelberg and Mayhew, 1978; Pagano and Weinstein, 1978; Papahadjopoulos *et al.*, 1981; Fraley and Papahadjopoulos, 1982). Since some methods of liposome preparation allow efficient capture of solutes of very high relative molecular mass, purified genes and conceivably chromosomes can be encapsulated and introduced into cells (reviewed in Fraley and Papahadjopoulos, 1982).

To realize the potential benefits of liposome encapsulation for intracellular delivery of membrane-impermeant compounds, it is necessary to understand the mechanisms by which liposomes interact with and deliver their contents to cells. The mechanisms supported by various types of data include liposome fusion with the plasma membrane, endocytosis or phagocytosis, and appositional transfer, whereby liposome contents enter cells after local release from liposomes bound to the cell membrane (for review see Tyrrell *et al.*, 1976; Finkelstein and Weismann, 1978; Pagano and Weinstein, 1978; Poste, 1980). In addition, various components of the liposome, such as sterols, phospholipids, or other lipoid components incorporated into the liposome membrane may transfer to cells without cellular delivery of liposome contents (Struck *et al.*, 1981). A number of recent studies have discounted liposome fusion with the plasma membrane as a major mechanism by which liposome contents enter cells (Szoka *et al.*, 1979, 1980; Struck *et al.*, 1981) and have implicated endocytosis as a major mechanism of liposome uptake (Heath *et al.*, 1983; Straubinger *et al.*, 1983b; Truneh *et al.*, 1983). Other studies have elucidated a number of parameters that alter the efficiency of liposome-mediated delivery of biologically active molecules (Wilson *et al.*, 1979; Fraley *et al.*, 1980, 1981).

II. EARLIER WORK

To summarize a great deal of work on liposome–cell interaction, it appears that the best vesicle lipid composition for delivery of aqueous contents to cells includes high mole percentages of negatively charged phospholipid (customarily phosphatidylserine) and cholesterol. Such vesicles bind avidly to cells, and cholesterol reduces leakage of liposome contents (Papahadjopoulos *et al.*, 1972, 1973; Mayhew *et al.*, 1979; Gregoriadis and Davis, 1979; Fraley *et al.*, 1981; Van Renswoude and Hoekstra, 1981; Allen *et al.*, 1981). The cellular events inducing loss of liposome contents are still unclear. While the cellular binding site is unknown, 10^3–10^4 liposomes bound saturate the capacity of cells to internalize liposome contents (Wilson *et al.*, 1979; Fraley *et al.*, 1981). Those studies also showed that liposome binding to cells was rapid, and the latter showed that competition by buffer-loaded liposomes can reduce the efficiency of delivery by DNA-loaded liposomes. Although delivery can be relatively efficient, it is statistically infrequent. As a result, it has been difficult to determine the mechanism by which very large, liposome-entrapped molecules gain access to the cell interior. A growing body of evidence (Szoka *et al.*, 1979; Struck *et al.*, 1981) suggests that in most cases, liposomes do not fuse with the plasma membrane. Under certain experimental conditions, liposome-mediated delivery of DNA requires energy-dependent events, as well as exposure to an acidic intracellular compartment (Fraley *et al.*, 1981). More recent studies to explore the role of endocytosis in liposome-mediated delivery (Straubinger *et al.*, 1983b) show that negatively charged liposomes are endocytosed in coated pits and proceed intracellularly through the well-defined coated vesicle endocytic pathway (Goldstein *et al.*, 1979; Helenius *et al.*, 1980; Pastan and Willingham, 1981). Eventually, much liposome-delivered material which remains in the cell can be found in the trans-Golgi region, either in dense bodies (secondary lysosomes), or in other vesicles. However, liposomes may subvert existing pathways by which cells process endocytosed macromolecules, and thereby deliver their contents.

There have been several efforts to correlate functional delivery of nucleic acids with cell-association of vesicle lipid and contents. From them, it was possible to estimate the comparative significance of several of the processes mentioned earlier (Papahadjopoulos *et al.*, 1980). Using ^{3}H-labelled phospholipid as a marker for vesicle lipid, ^{32}P poliovirus RNA as a marker for vesicle contents, and the appearance of progeny poliovirus as a marker for intracellular delivery (Wilson *et al.*, 1979), it was found that approximately 10^4 vesicles per cell must be added in order to insure expression of the encapsulated RNA by every cell (roughly 100 nmol phospholipid per 10^6 cells, assuming a mean vesicle diameter of 400 nm, a bilayer thickness of 3.5 nm, and an area of 7 nm^2 per phospholipid molecule). Approximately 10% of the vesicle lipid became cell-associated while only 1% of the RNA was cell-bound. Thus, each cell bound or internalized about 10^3 vesicles when a saturating concentration of vesicles was applied, and only 100 of those vesicles retained their contents. From the infectivity of the RNA, it was apparent that the vesicles that retained their contents were sufficient to ensure infection of virtually all the cells in a vesicle-exposed population, whether of primate (HeLa) or of rodent (L, CHO) origin, and that infectivity of the entrapped RNA was comparable to that of a high titre stock of whole poliovirus (one plaque per 100 particles).

III. MANIPULATION OF INCUBATION CONDITIONS TO ENHANCE DELIVERY

Dimethylsulphoxide (DMSO), glycerol, and polyethylene glycol (PEG) increase the functional delivery of liposome-entrapped DNA (Fraley *et al.*,

1981). PEG (44% w/v for 90 s) and DMSO (25% v/v for 4 min) increase the infectivity of entrapped SV40 DNA by a factor of 10. Glycerol has been the most effective agent for increasing DNA delivery, especially for negatively charged liposomes (100- to 200-fold enhancement). The effect is dose- and time-dependent, and useful with a variety of cell types (cf. Straubinger and Papahadjopoulos, 1983). However, viability after glycerol treatment varies with cell type and should be checked.

The effect of similar treatments to increase the delivery and expression of encapsulated nucleic acids was also observed with plant protoplasts. Although glycerol is toxic to *Nicotiana* protoplasts, treatment with PEG or polyvinyl alcohol increases the functional delivery of liposome-encapsulated Tobacco Mosaic Virus RNA by 200-fold or more (Fraley *et al.*, 1982).

While many studies show that liposome delivery of large molecules occurs without exposure of the contents to the external medium, such observations offer no definitive evidence for the mechanism of the delivery event. Although it is not inconsistent with the hypothesis of liposome fusion with the plasma membrane, the same result could be explained by endocytosis of liposomes and intracellular processing of the contents through a pathway that allows 1% of the internalized material to escape lysosomal degradation.

Agents that inhibit a variety of cellular functions offer an indication of one mechanism by which liposomes may deliver DNA (Fraley *et al.*, 1981). Short incubations of cytochalasin B, colchicine, chloroquine, or azide and 2-deoxyglucose do not alter the basal level or polyethylene glycol enhancement of SV40 DNA delivery, although electron microscopic examination shows liposomes bound to coated pits and in intracellular vesicles (Straubinger *et al.*, 1983b). It may be that passage of DNA-bearing liposomes through the drug-inhibited steps may proceed when the relatively short inhibitor treatments are terminated. However, the effect of glycerol is quite sensitive to azide and deoxyglucose and partially to cytochalasin B. This and several other lines of evidence suggest that glycerol increases liposome uptake by promoting a process that resembles macropinocytosis. Chloroquine, ammonium chloride, and several other agents (Miller and Lenard, 1981) with lysosomotropic activity (DeDuve *et al.*, 1974) enhance the glycerol effect, so lysosomal degradation may be the ultimate fate of at least some liposome-delivered DNA. The lysosomotropic amines may exert their effect during the initial period of liposome internalization, by inhibiting phagolysosome function, thus increasing the probability that intact DNA may escape to the cytoplasm. Alternatively, they may inhibit autophagic (Stacey and Allfrey, 1977; Marzella *et al.*, 1982) processing of intracellular DNA and increase the probability of nuclear access.

IV. NEWER STRATEGIES TO INCREASE INTRACELLULAR DELIVERY OF MACROMOLECULES

In previous work we found that negatively charged liposomes are endocytosed by the coated vesicle pathway, and that large or highly charged molecules can remain sequestered in intracellular vacuoles such as secondary lysosomes (Straubinger *et al.*, 1983b). Certain encapsulated molecules that become membrane-permeant at low pH, such as weakly acidic compounds, can gain access to the cytoplasm efficiently. Other molecules that are unable to exploit the low-pH environment of the endocytic pathway may escape to the cytoplasm with much lower frequency, and a significant fraction of the liposome-delivered molecules may be degraded in lysosomes.

Some lipid-enveloped viruses, including Semliki forest, fowl plague, and vesicular stomatitis virus, are likewise endocytosed by the coated vesicle system. However, acidification of the endocytic vesicle lumen may liberate the nucleocapsid into the cytoplasm through fusion of the viral envelope with the vacuole membrane (Helenius *et al.*, 1980; Miller and Lenard, 1980; White *et al.*, 1981; reviewed in White *et al.*, 1983). Considering such viruses a paradigm for pH-dependent cytoplasmic delivery, our aim has been to design liposomes that become unstable and/or fusion-prone at mildly acidic pH and to examine the ability of such liposomes to deliver charged or large molecules to the cytoplasm of cultured cells. Other groups are also currently pursuing various aspects of pH-dependent destabilization or fusion of liposomes (e.g. Yatvin *et al.*, 1980; Connor *et al.*, 1984; Ellens *et al.*, 1984; Uster and Deamer, 1985).

Our strategy was to use the zwitterionic phospholipid phosphatidylethanolamine (PE) as the principal liposome constituent (Düzgüneş *et al.*, 1983a, 1985; Straubinger *et al.*, 1983a, 1985). The protonated species of PE (p$K \geq$ pH 8; Papahadjopoulos, 1968) is unable to form bilayer vesicles near neutral pH (Papahadjopoulos and Watkins, 1967), although vesicles can be formed above pH 9 (Kolber and Haynes, 1979). Moreover, the presence of PE in liposome membranes facilitates membrane fusion induced by divalent cations (Düzgüneş *et al.*, 1981). To enable formation of stable PE-rich liposomes near neutral pH, we chose oleic acid (OA; *cis* 18:1) as it is a negatively charged amphiphile with a p*K* close to neutral when incorporated into phospholipid membranes (von Tscharner and Radda, 1981). Protonation of OA at a pH within the range expected for the endocytic pathway (6.5 > pH > 4.5; DeDuve *et al.*, 1974; Ohkuma and Poole, 1978) should result in destabilization of a bilayer rich in PE, leading to liposome collapse and/or membrane–membrane fusion. OA also imparts a net negative charge on the liposomes at pH 7.4. Considerable evidence suggests that negatively charged liposomes are superior to neutral and positively charged liposomes in functional delivery of a variety of materials to cells (Fraley *et al.*, 1981, 1982; Schäfer-Ridder *et al.*, 1982; Heath *et al.*, 1985. Similar strategies for creating pH-sensitive liposomes, namely by the inclusion of a titrable acidic amphiphile in phosphatidylethanolamine-rich liposomes, have been employed by others (Connor *et al.*, 1984; Ellens *et al.*, 1984).

Detailed studies on the biophysical properties of OA:PE (3:7 mole ratio) liposomes (Düzgüneş *et al.*, 1983a, 1985) show that pH < 6.5 leads to irreversible vesicle aggregation, observed as changes in light scattering and turbidity. In addition, OA:PE liposomes grow in size and membrane components intermix, as detected by freeze-fracture electron microscopy and by assays of resonant fluorescence energy transfer between phospholipid probes (Struck *et al.*, 1981). Such lines of evidence support the conclusion that OA:PE liposomes, but not control liposomes of OA:PC or PS:PE, undergo proton-induced membrane fusion at pH ≤ 6. The threshold for pH-induced leakage of liposome contents, however, is approximately pH 6.5–6.7. Nevertheless, both loss of contents and membrane fusion occur within the pH range reported for the endocytic pathway (DeDuve *et al.*, 1974; Ohkuma and Poole, 1978; Tycko and Maxfield, 1980).

To examine the ability of pH-sensitive liposomes to deliver macromolecules to the cytoplasm, we chose calcein (CAL) and fluorescein thiocyanyl dextran (FTC-D) as model compounds for highly charged and large molecules, respectively. Previous work showed that both compounds accumulate to a significant degree in vesicles of the endocytic pathway, and that neither is found in appreciable concentrations in the cytoplasm (Straubinger *et al.*, 1983b).

We found that liposomes of OA:PE delivered detectable amounts of CAL to the cytoplasm of CV-1 cells. Efficiency of delivery varied with cell confluence, but under optimal conditions 35–70% of the cells showed unambiguous cytoplasmic CAL fluorescence (Straubinger *et al.*, 1983a, 1985). Brief glycerol treatment (Norberg, 1970; Fraley *et al.*, 1981) increased drastically the intensity of diffuse, cytoplasmic CAL fluorescence from pH-sensitive liposomes but not from control liposomes. The presence of cholesterol (CH) in OA:PE liposomes (mole ratio 3:7:3 OA:PE:CH) did not interfere with the pH-sensitivity of the liposomes and seemed to increase the intensity of intracellular fluorescence. Such a result is anticipated from the well-documented effect of cholesterol to reduce liposome permeability in the presence or absence of cells (Papahadjopoulos *et al.*, 1973; Gregoriadis and Davis, 1979; Mayhew *et al.*, 1979; Allen *et al.*, 1981; Fraley *et al.*, 1981; Van Renswoude and Hoekstra, 1981).

Our results suggest that pH-sensitive liposomes can deliver membrane-impermeant molecules to the cytoplasm, and suggest the utility of such liposomes for microinjection of macromolecules into cells. The number of cells that can be exposed to liposomes is virtually unlimited; with a 1% to 50% frequency of injection, as suggested by the fluorescence results, we would expect cytoplasmic delivery to 10^4 to 10^6 cells out of the 2–4 × 10^6 cells per dish used in the experiments presented here. Such frequencies of injection would not be achieved easily with other methods, such as needle microinjection, and the number of cells exposed to liposomes could be increased 10- to 100-fold over the number used here. We are currently extending this work by examining functional delivery of another macromolecule, SV40 DNA. Preliminary results have verified the relative differences reported here for pH-sensitive and -insensitive liposomes, and suggest that OA:PE liposomes are more efficient for functional DNA delivery than any liposome composition previously examined (Fraley *et al.*, 1980, 1981).

V. METHODOLOGY FOR LIPOSOME PREPARATION AND INCUBATION WITH CELLS

A. Liposome types, preparation and encapsulation

Liposomes can be made by many procedures and composed of a variety of amphipathic molecules (Deamer and Uster, 1980; Szoka and Papahadjopoulos, 1980), and it is beyond the scope of this chapter to give a complete description of the various methods used. Many of the important considerations in liposome preparation, separation from unencapsulated material, and interaction with cells, have been considered in detail elsewhere (Straubinger and Papahadjopoulos, 1983). Therefore, the aim of this chapter is to summarize the most important principles, as deduced from experiments on liposome–cell interaction, and to give the reader an idea of the directions in which liposome technology may evolve in improving the efficiency of intracellular delivery of macromolecules.

Multilamellar vesicles (MLV) can be prepared from a wide variety of phospholipids. A heterogeneous population of particles is produced (0.1–5.0 μm diameter) and they are composed of multiple, concentric lamellae separated by aqueous layers (Bangham *et al.*, 1964). To make MLV, a thin film of lipid is deposited on the walls of a glass tube by evaporation of the lipid from organic solvent. The lipid is then hydrated with a solution of the material to be encapsulated. Vigorous agitation usually is necessary to resuspend most of the lipid, although slow hydration with gentle agitation can be used to produce large liposomes (Olson *et al.*, 1979). The ratio of entrapped volume to lipid typically is 3–7 μl/μmol (Papahadjopoulos and Vail, 1978) and the fraction of aqueous volume is only 3–7% of the original aqueous volume. Such a low capture efficiency can be a disadvantage when dealing with small quantities of relatively precious solutes. For some solutes such as DNA, there is evidence that encapsulation of liposome-associated material is not complete, since nucleases may digest some MLV-associated material (Hoffman *et al.*, 1978; Lurquin, 1979).

Extended sonication of a lipid suspension (such as MLV) produces a relatively homogeneous population of small (0.025–0.05 μm diameter), unilamellar liposomes (SUV; Papahadjopoulos and Miller, 1967; Papahadjopoulos and Watkins, 1967) that capture less than 1% of the initial aqueous medium. Solutes to be encapsulated may be added to a suspension of preformed MLV, and trapped as sonication disrupts the large vesicles and smaller vesicles form. SUV have been used to entrap small DNA fragments (Wong *et al.*, 1980) as well as a great variety of small, water soluble molecules, but the need for extended sonication makes it unlikely that large molecules, such as gene-sized nucleic acid fragments, are encapsulated intact. SUV also have the smallest internal aqueous volume (0.2–0.5 μl/μmol; Huang, 1969) making the procedure unsuitable for efficient encapsulation of high relative molecular mass molecules.

A number of methods produce large unilamellar vesicles (LUV) that capture a comparatively great aqueous volume (up to 14 μl/μmol; Szoka and Papahadjopoulos, 1980). The most commonly used for nucleic acid encapsulation include Ca^{2+}-EDTA chelation (Papahadjopoulos *et al.*, 1975; Wilson *et al.*, 1979), ether injection (Deamer and Bangham, 1976; Ostro *et al.*, 1977; Fraley *et al.*, 1979), detergent dialysis (Enoch and Strittmatter, 1979), and reverse-phase evaporation (REV; Szoka and Papahadjopoulos, 1978; Fraley *et al.*, 1980; Schäfer-Ridder *et al.*, 1982; Nicolau *et al.*, 1983). The REV procedure has received the most detailed examination in this laboratory, as it is well suited to encapsulating the nucleic acid probes used to study the mechanisms of liposome-mediated delivery. A relatively homogeneous population of liposomes is produced, with a mean diameter of approximately 0.45 μm (Szoka and Papahadjopoulos, 1978). Subsequent extrusion of the vesicles through polycarbonate filters of defined pore diameter can be used to ensure sterility (Fraley *et al.*, 1980) or to limit the maximum liposome diameter (Olson *et al.*, 1979; Szoka *et al.*, 1980). The efficiency of solute capture depends on a number of parameters, including the ionic strength of the aqueous medium, the lipids used in liposome preparation (Szoka and Papahadjopoulos, 1978), and liposome diameter. The capture by REV is consistently high, ranging from 20% to 50%, depending on encapsulation conditions. Furthermore, the preparation can be scaled to virtually any volume, so that high ratios of solute to lipid may be achieved using a minimum of material. The efficiency of encapsulation by the REV method is essentially independent of solute relative molecular mass, and as a result, the procedure has been widely used for encapsulation of nucleic acids.

B. Lipids used in liposome preparation

While it may be possible to form liposomes in the presence of common lipid contaminants such as lyso compounds and metal ions, the vesicles produced may be unstable cytotoxic, or of a different electrostatic charge than expected for the pure lipid. Lipids of high purity can be obtained from commercial suppliers, but purity should be checked by thin layer chromatography in several solvent systems (Kates, 1972). Furthermore, it is advisable to store all lipid products under an inert atmosphere, such as argon or nitrogen, at low temperature (−70°C). These storage conditions are especially important for the many naturally occurring phospholipids that contain readily peroxidized polyunsaturated fatty acids.

The concentration of lipid constituents is important in the REV procedure, as well as in other methods. Lipid phosphorus quantitation is convenient for phospholipids (Bartlett, 1959), and a variety of methods exist for quantitation of cholesterol and other lipids (Kates, 1972).

The acidic phospholipids, such as phosphatidylglycerol and phosphatidylserine, are often used for encapsulation and intracellular delivery, as liposomes of negative charge have generally shown the highest efficiency of intracellular delivery (Wilson *et al.*, 1979; Fraley *et al.*, 1980, 1981, 1982; Dahl *et al.*, 1981; Schaefer-Ridder *et al.*, 1982; Heath *et al.*, 1985). One major source of difficulty encountered with these lipids arises from the fact that they sometimes are supplied as the acid, rather than as the sodium salt. In addition, acidic phospholipids also may contain significant quantities of divalent cations. Low pH and divalent cations alter significantly the physical properties of these lipids (Papahadjopoulos *et al.*, 1976), so it is important to ensure that they have been washed with EDTA (ethylenediaminetetraacetate) and NaCl (Papahadjopoulos *et al.*, 1973; Papahadjopoulos and Kimelberg, 1973).

C. Encapsulation by the REV method

The reverse-phase evaporation method (Szoka and Papahadjopoulos, 1978) refers to a critical physical step in liposome formation. A stable water-in-oil emulsion is produced first by brief sonication of phospholipids and aqueous buffer in a larger volume of organic solvent, and the phases are subsequently reversed by evaporation of the organic solvent, leaving a stable liposome emulsion. Important parameters include: the type of organic solvent, the type of phospholipid, its solubility in the organic solvent, and the initial ratio of the aqueous phase to the lipid phase. The original procedure (Szoka and Papahadjopoulos, 1978) used 1.5 ml aqueous phase and 50 or 100 μmol phospholipid in 5 ml ether. However, we routinely scale down the preparation to use 0.175 ml aqueous phase with 5 μmol lipid and 0.6 ml ether. The quantities can be reduced further to as little as 0.035 aqueous and 1.0 μmol lipid, although characteristics of the resulting liposomes have not been verified in the case of such small volumes. To adapt the procedure to volumes other than those given here, the aqueous volume determines the amount of lipid and ether added to maintain the aqueous:lipid:solvent ratio given below.

Five μmol of lipid (usually phosphatidylserine:cholesterol in a 2:1 mol ratio) is transferred to a 10 mm × 100 mm screw cap glass tube. If the material for encapsulation is not soluble in aqueous media, it would be dissolved in organic solvent and added to the lipid mixture at this point. Standard rotary evaporator glassware can be used in the procedure, but the 10 mm × 100 mm tube reduces the amount of material lost during small-scale preparations, and makes sterility easier to maintain. The dimensions of the screw cap tube are chosen so that it can be inserted into the larger tube commonly used on rotary evaporators. A small amount of glycerol or H_2O is added to the larger tube to ensure thermal contact between the sample tube and the evaporator bath.

A thin film of lipid is deposited on the walls of the tube as the original organic solvent is removed by rotary evaporation. Once the lipid has dried, 0.6 ml of diethyl or isopropyl ether is added to resuspend the lipid. It is essential to ensure that the ether is peroxide free, especially in the case of isopropyl ether. In addition to its deleterious effect on phospholipids, the formation of peroxide in anhydrous ether represents a serious safety hazard. Redistillation or extraction with aqueous bisulphide are two ways to eliminate peroxide from the ether. A benefit of the aqueous extraction method is that the ether remains hydrated, and may thus aid in resuspension of well-dried lipids. Often, the choice of ether is arbitrary. However, phospholipids must be in the liquid-crystalline state for vesicle formation, so lipids with a high transition temperature may require warming above the boiling point of diethyl ether. In such cases the higher boiling point of isopropyl ether makes it the solvent of choice.

The solute for encapsulation is added to the ether:lipid mixture in 0.175 ml aqueous buffer. NaCl 150 mM; Tris 10 mM; EDTA 0.1 mM; pH 7.4 is an example of a commonly used buffer. The buffer should have a pH in the range of 7 to 8; Tris [tris(hydroxymethyl)aminomethane], Tes [*N*-tris(hydroxymethyl) methyl-2-aminomethane sulphonic acid], Hepes [*N*-2-(hydroxyethyl) piperazine-*N*′-2-ethane sulphonic acid], or phosphate buffers are acceptable. The buffer must not contain millimolar concentrations of divalent cations if acidic phospholipids are used in the preparation, since divalent cations will precipitate these phospholipids. EDTA (pH 7–8) may be included to ensure that the divalent cation concentration is low. The liposomes produced are osmotically sensitive, so the buffer must be isotonic with respect to the final buffer in which the incubation with cells will take place. If high osmolality is required, it is recommended that sucrose (Fraley *et al.*, 1980, 1982), mannitol (e.g. Mannitol 400 mM; NaCl 50 mM; Tris 5 mM; EDTA 0.1 mM; pH 7.4), or other sugars be used instead of NaCl or KCl for raising the tonicity. Negatively charged liposomes aggregate in high concentrations of Na^+ or K^+. Finally, a small amount of a radioactive tracer such as sucrose, inulin or polyadenylic acid may be included in the buffer to allow measurement of the final captured volume, a useful indicator of the encapsulation efficiency.

Brief sonication of the two-phase system generates a stable emulsion that would not coalesce if allowed to stand for 20–30 min. A bath-type sonicator allows the sonication to be done in a closed tube purged with inert gas. Thus the preparation remains sterile, the aerosols generated are contained and lipid peroxidation is avoided. The original method (Szoka and Papahadjopoulos, 1978) calls for 2–5 min of sonication, but the small volumes used here can be emulsified in as little as 5–7 s of sonication. Low-power or poorly-tuned bath sonicators may necessitate much longer irradiation and may thus cause degradation or denaturation of large macromolecules.

Most of the ether is removed by rotary evaporation under low vacuum (300–400 mm Hg), the pressure at which the sample bubbles in a controlled way. Pressure in the rotary evaporator is most conveniently regulated by means of a bleed valve attached to the evaporator's air inlet. In this laboratory, argon or nitrogen is vented into the rotary evaporator to reduce exposure of the lipids to air. A viscous gel forms when the bulk of the ether has evaporated. At this point, the sample tube is removed from the evaporator, vortexed briefly, and then returned to a higher vacuum (500–600 mm Hg). Vortex mixing promotes breakdown of the gel without resorting to high vacuum (>650 mm Hg). Stable gels may break down suddenly under high vacuum and eject the sample from the tube. The mixture may froth and bubble until the gel breaks and the slightly turbid vesicle suspension forms. During the frothing, the vacuum is regulated so that material is not lost from the sample tube. Residual ether can be removed in several minutes at high vacuum (700–750 mm Hg), but care must be taken to ensure that small-volume preparations do not evaporate. An additional volume of buffer may be added to the sample after the gel breaks (e.g. 0.3 ml) to prevent dehydration. At this point, encapsulation of the material is complete, and the preparation may be stable for months under an inert atmosphere at 4°C.

D. Separation of liposomes from free material

Although some applications may not require that free and liposome-entrapped material be separated, there are a number of reasons for doing so. Separation allows calculation of the efficiency of encapsulation, which is necessary when one is interested in maximizing delivery of the encapsulated material under specific conditions. Also, some methods of separation allow reclamation of the 50–65% of the material that is not encapsulated. There are many methods for separation of liposomes from unencapsulated material; only a few will be mentioned here. Gel chromatography is a common method, since large liposomes are excluded by most gels. Sepharose (2-B or 4-B) or BioGel (A1.5M) exclude LUV, but enzymatic digestion of unentrapped material is necessary with such large macromolecules as DNA fragments of >200000 Da. Disadvantages of column chromatography are degradation of unencapsulated material, sample dilution, difficulty in maintaining sterility, and lipid adsorption to polyacrylamide (F. J. Martin, unpublished observation, 1979) or agarose gels (Huang, 1969).

A large proportion of LUV will pellet if centrifuged at 120000 × *g* for 30 s. Therefore, differential centrifugation is a method of sterile separation that allows reclamation (Wilson *et al.*, 1977; Schäfer-Ridder *et al.*, 1982) of unentrapped material. However, good separation requires several washes, and 20–40% of the phospholipid may be lost in the supernatant.

Flotation of liposomes on discontinuous gradients is the most common separation method used in this laboratory (Fraley *et al.*, 1980; Heath *et al.*, 1981). By the flotation method, resolution of entrapped and free material is complete and rapid for all but low relative molecular mass solutes. The technique is adaptable to multiple samples, allows the maintenance of sterility and does not dilute the sample. For encapsulations in which some lipid loss is acceptable, both pelleting and flotation can be used in order to allow reclamation of unencapsulated material. A variety of gradient media are acceptable, including Metrizamide, Ficoll and dextran. The latter two are useful for negatively charged liposomes but can cause neutral vesicles to flocculate. Another disadvantage is that Ficoll and dextran precipitate in ethanol and are retained by most dialysis tubing, thus requiring dilution and centrifugation for reclamation of unentrapped molecules such as DNA. Metrizamide is useful with liposomes of most compositions and is dialysable, although it is more likely to enter liposomes in the presence of an osmotic gradient and thus hinder flotation.

The flotation method is detailed here; the first step, differential centrifugation, can be omitted if reclamation of the unencapsulated material is not desired. The sample is first diluted in the original encapsulation buffer and centrifuged once (20 min at 120000 × *g*, SW 50.1 Beckman rotor). The supernatant is removed and saved for reclamation of the unencapsulated material. The pellet is resuspended in a small volume of buffer (e.g. 0.5 ml).

The common gradient media used in this laboratory are: Dextran, 20% and 10% (average relative molecular mass 40000); or Ficoll, 25% and 10%; or Metrizamide, 10% and 5%. All percentages represent weight per volume of buffer. The gradient solutions usually are made in the original encapsulation buffer and are isotonic with the buffer in which the liposomes were prepared. Metrizamide undergoes reversible, concentration-dependent dimerization, so it is important to verify that the 10% solution becomes isotonic upon dilution with the volume of buffer in which the liposomes are suspended.

The liposome solution is diluted with buffer to a volume of 0.5 ml and mixed with 1.0 ml of the more concentrated gradient solution. These volumes and the volumes given below assume the centrifuge tube used it that for the SW 50.1 rotor, with capacity of 5.5 ml. Three ml of the less concentrated solution are overlaid, and 0.5 ml of encapsulation buffer forms the top gradient step. The gradient is centrifuged at 35000 rpm for 30 min, 20°C in the SW 50.1 rotor. If Metrizamide is used, the speed is increased to 45000 rpm, with no brake and minimal acceleration. After centrifugation, the liposomes can be pipetted from the buffer–polymer interface in a volume of 0.5 to 1.0 ml. A small quantity of the gradient medium may be included when the vesicle band is pipetted, but those mentioned here generally are regarded as non-toxic.

E. Liposome–cell incubation

The following is a general summary of the protocol for the incubation of liposomes with cells. It is used for both monolayer and suspension cultures; the only difference is that suspension cells are washed by low speed centrifugation. It is assumed that the composition of the liposomes includes acidic phospholipids.

Cells in growth medium are washed twice before liposome addition in order to remove serum and to assure that divalent cations are reduced to submillimolar concentrations. Calcium- and magnesium-free Tris- or phosphate-buffered saline commonly are used, with just enough divalent cations added to keep adherent cells attached to the substrate (usually 0.5 mM Ca^{2+} and 0.5 mM Mg^{2+}). Serum-free medium may be substituted for the buffers mentioned and may improve vesicle delivery by improving the metabolic state of the cells. If necessary, EDTA should be added to reduce the divalent cation concentration. If chloroquine is to be used, it is added to the cells 30–60 min before adding vesicles and is maintained in all buffers until the final post-liposome washes. Usually it is most convenient to add the drug to the original growth medium as a concentrated solution at physiological pH. Chloroquine is more toxic to some cells than to others, but most cell lines can tolerate a final concentration of 100 μM.

Liposomes are added to cells in a small volume in order to maximize cell–vesicle interaction; 200 μl may be sufficient for 5×10^6 cells. For most cells studied, the capacity for liposome uptake saturates at about 100 to 200 nmol (negatively charged) phospholipid per 1×10^6 cells, and there is likely to be little advantage to adding more material. In addition, high concentrations of liposomes (>500 μmol/ml), particularly those made with charged lipids, can be toxic to both animal and plant cells.

For negatively charged liposomes, the interaction relevant to nucleic acid delivery takes place in the first 30 min of incubation (Wilson *et al.*, 1979; Fraley *et al.*, 1982). Longer incubations may be undesirable because of effects on cellular metabolism. At the end of the incubation, cells are washed twice with drug-free medium or buffer and replated in the usual growth medium.

If polyethylene glycol or glycerol is to be used, it is added just before the post-incubation washes. The usual range of PEG concentrations that cells will tolerate is 25 to 50% (w/v) for 60 to 90 s, although toxicity is a dose- and time-dependent effect. There is no known advantage to PEG of any particular relative molecular mass or supplier, although PEG of 6000 Da or greater is difficult to wash away and may be toxic for that reason. For glycerol, the useful range of concentrations is 15 to 35% (v/v, buffer or medium) for 4 min or more. The effectiveness and the toxicity of glycerol both increase with the concentration and the length of exposure. At the end of the period of exposure, the glycerol (or polyethylene glycol) is diluted slowly, and cells are washed three times with medium or buffer before return to the normal growth medium.

F. Preparation of pH-sensitive liposomes

We present here the procedure for making pH-sensitive liposomes of oleic acid and phosphatidylethanolamine. As the procedure continues to evolve, a number of parameters are expected to change, including liposome composition, preparation and the incubation conditions used with cells. Nonetheless, the procedure is likely to be of considerable use as presented here.

A thin film of lipid is deposited onto the wall of a glass screw cap tube by rotary evaporation of a chloroform solution at 30°C. Ten μmol total lipid is used in a typical preparation. One-half ml of the aqueous solution to be encapsulated is added to the lipid at 30°C. The lipid is allowed to hydrate under argon for 20 min and then vortexed vigorously for 20 min. The multilamellar liposomes thus formed are incubated at 30°C for an additional 30 min, extruded through polycarbonate membranes (pore diameter 0.2 μm; Olson *et al.*, 1979), and vortexed briefly. Extrusion limits the maximum diameter of the liposome population produced and tends to produce uni- and oligolamellar liposomes (Olson *et al.*, 1979; Düzgüneş *et al.*, 1983b). Liposomes are separated from free material as described above.

G. Incubation of pH-sensitive liposomes with cells

Cells are washed twice with PBS supplemented with Ca^{2+} and Mg^{2+} as above. Liposomes are diluted in PBS-CM to 500 μM and a volume of 0.2 ml was added to each dish of cells. Cells are allowed to adsorb liposomes at room temperature for 10 min and then at 37°C in a humidified incubator for an additional 20 min. Cell monolayers can be exposed afterward to pre-warmed 21% (v/v PBS-CM) glycerol (Aldrich; spectrophotometric grade) for 5 min at 37°C. Subsequently, cells are washed twice with buffer, and either returned to the growth medium or analysed for delivery of the encapsulated probe.

A convenient fluorescent probe for verifying delivery is calcein, obtained from the Alfa Division of Ventron Corp., Danvers, MA. A relatively simple purification procedure is described in Straubinger *et al.* (1983b). The dye is adjusted to pH 7.6 and 300 mosmol/kg (or isotonic with the buffer in which incubation with cells takes place), and has a final concentration of roughly 60 mM, assuming a millimolar extinction coefficient of 72 at 490 nm. After exposure of cells to pH-sensitive liposomes, the cells are examined under a fluorescence microscope for diffuse, intracellular fluorescence.

VI. CONCLUSIONS

We have reviewed in detail two methods for making liposomes, as well as some of the considerations important in liposome preparation. The first method, the REV procedure, produces relatively large liposomes that capture a variety of solutes with high efficiency. Liposomes made by this procedure have been used to deliver molecules to cells in a number of studies, and many aspects of liposome–cell interaction have been examined. Thus, parameters governing the efficiency of delivery of biologically active molecules have been optimized in a number of systems.

The second method, which produces pH-sensitive liposomes, is less well characterized, but is included because of the promise it holds for high efficiency cytoplasmic delivery of large and membrane-impermeant molecules. Current work in this laboratory is directed toward improving the efficiency of solute capture during liposome preparation, as well as understanding the mechanism by which the aqueous contents of the pH-sensitive liposomes are delivered to the cytoplasm. Workers in several other laboratories are also examining various aspects of pH-dependent membrane fusion, and it is expected that the growing interest in this area will provide the basis for future development of a high efficiency intracellular delivery system.

REFERENCES

Allen, T. M., McAllister, L., Mausolf, S. and Gyoffry, E. (1981). *Biochim. Biophys. Acta* **643**, 346.

Bangham, A. D. (1983). *In* "Liposomes" (M. J. Ostro, ed.) p. 1. Marcel Dekker, New York.

Bangham, A. D. and Horne, R. W. (1964). *J. Mol. Biol.* **8**, 660.

Bangham, A. D., Standish, M. and Watkins, J. (1964). *J. Mol. Biol.* **13**, 238.

Bartlett, G. (1959). *J. Biol. Chem.* **234**, 466.

Connor, J., Yatvin, M. B. and Huang, L. (1984). *Proc. Natl. Acad. Sci. USA* **81**, 1715.

Dahl, G., Azarnia, R. and Werner, R. (1981). *Nature* **289**, 683.

Deamer, D. and Bangham, A. (1976). *Biochim. Biophys. Acta* **443**, 629.

Deamer, D. and Uster, P. (1980). *In* "Introduction of Macromolecules into Viable Mammalian Cells" (R. Baserga, C. Croce and G. Roueza, eds) p. 205. Alan Liss, New York.

DeDuve, C., de Barsy, T., Poole, B., Trouet, A., Tulkens, P. and van Hoof, F. (1974). *Biochem. Pharmacol.* **23**, 2495.

Düzgüneş, N., Wilschut, J., Fraley, R. and Papahadjopoulos, D. (1981). *Biochim. Biophys. Acta* **642**, 182

Düzgüneş, N., Straubinger, R. M. and Papahadjopoulos, D. (1983a). *J. Cell Biol.* **97**, 178a.

Düzgüneş, N., Wilschut, J., Hong, K., Fraley, R., Perry, C., Friend, D. S., James, T. L. and Papahadjopoulos, D. (1983b). *Biochim. Biophys. Acta* **732**, 289.

Düzgüneş, N., Straubinger, R., Baldwin, P. and Papahadjopoulos, D. (1985). *Biochemistry* **24**, 3091.

Ellens, H., Bentz, J. and Szoka, F. C. (1984). *Biochemistry* **23**, 1532.

Enoch, H. and Strittmatter, P. (1979). *Proc. Natl. Acad. Sci. USA* **76**, 145.

Finkelstein, M. and Weissmann, G. (1978). *J. Lipid Res.* **18**, 289.

Fraley, R., Fornari, C. S. and Kaplan, S. (1979). *Proc. Natl. Acad. Sci. USA* **76**, 3348.

Fraley, R., Subramani, S., Berg, P. and Papahadjopoulos, D. (1980). *J. Biol. Chem.* **255**, 10431.

Fraley, R., Straubinger, R. M., Rule, G., Springer, E. L. and Papahadjopoulos, D. (1981). *Biochemistry* **20**, 6978.

Fraley, R., Dellaporta, S. and Papahadjopoulos, D. (1982). *Proc. Natl. Acad. Sci. USA* **79**, 1859.

Fraley, R. and Papahadjopoulos, D. (1982). *In* "Current Topics in Microbiology and Immunology: Gene Cloning in Organisms Other Than *E. coli*" (P. H. Hofschneider and W. Goebel, eds) Vol. 96, p. 171. Springer-Verlag, Heidelberg.

Goldstein, J. L., Anderson, R. G. W. and Brown, M. S. (1979) *Nature* **279**, 679.

Gregoriadis, G. and Davis, C. (1979). *Biochem. Biophys. Res. Commun.* **89**, 1287.

Heath, T. D., Fraley, R. and Papahadjopoulos, D. (1980). *Science* **210**, 539.

Heath, T. D., Lopez, N. G. and Papahadjopoulos, D. (1985). *Biochim. Biophys. Acta* (in press).

Heath, T. D., Macher, B. A. and Papahadjopoulos, D. (1981). *Biochim. Biophys. Acta* **640**, 66.

Heath, T. D., Montgomery, J. A., Piper, J. R. and Papahadjopoulos, D. (1983). *Proc. Natl. Acad. Sci. USA* **80**, 1377.

Helenius, A., Kartenbeck, J., Simons, K. and Fries, E. (1980). *J. Cell Biol.* **84**, 404.

Hoffman, R., Margolis, P. and Bergelson, L. (1978). *FEBS Lett.* **93**, 365.
Huang, C. (1969). *Biochemistry* **8**, 344.
Huang, A. C., Huang, L. and Kennel, S. J. (1980). *J. Biol. Chem.* **255**, 8015
Kates, M. (1972). *In* "Laboratory Techniques in Biochemistry and Molecular Biology" (T. S. Work and E. Work, eds). North Holland, New York.
Kimelberg, H. K. and Mayhew, E. G. (1978). *CRC Crit. Rev. Toxicol.* **6**, 25.
Kolber, M. A. and Haynes, D. H. (1979). *J. Membrane Biol.* **48**, 95.
Leserman, L., Barbet, J., Kourilsky, R. and Weinstein, J. (1980). *Nature* **288**, 602.
Lurquin, P. (1979). *Nucl. Acid Res.* **6**, 3773.
Lurquin, P. (1981). *Nucl. Acid Res.* **12**, 3773.
Martin, F., Hubbel, W. and Papahadjopoulos, D. (1981). *Biochemistry* **20**, 4429.
Marzella, L., Ahlberg, J. and Glaumann, H. (1982). *J. Cell Biol.* **93**, 144.
Matthay, K. K., Heath, T. D. and Papahadjopoulos, D. (1984). *Cancer Res.* **44**, 1880.
Mayhew, E., Rustum, Y., Szoka, F. and Papahadjopoulos, D. (1979). *Cancer Treatment Rep.* **63**(11–12), 1923.
Miller, D. K. and Lenard, J. (1980). *J. Cell. Biol.* **84**, 430.
Miller, D. K. and Lenard, J. (1981). *Proc. Natl. Acad. Sci. USA* **78**, 3605.
Nicolau, C., Le Pape, A., Soriano, P., Fargette, F. and Juhel, M. F. (1983). *Proc. Natl. Acad. Sci. USA* **80**, 1068.
Norberg, B. (1970). *Exp. Cell Res.* **59**, 11.
Ohkuma, S. and Poole, B. (1978). *Proc. Natl. Acad. Sci. USA* **75**, 3327.
Olson, F., Hunt, C. A., Vail, W. and Papahadjopoulos, D. (1979). *Biochim. Biophys. Acta* **557**, 9.
Ostro, M. J., Giacomoni, D. and Dray, S. (1977). *Biochem. Biophys. Res. Commun.* **76**, 836.
Pagano, R. E. and Weinstein, J. N. (1978). *Ann. Rev. Biophys. Bioeng.* **7**, 435.
Papahadjopoulos, D. (1968). *Biochim. Biophys. Acta* **163**, 240.
Papahadjopoulos, D. and Kimelberg, H. (1973). *In* "Progress in Surface Science" (S. G. Davidson, ed.) Vol. 4, pp. 141–232. Pergamon Press, New York.
Papahadjopoulos, D. and Miller, W. (1967). *Biochim. Biophys. Acta* **135**, 624.
Papahadjopoulos, D. and Vail, W. J. (1978). *Ann NY Acad. Sci.* **308**, 259.
Papahadjopoulos, D. and Watkins, J. C. (1967). *Biochim. Biophys. Acta* **135**, 639.
Papahadjopoulos, D., Nir, S. and Ohki, S. (1972). *Biochim. Biophys. Acta* **266**, 561.
Papahadjopoulos, D., Jacobson, K., Nir, S. and Isac, T. (1973). *Biochim. Biophys. Acta* **311**, 340.
Papahadjopoulos, D., Vail, W., Jacobson, K. and Poste, G. (1975). *Biochim. Biophys. Acta* **394**, 483.
Papahadjopoulos, D., Vail, W., Pangborn, W. and Poste, G. (1976). *Biochim. Biophys. Acta* **448**, 265.
Papahadjopoulos, D., Wilson, T. and Taber, R. (1980). *In Vitro* **16**, 49.
Papahadjopoulos, D., Fraley, R., Heath, R. and Straubinger, R. M. (1981). *In* "Techniques in Cellular Physiology" (P. F. Baker, ed.) p. 1. Elsevier North Holland, New York.
Pastan, I. H. and Willingham, M. C. (1981). *Ann. Rev. Physiol.* **43**, 239.
Poste, G. (1980). *In* "Liposomes in Biological Systems" (G. Gregoriadis and A. Alison, eds) p. 101. John Wiley, New York.
Schäfer-Ridder, M., Wang, Y. and Hofschneider, P. H. (1982). *Science* **215**, 166.
Stacey, D. W. and Allfrey, V. G. (1977). *J. Cell Biol.* **75**, 807.
Straubinger, R. and Papahadjopoulos, D. (1983). *Methods Enzymol.* **101**, 512.

Straubinger, R. M., Düzgüneş, N. and Papahadjopoulos, D. (1983a). *J. Cell Biol.* **97**, 109a.

Straubinger, R. M., Hong, K., Friend, D. S. and Papahadjopoulos, D. (1983b). *Cell* **32**, 1069.

Straubinger, R. M., Düzgüneş, N. and Papahadjopoulos, D. (1985). *FEBS Lett.* **179**, 148.

Struck, D. K., Hoekstra, D. and Pagano, R. E. (1981). *Biochemistry* **20**, 4093.

Szoka, F. and Papahadjopoulos, D. (1978). *Proc. Natl. Acad. Sci. USA* **75**, 145.

Szoka, F. and Papahadjopoulos, D. (1980). *Ann. Rev. Biophys. Bioeng.* **9**, 467.

Szoka, F., Jacobson, K. and Papahadjopoulos, D. (1979). *Biochim. Biophys. Acta* **551**, 295.

Szoka, F. C., Jacobson, K., Derzko, Z. and Papahadjopoulos, D. (1980). *Biochim. Biophys. Acta* **600**, 1.

Truneh, A., Mishal, Z., Barbet, J., Machy, P. and Leserman, L. D. (1983). *Biochem. J.* **214**, 189.

Tycko, B. and Maxfield, F. R. (1980). *Cell* **28**, 643.

Tyrrell, D., Heath, T., Colley, C. and Ryman, B. (1976). *Biochim. Biophys. Acta* **457**, 259.

Uster, P. and Deamer, D. (1985). *Biochemistry* **24**, 1.

Van Renswoude, J. and Hoekstra, D. (1981). *Biochemistry* **20**, 540.

von Tscharner, V. and Radda, G. K. (1981). *Biochim. Biophys. Acta* **643**, 435.

White, J., Matlin, K. and Helenius, A. (1981). *J. Cell Biol.* **89**, 674.

White, J., Kielian, M. and Helenius, A. (1983). *Q. Rev. Biophys.* **16**, 151.

Wilson, T., Papahadjopoulos, D. and Taber, R. (1977). *Proc. Natl. Acad. Sci. USA* **74**, 3471.

Wilson, T., Papahadjopoulos, D. and Taber, R. (1979). *Cell* **17**, 77.

Wong, T.-K., Nicolau, C. and Hofschneider, P. (1980). *Gene* **10**, 87.

Yatvin, M. B., Kreutz, W., Horwitz, B. A. and Shinitzky, M. (1980). *Science* **210**, 1253.

8

Liposomes in Drug Targeting

G. Gregoriadis, J. Senior and B. Wolff

I. INTRODUCTION

Specific interaction of liposomes with cells *in vitro* via antibodies and other receptor recognizing molecules on the liposomal surface, has been demonstrated repeatedly (Toonen and Crommelin, 1983) since initial reports on liposome targeting were published (Gregoriadis, 1974; Gregoriadis and Neerunjun, 1975). It is now established that binding of targeted liposomes to cells can lead to the interiorization of the carrier and its drug contents and eventual drug action (Toonen and Crommelin, 1983). In this way a variety of drugs, including genetic material, can be introduced selectively into the cell's interior (see also Chapter 9). Furthermore, techniques are now being developed by which entry of liposomal contents will favour a given intracellular compartment (Connor *et al.*, 1984; see also Chapter 7). This is of particular importance in the introduction of genetic material into specific cells where the lysosomal apparatus must probably be avoided. Nonetheless, in the few experiments suggesting gene expression *in vitro* with gene-containing liposomes (see Chapter 9), the latter were conventional vesicles (i.e. non-targeted) and expected to be phagocytosed. Although there has been a considerable amount of work with targeted liposomes in cell culture (Toonen and Crommelin, 1983), information on liposome targeting *in vivo* and conditions favouring it is scarce.

It is well established (Ryman and Tyrrell, 1980; Gregoriadis, 1981) that following intravenous injection, liposomes and entrapped drugs are taken up mostly by the fixed macrophages of the reticuloendothelial system (RES). Extent and rate of uptake by particular tissues of the RES depend on the size, surface charge and lipid composition of the vesicles, amount of lipid given, animal species injected and physiological state. For instance, a large vesicle size and/or a negative surface charge will promote rapid uptake by tissues. Also, depending on the lipid composition of liposomes, plasma high

Microinjection and Organelle Transplantation Techniques

ISBN: 0-12-164722-6
ISBN: 0-12-164723-4 Pbk

density lipoproteins (HDL) can remove phospholipid molecules and destabilize vesicle structure with entrapped drug being released into the circulation. Thus, tissues will take up vesicles in various stages of destabilization and with a portion of their drug content lost. Hepatic parenchymal cells are the only other cell type which liposomes can reach to a significant extent. However, vesicle size must be small enough to allow passage through the fenestrations.

Targeting of liposomes to accessible alternative cells *in vivo* require that a number of conditions must be satisfied. Among these, the following appear especially important: liposomes must (a) be endowed with target selectivity by means of ligands attached on their surface and capable of binding to respective receptors on target cells; (b) retain quantitatively both targeting ligand and entrapped drug *en route* to their destination; and (c) avoid interception by the RES for periods of time long enough to enable vesicles to seek and interact with their target efficiently. Recent work in this laboratory (Kirby and Gregoriadis, 1980; Senior and Gregoriadis, 1982a, b; Gregoriadis, 1983; Wolff and Gregoriadis, 1984) suggest that such liposomal properties are attainable and operative *in vivo*.

II. DRUG RETENTION BY LIPOSOMES IN THE PRESENCE OF BLOOD

The problem of massive drug loss from liposomes upon exposure to blood, encountered in the early days of liposome research, has now been resolved (at least for polar drugs) and will be considered here first since it applies to liposomes regardless of whether or not they bear receptor-recognizing ligands. Appreciation (Krupp *et al.*, 1976; Scherphof *et al.*, 1978; Kirby *et al.*, 1980a, b; Allen, 1981) of the role of plasma HDL in vesicle destabilization, helped to reason (Gregoriadis and Davis, 1979; Kirby *et al.*, 1980b; Senior and Gregoriadis, 1982a) that packing of the liposomal bilayer with excess cholesterol and/or the inclusion of phospholipids with a high liquid-crystalline transition temperature (T_c), may prevent the removal of phospholipids by HDL. We were thus able to show (Gregoriadis, and Senior, 1980; Senior and Gregoriadis, 1982a, b) that cholesterol equimolar to total phospholipid, prevents solute loss in the presence of blood, plasma or serum to an extent dependent on the nature of the phospholipid used. A striking example of this is shown in Fig. 1. where an increasing proportion of sphingomyelin (SM) relative to egg phosphatidylcholine (PC) in cholesterol-rich liposomes is paralleled by increasing solute retention. Retention in the presence of blood plasma at 37°C reached 100% when at least 77% of the total phospholipid was SM. Even more stable liposomes (100% solute retention for at least 48

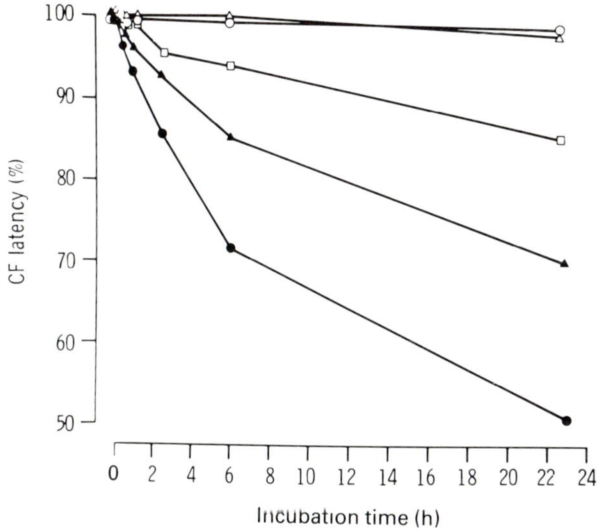

Fig. 1. The effect of phospholipid composition of liposomes on their permeability in plasma. Small unilamellar liposomes containing quenched CF and composed of: SM (○); 77% SM, 23% PC (△); 47% SM, 53% PC (□); 23% SM, 77% PC (▲); and PC (●) were incubated in the presence of mouse plasma at 37°C. All liposomal preparations contained cholesterol, equimolar to total phospholipid. CF latency values are percentage of total CF present (from Senior and Gregoriadis, 1982b).

h) are obtained with equimolar distearoyl phosphatidylcholine (DSPC) and cholesterol (Senior and Gregoriadis, 1982b).

Using liposomes containing radiolabelled phospholipids (Kirby *et al.*, 1980a, b; Kirby and Gregoriadis, 1980; Senior *et al.*, 1983) it was shown that such manipulations of lipid composition do indeed reduce or abolish altogether loss of phospholipid to HDL in the presence of plasma. Thus, increasing presence of SM in small unilamellar liposomes (which, as discussed already, parallels increasing solute retention; Fig. 1) is associated with decreasing elution of the radiolabelled lipid together with HDL (Gregoriadis, *et al.*, 1985). Additional support for this role of HDL in removing phospholipids has come from work in which cholesterol-free PC liposomes were exposed to plasma from lipoprotein-deficient mice. There was virtually no transfer of ^{3}H-PC to the HDL (Senior *et al.*, 1983). Furthermore, when purified HDL, low and intermediate density (LDL + IDL) or very low density (VLDL) mouse lipoproteins were added to lipoprotein-deficient mouse plasma in increasing quantities to cover physiological levels of the lipoproteins, only HDL had a destabilizing effect on liposomes (Senior *et al.*, 1983).

It should be noted here that although polar solutes (Kirby and Gregoriadis, 1981; Wolff and Gregoriadis, 1984) are retained quantitatively by cholesterol-rich liposomes in the presence of plasma, other solutes of lipophilic nature do not behave similarly (Kirby and Gregoriadis, 1983). Although the presence of cholesterol and the correct choice of phospholipid influence lipophilic solute retention, the effect is less pronounced.

III. DRUG RETENTION BY CIRCULATING LIPOSOMES AND LIPOSOME CLEARANCE

Liposomes retaining their drug contents quantitatively in the presence of plasma *in vitro* at 37°C, also do so in the bloodstream after injection (Kirby *et al.*, 1980b; Kirby and Gregoriadis, 1980, 1983; Senior and Gregoriadis, 1982a, b). Clearance of liposomes in intact form has been followed by the measurement in blood of both radioactive lipid label and entrapped solute and also by the monitoring of lipid label transfer to HDL. For very stable liposomes the two markers are cleared from the circulation at the same rate and there is virtually no transfer of phospholipid to HDL (Senior and Gregoriadis, 1982a). Another indication that liposomes retain their structural integrity in the blood is the persistence of highly quenched carboxyfluorescein (CF) in blood samples taken at time intervals after injection of quenched CF-containing liposomes (Gregoriadis and Senior, 1980; Senior and Gregoriadis, 1982a, b): leaking of CF from destabilized liposomes would have led to its dilution in the plasma and fluorescence.

A direct relationship between solute retention by liposomes in the presence of blood and the rate of vesicle clearance from the circulation was observed recently (Senior and Gregoriadis, 1982b). This is demonstrated in Fig. 2 where clearance rates of five preparations of small unilamellar liposomes (SUV), shown to be increasingly stable in plasma at 37°C (see Fig. 1), show increasingly longer half-lives after intravenous injection, ranging from about 2 h for PC cholesterol-rich liposomes to about 11 h for cholesterol-rich SM liposomes. A similar relationship was observed (Senior and Gregoriadis, 1982b) in the case of two preparations of distearoyl phosphatidylcholine, one without and the other with (equimolar) cholesterol (Fig. 3). In the latter case half-life after intravenous injection was 20 h. It has been claimed (Patel *et al.*, 1984) that the slower clearance of cholesterol-rich liposomes is due to the inhibition (by cholesterol) of liposome uptake by the liver. This, however, is not supported by observations made with a number of cholesterol-rich preparations of differing phospholipid composition (1:1 phospholipid:cholesterol molar ratio) exhibiting a wide range of half-lives of 0.1 h to 20 h (Gregoriadis and Senior, 1980;

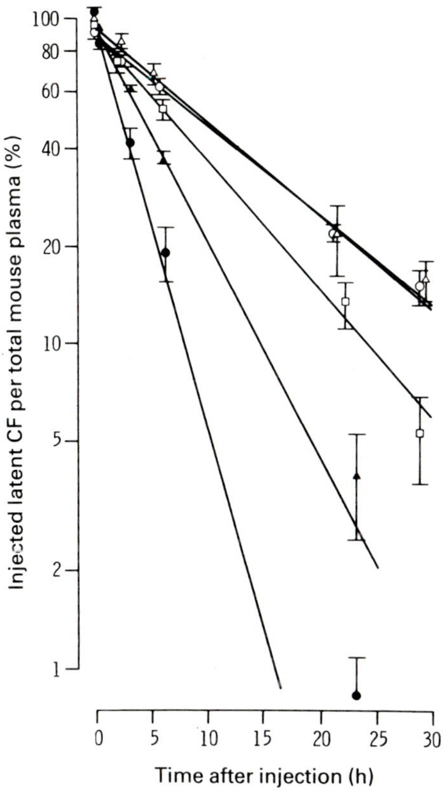

Fig. 2. The effect of phospholipid composition of liposomes on their clearance from the circulation. Liposomes composed as described in Fig. 1 were injected intravenously into mice. Latent CF values (mean ± s.d.; 3–6 mice) are percentage of injected latent CF per total mouse plasma. Symbols as in Fig. 1 (from Senior and Gregoriadis, 1982b).

Senior and Gregoriadis, 1982a, b; Hwang *et al.*, 1980; see also Fig. 2). A more likely explanation for the direct relationship between vesicle clearance rate and vesicle permeability in the presence of plasma may be that the greater the vesicle permeability is the less packed the bilayers are and the easier for plasma proteins (such as opsonins) implicated in the elimination of foreign matter from the circulation to adsorb onto or insert themselves into the vesicles, and so to render the latter recognizable by the RES.

A longer half-life, however, does not seem to facilitate escape of liposomes from the RES to any significant extent. Nor does the prolonged presence of such liposomes in the circulation lead to their interaction with intravascular tissues or escape into the vascular compartment. Our recent

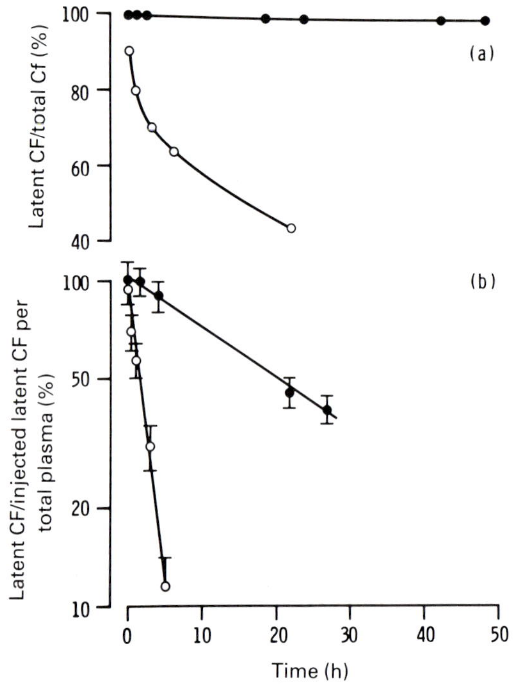

Fig. 3. Stability of DSPC-liposomes in mouse plasma and clearance from the circulation. Small unilamellar liposomes containing quenched CF and composed of DSPC (○) or equimolar DSPC and cholesterol (●) were (a) incubated in the presence of mouse plasma at 37°C or (b) injected intravenously into four mice. Values are percentage of latent CF of total CF present or percentage (mean ± s.d.) of latent CF of injected latent CF per total mouse plasma (from Senior and Gregoriadis, 1982b).

work (Senior *et al.*, 1985) in which the fate of very stable (e.g. Fig. 4) ^{111}In-bleomycin-containing small unilamellar liposomes of varying half-lives in intravenously injected mice or rats was followed for up to 72 h, shows that whilst uptake by the hepatic and splenic moieties of the RES is diminished, much of the remainder of the dose eventually accumulates in the bones, presumably the bone marrow (Figs 5 and 6).

It would appear, therefore, that in choosing liposomes which can exhibit long half-lives, one must look for preparations capable of quantitatively retaining entrapped solutes in the presence of plasma. Unfortunately, however, half-lives achieved for larger liposomes, even for the most stable vesicles (Table I, showing stability), are only modestly long (about 60 and 20 min for liposomes of about 0.2 and 0.4 m diameter, respectively; Senior *et al.*, 1985). We are at present investigating ways by which such short half-lives of large liposomes could be improved upon. These include modifi-

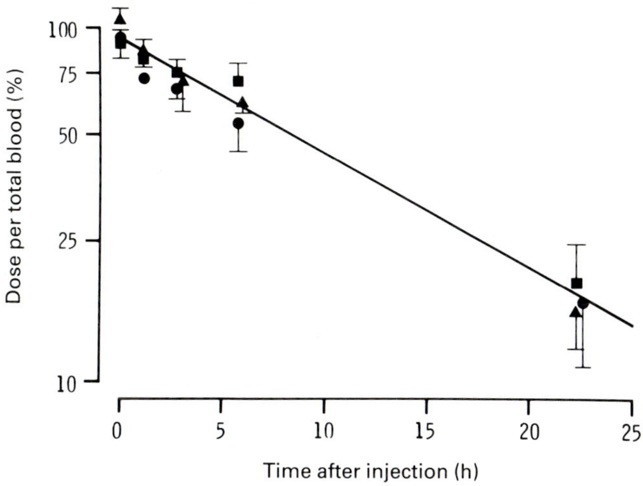

Fig. 4. Clearance of cholesterol-rich DSPC liposomes from the circulation. Mice (five animals) were injected intravenously with 0.2 ml SUV composed of equimolar DSPC and cholesterol (43.4 mg phospholipid per kg body weight). Liposomes contained 0.2 M carboxyfluorescein and tracer ^{111}In-bleomycin (5.2 × 10^4 cpm) in the aqueous phase and tracer [^{14}C]DSPC (9 × 10^4 cpm) in the lipid phase. Values are percentage ± s.d. of administered quenched carboxyfluorescein or radioactivity per total blood at time intervals after injection (from Senior *et al.*, 1985).

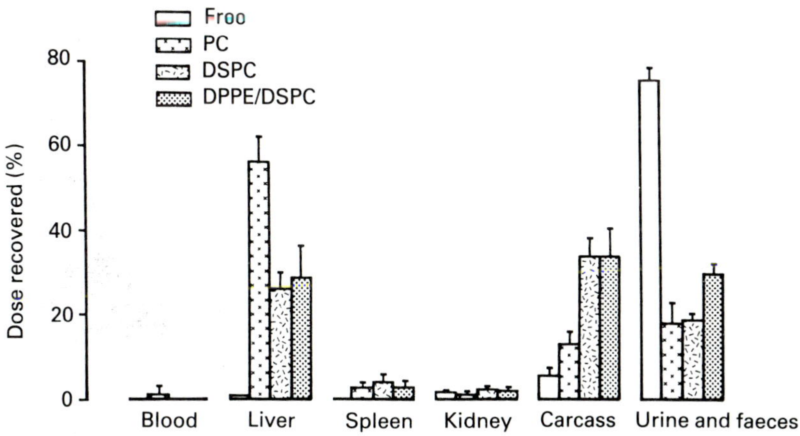

Fig. 5. Tissue distribution of cholesterol-rich liposomes after intravenous injection. Mice in groups of six were injected with 0.2 ml ^{111}In-bleomycin, free (4 × 10^4 cpm) or entrapped (1.7–13.8 × 10^4 cpm) in SUV composed to equimolar PC and cholesterol (25.0 mg phospholipid per kg body weight), equimolar DSPC and cholesterol (27.2 mg phospholipid per kg body weight) or DSPC, DPPE and cholesterol (25.4 mg phospholipid per kg body weight, 0.8:0.2:1, molar ratios). At 26 h (free and PC SUV) or 72 h (other SUV) after injection, animals were killed, and radioactivity was measured in blood, liver, spleen, kidney, the carcass and urine and faeces. Values are percentage of dose per total blood, total tissues, or collected 26–72 h urine and faeces (from Senior *et al.*, 1985).

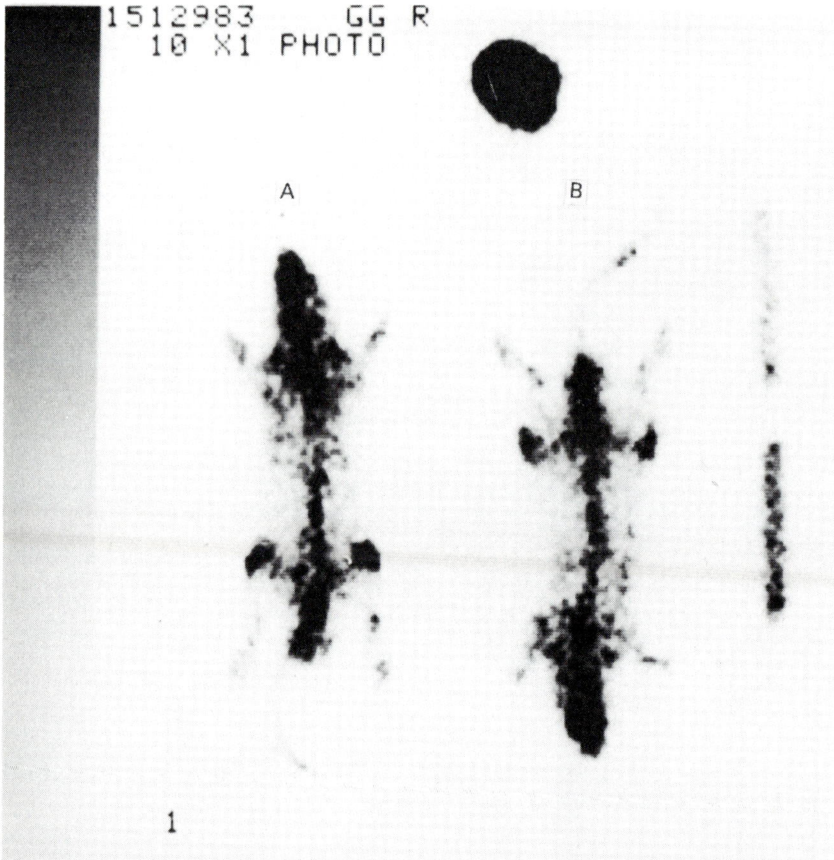

Fig. 6. Scans of the carcass of rats injected with 1.0 ml radiolabelled cholesterol-rich SUV. Two rats (A, 188 g; B, 207 g body weight) were injected intravenously with SUV (10 mg phospholipid) composed of equimolar DSPC and cholesterol and containing ^{111}In-bleomycin (5.3×10^6 cpm). At 72 h after injection, the rats were killed and scanned after the removal of all tissues including the stomach and large and small intestines. Radioactivity distribution (percentage of total in the carcass) in the bones of various areas in the two rats (A and B) was as follows: head, 14.5 and 13.9; thorax, 23.2 and 26.8; top of legs and pelvis, 28.9 and 29.6; tail, 4.3 and 2.8. Radioactivity (percentage of dose for each animal) in total blood was 3.2 (A) and 1.2 (B), and in skeletal muscle 0.1 and 0.1 per g tissue. Carcass radioactivity was 25.1% (A) and 26.1% (B) of the injected dose. Rats are placed in the figure with head (A) and tail (B) at the top (from Senior *et al.*, 1985).

Table I. Retention of solutes by liposomes in the presence of plasma.

Liposomes	^{111}In retention (%)	CF retention (%)
SUV		
PC, Chol	92.6 (2 h)	
	51.2 (24 h)	
DSPC, Chol	99.5 (24 h)	100.0 (24 h)
DSPC, DPPE, Chol	97.4 (24 h)	
REV		
PC, Chol		90.5 (10 min)
		46.6 (24 h)
DSPC, Chol		98.5 (24 h)

SUV or REV (passed through a nucleopore filter of 0.4 μm pore diameter) composed of equimolar total phospholipid and cholesterol (Chol) and containing ^{111}In-bleomycin or 0.2 M carboxyfluorescein (CF) were incubated in the presence of 5 volumes of mouse plasma at 37°C. At time intervals (shown in parentheses) samples were chromatographed. Values denote solute recovered with the eluted liposome fractions and is expressed as percentage of that recovered (from Senior *et al.*, 1985).

cation of the liposomal surface with agents which would render it more hydrophilic, a state which apparently (van Oss *et al.*, 1974) discourages opsonin adsorption. Prolongation of the circulation time of large liposomes would be a considerable achievement towards their use in drug targeting *in vivo*. Because of their size, large liposomes can carry much more drug per lipid unit weight and are, in addition, easier to prepare. Indeed, in a recent simple method developed in this laboratory (Kirby and Gregoriadis, 1984a,b,c), liposomes are prepared under mild conditions in the absence of organic solvents, sonication or detergent and entrap drugs, proteins or nucleic acids in amounts of up to 60–70% of the original materials. Such liposomes, named dehydration–rehydration vesicles (DRV) because of the dehydration and rehydration steps in their formation, are obviously suitable for the rapid delivery of drugs, including genetic material, to the macrophages of the RES but would also be ideal for targeting to alternative tissues if ways could be found to delay their rapid clearance from the circulation.

IV. TARGETING OF LIPOSOMES

Liposomes composed of equimolar DSPC and cholesterol combine both great stability in plasma and prolonged survival in the circulation and thus qualify as a highly appropriate preparation for drug targeting within the vascular system. Preparation of targeted liposomes, however, requires their association with molecules such as antibodies and glycoproteins which are expected to mediate vesicle binding to respective antigens and receptors on the surface of target cells (Gregoriadis, 1981; Toonen and Crommelin, 1983).

Initial attempts to target liposomes (Gregoriadis, 1974; Gregoriadis and Neerunjun, 1975) were made with preparations sonicated in the presence of protein which ended up partially exposed on the vesicle's surface. Amino groups of the protein and of the targeting molecule, in this instance asialofetuin which binds selectively to the galactose receptors in the liver (Morell *et al.*, 1971), were coupled via gluteraldehyde (Gregoriadis, 1974). Alternatively, liposomes were sonicated in the presence of anti-target cell IgG which again appeared partially on the vesicle's surface. Such antibody-bearing liposomes were shown to interact selectively with a variety of cell targets (Gregoriadis and Neerunjun, 1975; Gregoriadis *et al.*, 1977).

The same procedure was applied later (Gregoriadis *et al.*, 1981) in the preparation of (affinity chromatography-purified) antibody-bearing small unilamellar liposomes. In an alternative procedure, antibody against IgG was incorporated into liposomes as above and then interacted with anti-target purified IgG, which retained its ability to interact with the target (Gregoriadis *et al.*, 1981). These latter studies demonstrated that antibody-bearing liposomes can interact extensively and selectively with circulating antigens in the blood *in vivo* after intravenous injection (Gregoriadis *et al.*, 1981). Further *in vitro* work with lymphocytes coated with antigen via $CrCl_3$ and exposed to liposomes bearing the respective purified antibody revealed the significance of antibody and antigen concentrations on the liposomal and cellular surfaces respectively (Gregoriadis and Meehan, 1981).

We have recently attempted to target liposomes by coupling targeting macromolecules on the liposomal surface via a heterobifunctional reagent (Gregoriadis and Senior, 1984; Wolff *et al.*, 1984). Liposomes used were composed of DSPC, cholesterol and dipalmitoyl phosphatidylethanolamine (DPPE), which provides the amino groups needed for coupling. We established (Gregoriadis *et al.*, 1985) that the presence of up to 50% DPPE (of total phospholipid) in the liposome structure did not alter liposomal stability significantly upon incubation at 37°C in plasma for at least 50 h. Maintenance of stability in the presence of plasma was also observed when the DPPE component of liposomes was modified with the heterobifunctional reagent *N*-succinimidyl 3-(2-pyridyldithio) propionate (SPDP) to give PDP-DPPE. However, when liposomal PDP-DPPE was coupled to the targeting ligand, stability (in plasma) in terms of entrapped solute and targeting ligand retention by the carrier was reduced, albeit modestly (see below).

A. Targeting of liposomes to the galactose receptor *in vivo*

Specific interaction of liposomes with cells *in vivo* was first demonstrated by using multilamellar liposomes with asialofetuin adsorbed on their surface (Gregoriadis and Neerunjun, 1975). More recent studies have been carried out with small unilamellar liposomes incorporating lactosylceramide (Szoka and Mayhew, 1983; Spanjer and Scherphof, 1983) or asialoorosomucoid (Gregoriadis and Senior, 1984). Small liposomes were chosen because of previous findings (Ashwell and Morell, 1974) that the galactose receptor is located on the surface of the hepatic parenchymal cells, access to which (through the fenestrae) is possible only for vesicles with a diameter smaller than about 100 nm. It has been recently claimed (Teradaira *et al.*, 1983) that the galactose receptor also exists on the surface of the Kupffer cells and that this receptor binds galactose-terminating molecules in both the particulate and free forms. Therefore, for these cells large liposomes would also be suitable.

Liposomes (small unilamellar) composed of DSPC, cholesterol and DPPE modified with SPDP to give PDP-DPPE (1:1:0.15 molar ratios) contained 0.2 M (quenched) CF and tracer ^{111}In-labelled bleomycin. These liposomes were subsequently interacted with SPDP-modified ^{125}I-labelled orosomucoid (Gregoriadis and Senior, 1984). The preparation was divided into two parts, one part being desialylated so as to expose the penultimate galactose residues of the protein. The two liposomal preparations, bearing orosomucoid and asialoorosomucoid, were then used for *in vivo* work. Mice were injected intravenously with orosomucoid-bearing liposomes, asialoorosomucoid-bearing liposomes or with free asialoorosomucoid followed by asialoorosomucoid-bearing liposomes.

Clearance rates of both markers (latent CF and ^{111}In) for orosomucoid liposomes from the circulation were almost identical, exhibiting a half-life of about 4.5–5 h (Fig. 7). This half-life is less than that expected from cholesterol-rich DSPC liposomes injected at a similar dose of 0.8 mg lipid per mouse (Senior *et al.*, 1985) and is likely to reflect the chemical modification of their surface after coupling with orosomucoid via SPDP. Following injection of the desialylated preparation, half-life was reduced to less than 30 min, presumably because of rapid binding of the vesicles to the galactose receptor. Confirmation of such selective binding came from patterns of clearance obtained by administering free asialoorosomucoid which competes for binding sites with asialoorosomucoid-bearing liposomes given later on: rates of clearance for both markers returned to those originally seen with orosomucoid liposomes (Fig. 7). The use of free intact orosomucoid in a similar competition experiment did not have the same effect.

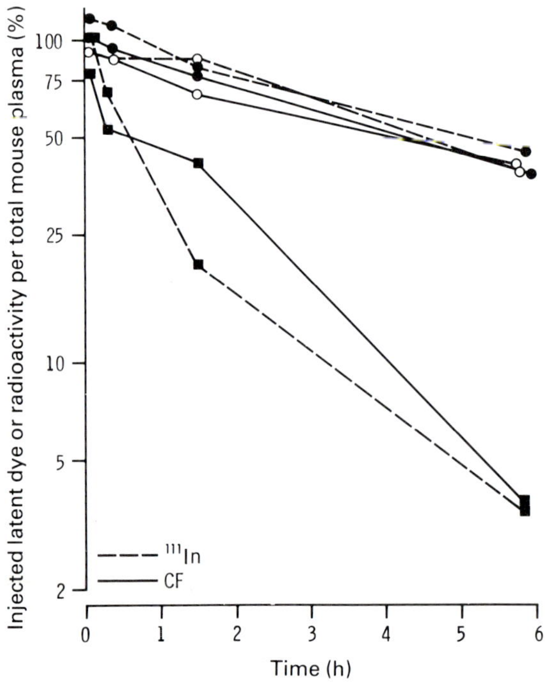

Fig. 7. Plasma clearance of asialoorosomucoid liposomes. Mice in groups of four were injected intravenously with orosomucoid liposomes (●), asialoorosomucoid liposomes (■) or 4 mg of free asialoorosomucoid followed 12 min later with asialoorosomucoid liposomes (○). Values (at time intervals after injection) of latent CF (continuous lines) and ^{111}In (broken lines) are percentage of injected latent dye or radioactivity per total mouse plasma (from Gregoriadis and Senior, 1984).

On the basis of ^{111}In level in the tissues at 6 h post-injection (Fig. 8), 68% of the injected asialoorosomucoid-bearing liposomes was recovered in the liver. Hepatic uptake of ^{111}In from orosomucoid liposomes was 29% of the dose at 6 h, with the difference (39%) between the two values assumed as the minimum proportion of the dose interacted with the galactose receptor. Unexpectedly, however, in the competition experiment where excess free asialoorosomucoid was given prior to asialoorosomucoid-bearing liposomes (Fig. 7), hepatic values did not return to the "normal" level of 29% but, instead, diminished further to 15% (Fig. 8). It is therefore conceivable that the difference (53%) between the values of hepatic uptake of asialoorosomucoid liposomes given in the absence and presence of free asialoorosomucoid represents more truly the extent of binding of liposomes to the galactose receptor. This is because asialoorosomucoid liposomes may not be intercepted by the RES as readily as orosomucoid liposomes.

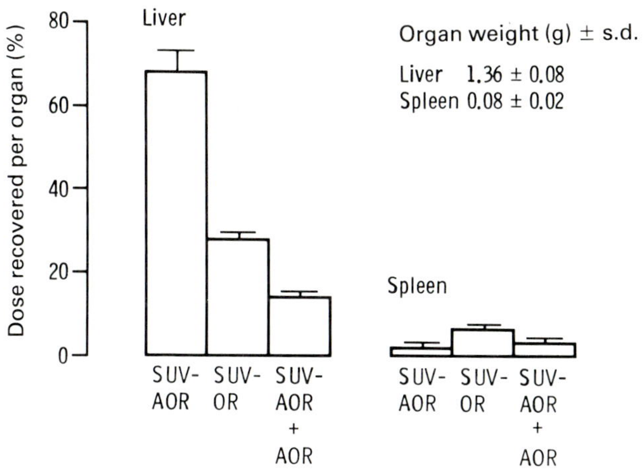

Fig. 8. Uptake of asialoorosomucoid liposomes by tissues. Mice from experiments described in Fig. 7 were killed 6 h post-injection and ^{111}In-radioactivity measured in the liver and spleen. SUV-AOR, mice given asialoorosomucoid liposomes; SUV-OR, mice given orosomucoid liposomes; SUV-AOR + AOR, mice given free asialoorosomucoid followed by asialoorosomucoid liposomes. Values are percentage ± s.d. of the dose recovered per organ.

Furthermore, in view of the possibility that free asialoorosomucoid may not suppress completely binding of liposomes to the receptor, some of the observed hepatic uptake in the competition experiment could be attributed to specific binding by the receptor. Fig. 8 also shows that the shift of non-specific uptake of orosomucoid liposomes by the liver to desialylation-induced specific uptake by cells expressing the galactose receptor, is reflected in the changes of radioactivity values in the spleen. Thus, although 6.5% of the dose is recovered in the tissue after injection of orosomucoid liposomes, this value is reduced to 2.0% for asialoorosomucoid liposomes. Interestingly, it remains low (3.1%) in the competition experiment, supporting the notion above that asialoorosomucoid liposomes may have a reduced affinity for the RES.

B. Targeting of liposomes via monoclonal anti-Thy$_1$ IgG$_1$

The great target versatility of antibodies has rendered them the ligand of choice in most targeting work with liposomes. Furthermore, there is evidence that targeting of liposomes with antibodies may, in some instances, have certain advantages over the use of antibodies coupled to drugs directly (Gregoriadis, 1983). For instance, liposomes can incorporate large quantities of a wide range of drugs including genetic material, keep drugs in isolation from the biological milieu (e.g. blood) and deliver them to cells, potentially by a single immunoglobulin molecule per vesicle. In addition, a firmer and more specific binding to cells may be achieved with liposomes bearing antibodies against more than one type of antigenic determinant.

Successful use of antibody-bearing liposomes *in vivo* is dependent on at least two conditions: Firstly, it is, as already discussed, logical to expect that binding of liposomes to cells will occur more effectively when the former retain both their drug and ligand components in the presence of blood and circulate in it for periods long enough to ensure sufficient exposure to the target. As shown above, vesicle stability and half-life in the circulation can be considerably augmented by the correct choice of lipids. Secondly, although recent findings suggest that transcapillary passage of small liposomes may be possible with some tumours (Proffitt *et al.*, 1983; Hashimoto *et al.*, 1983; Mayhew and Rustum, 1983), it is more likely that *in vivo* liposomes will preferentially target to cells within the vasculature or in tissues containing sinusoidal capillaries (Poste, 1983). Both these aspects were taken into account in work described below and, in more detail, elsewhere (Wolff *et al.*, 1984).

(1) Coupling of anti-Thy$_1$ IgG$_1$ onto liposomes

Small unilamellar liposomes containing quenched CF alone, or together with tracer ^{111}In-Ca-diethylene triaminepentaacetic acid (^{111}In-Ca-DPTA) were composed of DSPC, DPPE and cholesterol (molar ratio of total phospholipid to cholesterol, 1:1). Heterobifunctional reagents used to activate DPPE before or after its incorporation into liposomes were *N*-hydroxysuccinimide ester of iodoacetic acid (NHIA), *N*-succinimidyl-4-(2-bromoacetylamino) benzoate (SBAB) and SPDP. ^{125}I-labelled rat anti-Thy$_1$

Table II. Anti-Thy$_1$ IgG$_1$ on the surface of liposomes.

IgG-bearing liposomes	IgG$_1$ bound (μg/μmol phospholipid)	IgG$_1$ molecules per vesicle
IgG (SUV-IA)	4.2	0.6
IgG (SUV-BAB)	6.7	0.9
	9.2	1.3
	17.1	2.3
IgG (PDP-DPPE SUV)	30.0	4.1
	32.0	4.3
	49.3	6.7
	57.4	7.9

Estimation of the number of IgG molecules (assumed relative molecular mass 150000) per vesicle was based on an average vesicle diameter of 60 nm, a surface of the phospholipid/cholesterol unit of 0.83 nm^2 and on the localization of two-thirds of the phospholipid in the outer bilayer. IgG-bearing liposomes were composed of DSPC, activated DPPE and cholesterol (0.99:0.01:1 or 0.9:0.1:1) (from Wolff and Gregoriadis, 1984).

IgG_1 was activated with SPDP prior to its use with all three types of activated liposomes. Liposomes activated with SPDP gave best values in terms of extent of binding (Table II).

(2) Binding of anti-Thy$_1$ IgG$_1$-bearing liposomes to AKR-A cells in vitro Liposomes used were made of DSPC, DPPE (modified with SPDP prior to its incorporation into liposomes) and cholesterol (molar ratios 0.9:0.1:1 or 0.99:0.01:1) or DSPC, DPPE (modified with SBAB after its incorporation into liposomes) and cholesterol (molar ratios 0.9:0.1:1). Exposure of an increasing number of AKR-A cells expressing the cross-reacting mouse $Thy_{1.1}$ antigen on their surface to anti-Thy_1 IgG_1-bearing liposomes revealed that at least 69.5% of the liposomes used contained enough IgG on their surface to ensure binding to cells (Table III). The role of the anti-Thy_1 IgG_1 in promoting association of the liposomal moiety with the AKR-A cells specifically was also supported by the low association values observed for liposomes devoid of IgG and from experiments where anti-Thy_1 IgG_1-bearing liposomes presented to AKR-A cells and to another cell line (EL4-Tc) which does not express the $Thy_{1.1}$ antigen, bound considerably more (3- to 4-fold) to the former cells (Wolff *et al.*, 1984). Interestingly, binding of the IgG_1-bearing liposomes to AKR-A cells was equally effective with both types of liposomes used, one activated with SBAB, the other with SPDP, in spite of the reduced amount of IgG (1.3–2.3 molecules per vesicle, Table II) in the SBAB-activated liposomes.

Table III. Effect of cell number on the binding of free and liposomal anti-Thy_1 IgG_1 to AKR-A cells.

Preparation	Cell number	IgG bound (% of added)	CF bound (% of added)
Free IgG	10^6	6.8 ± 0.6	—
	7.5×10^6	35.5 ± 0.3	—
	10^7	56.4 ± 3.9	—
	1.5×10^7	59.6 ± 1.9	—
IgG (PDP-DPPE SUV)*	10^6	15.2 ± 2.0	14.3 ± 1.6
	10^7	68.2 ± 7.0	69.5 ± 6.9
IgG (PDP-DPPE SUV)†	10^6	14.2 ± 0.5	11.9 ± 0.9
	10^7	68.1 ± 4.5	60.0 ± 3.6
PDP-DPPE SUV†	5×10^6		7.7 ± 1.2

AKR-A cells were incubated at 4°C for 1 h with 1 μg of anti-Thy_1 ^{125}I-IgG_1, free or coupled to CF-containing liposomes composed of DSPC, PDP-DPPE and CHOL (0.99:0.01:1 or 0.9:0.1:1) or with similar liposomes devoid of IgG. All values are means ± s.d. from three separate experiments (from Wolff and Gregoriadis, 1984).

* Liposomes contained 10% (of total phospholipid) DPPE.

† Liposomes contained 1% (of total phospholipid) DPPE.

Table IV. Effect of plasma on the binding of free and liposomal anti-Thy$_1$ ^{125}I-IgG$_1$ to AKR-A cells.

	Incubation buffer		Plasma	
Preparation	^{125}I-IgG (bound)	CF (bound)	^{125}I-IgG (bound)	CF (bound)
Free IgG	56.4 ± 3.9*	—	55.4 ± 4.1*	—
IgG-SUV†	68.1 ± 4.5	60 ± 3.6*	51.3 ± 2.2	48.7 ± 0.2*

AKR-A cells (10^7) were incubated at 4°C for 1 h in incubation buffer or in mouse plasma with free (1 μg) or liposomal (0.86–0.90 μg) anti-Thy$_1$ ^{125}I-IgG$_1$. Liposomes were composed of DSPC, PDP-DPPE and cholesterol (0.99:0.01:1). Values are means ± s.d. from three separate experiments. (From Wolff and Gregoriadis, 1984).

* Values denote percentage of added that is bound.

† IgG (PDP-DPPE SUV).

The effect of plasma on the binding of IgG-bearing liposomes to the AKR-A cells was investigated (Table IV). As already noted with other targeted liposomes (Gregoriadis *et al.*, 1981; Heath *et al.*, 1980) the presence of plasma reduced binding of liposomes to the cells only modestly. Although it is conceivable that a variety of plasma components may adhere to or interact with uncoupled pyridyldithiopropionyl groups on the surface of liposomes and, in this way, mask the antigen recognition sites of the IgG, it is also possible that there may have been some cleavage of the disulphide bond between the (SPDP-modified) IgG and liposomes by plasma reducing agents. The latter possibility is enhanced by data presented in Table V from experiments in which control (IgG free) and IgG-bearing liposomes were chromatographed following their exposure to plasma. Although loss of IgG after 0.5 h was only 15%, it increased to nearly 50% on longer (24 h) incubation. Table V also shows that cholesterol-rich DSPC liposomes, known to retain entrapped solutes fully upon extensive incubation with plasma (Fig. 3), behave similarly when SPDP-modified DPPE replaces some of the DSPC component. On the other hand, the coupling of IgG onto the liposomal surface does lead to some loss of vesicle stability (CF and ^{111}In markers) in the presence of plasma, but only upon prolonged (24 h) exposure (Table V).

(3) Targeting of anti-Thy$_1$ IgG$_1$-bearing liposomes to AKR-A cells in vivo

Interaction of anti-Thy$_1$ ^{125}I-IgG$_1$-bearing liposomes with AKR-A cells *in vivo* (Fig. 9) was studied with vesicles composed of DSPC, a small proportion of DPPE (in the form of PDP-DPPE) and cholesterol (molar ratios 0.99:0.01:1) and containing quenched CF and ^{111}In-Ca-DTPA. Since it was

Table V. Stability of liposomes in the presence of plasma.

Incubation time (h)	Liposomes Latent CF (%)	Liposomes Retained ^{111}In (%)	IgG-liposomes Latent CF (%)	IgG-liposomes Retained ^{111}In (%)	IgG-liposomes Retained ^{125}I (%)
0.5	99.8	96.0	100.0	95.5	85.3
5.5	99.3	95.1	99.6	93.3	78.5
24.0	98.2	91.0	72.8	71.9	54.3

IgG-free or anti-Thy$_1$ ^{125}I-IgG$_1$-bearing liposomes composed of DSPC, PDP-DPPE and CHOL (0.99:0.01:1) contained CF and ^{111}In-Ca-DTPA. Incubation with mouse plasma was carried out as described (Wolff and Gregoriadis, 1984). CF latency is expressed as percentage of latency in the original preparations (97.9–98.1%). ^{111}In and ^{125}I radioactivity retained by liposomes upon incubation with plasma was estimated after passing samples of the incubation mixtures through CL-4B Sepharose minicolumns and expressed as percentage of the applied radioactivity recovered with liposomes (from Wolff and Gregoriadis, 1984).

expected that liposomes given intravenously would only be able to reach and bind to target cells within the intravascular space, mice injected intravenously with AKR-A cells were chosen as a model system for targeting *in vivo*. It was assumed that after the injection of the cells, a proportion of these would be available in the circulation to interact with anti-Thy$_1$ IgG$_1$-bearing liposomes injected subsequently by the same route. In control experiments, either injection of AKR-A cells was omitted or liposomes were devoid of IgG. The preference as a control of IgG-free liposomes rather than liposomes bearing non-specific IgG has been justified elsewhere (Wolff and Gregoriadis, 1984).

Patterns of liposome clearance (Fig. 9) suggest the following:

(a) the presence of AKR-A cells in the circulation does not influence the clearance rates of IgG-free liposomes (CF and ^{111}In markers);

(b) clearance of the liposome-entrapped CF and ^{111}In-markers in both intact mice and in mice injected with AKR-A cells is more rapid for the anti-Thy$_1$ IgG$_1$-bearing vesicles than for vesicles devoid of IgG. This, also in agreement with the clearance pattern of the ^{125}I-IgG radioactivity (Fig. 9), probably results from the accumulative effect of the binding of the Fc portions of IgG to the Fc receptors in the reticuloendothelial system, the interaction of the anti-Thy$_1$ IgG$_1$-bearing liposomes with the Thy$_{1.1}$ antigen on the surface of T lymphocytes and, for mice injected with AKR-A cells, interaction of such liposomes with the Thy$_{1.1}$ antigen on the surface of AKR-A cells;

(c) anti-Thy$_1$ IgG$_1$-bearing liposomes (all three markers) are cleared from the circulation more rapidly when mice have been previously injected with

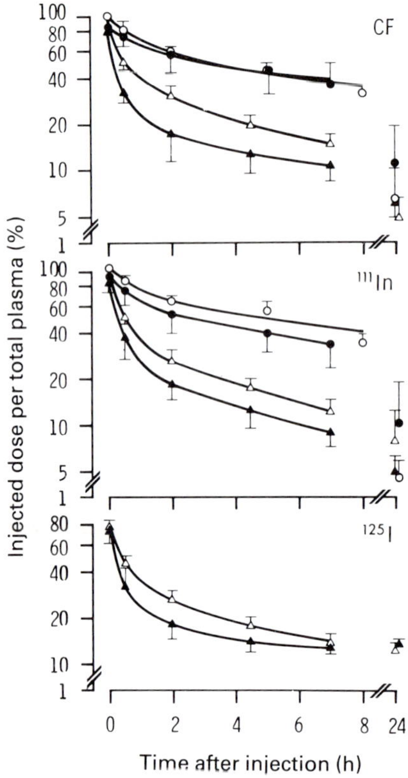

Fig. 9. Clearance of antibody-coated liposomes from the circulation of injected mice. AKR mice (four to five mice in each group) were injected intravenously with IgG-free liposomes (1.25 μmol phospholipid) (○) or anti-Thy_1 ^{125}I-IgG_1-bearing (△) liposomes (1.36 μmol phospholipid) composed of DSPC, PDP-DPPE and cholesterol (0.99:0.01:1) and containing CF and ^{111}In-Ca-DTPA. In other experiments, AKR mice (four to five mice in each group) were injected as above with 3.7–4.0 × 10^7 AKR-A cells followed 2–3 min later with similar IgG-free (●) or anti-Thy_1 ^{125}I-IgG_1-bearing (▲) liposomes. Plasma values for latent CF, ^{111}In and ^{125}I at time intervals after the injection of liposomes are expressed as percentage ± s.d. of the dose per total plasma. On the basis of latent CF, values of differences in clearance patterns between mice that had or had not been injected with AKR-A cells prior to receiving anti-Thy_1 IgG_1-bearing liposomes, were significant ($p < 0.001$–003) up to and including the 4.5 h time interval. Differences between mice treated with AKR-A cells prior to receiving IgG-free or IgG-bearing liposomes were significant ($p < 0.001$) up to and including the 7 h time interval. At 24 h, ^{111}In values (percentage ± s.d. of the injection; corrected for blood contamination) in the liver and spleen for mice injected successively with AKR-A cells and anti-Thy_1 IgG_1-bearing or IgG-free liposomes were respectively 51.7 ± 7.0 and 40.3 ± 4.5 (liver; $p < 0.001$) and 5.9 ± 1.6 and 4.9 ± 0.3 (spleen; $p < 0.03$) (from Wolff and Gregoriadis, 1984).

AKR-A cells (Fig. 9). This suggests that liposomes and cells associate to some extent in the circulation and that those vesicles that are cell-bound assume the rate of AKR-A cell clearance which is much greater than that of the small liposomes used in this study (Wolff and Gregoriadis, 1984).

Binding of anti-Thy$_1$ IgG$_1$-bearing liposomes to the macrophages (through the Fc receptors), T lymphocytes and circulating AKR-A cells occurs probably during the first phase (1–2 h post-injection) of the biphasic vesicle clearance (Fig. 9; all markers). The proportion of the dose cleared during this period, as a result of specific interaction of liposomes with the various cell targets was estimated (Wolff and Gregoriadis, 1984) to be about 45% and at least one-third of it relates to liposomes cleared specifically because of their interaction with circulating AKR-A cells. As discussed elsewhere (Wolff and Gregoriadis, 1984) however, this latter value could easily be an underestimate since anti-Thy$_1$ IgG$_1$-bearing liposomes may interact with the circulating AKR-cells in preference to T lymphocytes or fixed macrophages. The second phase of clearance of IgG$_1$-bearing liposomes is slower and similar to that observed for liposomes devoid of IgG, presumably because the remainder of the vesicles cannot interact specifically with target sites (Fig. 9). The existence of a population of IgG-deficient vesicles in liposomes bearing IgG is supported with data in Table III and has been demonstrated and discussed elsewhere (Gregoriadis and Neerunjun, 1975; Gregoriadis and Meehan, 1981).

V. CONCLUSIONS

There is little doubt that stability of liposomes can now be arranged in a way that, upon exposure to blood, it remains virtually unchanged, with entrapped drugs being retained quantitatively. In addition, liposome clearance from the circulation by the RES can be delayed for periods of time sufficiently long to ensure effective vesicle interaction with accessible targets. Other developments in liposome technology (Gregoriadis, 1984) have led to simple techniques for high yield drug entrapment, appropriate for scaled up preparations. These developments have contributed to the acceptance of liposomes as a delivery system for the treatment of microbial, viral and other diseases involving the RES, as immunological adjuvants in vaccines, as diagnostic agents *in vitro* and *in vivo* including the imaging of tissues, and for a multitude of other uses requiring a carrier system of such qualifications. More recently, gene delivery and expression *in vivo* using liposomes has been attempted (see also Chapter 9). It is becoming increasingly apparent that antibodies and other cytophilic molecules may serve as targeting devices to direct liposome-entrapped drugs to tissues other than those of the RES. It may be that gene manipulation will also be achieved in this way. However, prior to this, better understanding of the targeted liposome–cell interaction at the subcellular level and appropriate control of such interaction will be required.

ACKNOWLEDGEMENTS

We thank Miss Olivia Dansie for secretarial assistance. Barbara Wolff acknowledges support from the British Council.

REFERENCES

Allen, T. M. (1981). *Biochim. Biophys. Acta* **640**, 385–397.
Ashwell, G. and Morell, A. G. (1974). *Adv. Enzymol.* **41**, 99–128.
Connor, J., Yatvin, M. B. and Huang, L. (1984). *Proc. Natl. Acad. Sci. USA* **81**, 1715–1718.
Gregoriadis, G. (1974). *In* "Enzyme Therapy in Lysosomal Storage Diseases" (J. M. Tager, G. J. M. Hooghwinkel and W. Th. Daems, eds) pp. 131–148. North Holland, Amsterdam.
Gregoriadis, G. (1981). *The Lancet* **ii**, 241–247.
Gregoriadis, G. (1983). *TIPS* **4**, 304–307.
Gregoriadis, G. (ed.) (1984). "Liposome Technology," Vols I–III. CRC Press, Boca Raton.
Gregoriadis, G. and Davis, C. (1979). *Biochem. Biophys. Res. Commun.* **89**, 1287–1293.
Gregoriadis, G. and Meehan, A. (1981). *Biochem. J.* **200**, 211–216.
Gregoriadis, G. and Neerunjun, D. (1975). *Biochem. Biophys. Res. Commun.* **65**, 537–544.
Gregoriadis, G. and Senior, J. (1980). *FEBS Lett.* **119**, 43–46.
Gregoriadis, G. and Senior, J. (1984). *Biochem. Soc. Trans.* **12**, 337–339.
Gregoriadis, G., Neerunjun, D. and Hunt, R. (1977). *Life Sci.* **21**, 357–369.
Gregoriadis, G., Mah, M. M. and Meehan, A. (1981). *Biochem. J.* **200**, 203–210.
Gregoriadis, G., Kirby, C., Senior, J. and Wolff, B. (1985). *In* "Receptor-Mediated Targeting of Drugs" (G. Gregoriadis, G. Poste, J. Senior and A. Trouet, eds). pp. 243–266. Plenum Press, New York.
Hashimoto, Y., Sugawara, M., Masuko, T. and Hojo, H. (1983). *Cancer Res.* **43**, 5328–5334.
Heath, T. D., Fraley, R. T. and Papahadjopoulos, D. (1980). *Science* **210**, 539–541.
Hwang, K. J., Luk, K.-F. S. and Beaumier, P. L. (1980). *Proc. Natl. Acad. Sci. USA* **77**, 4030–4034.
Kirby, C. and Gregoriadis, G. (1980). *Life Sci.* **27**, 2223–2230.
Kirby, C. and Gregoriadis, G. (1981). *Biochem. J.* **199**, 251–254.
Kirby, C. and Gregoriadis, G. (1983). *Biochem. Pharmacol.* **32**, 609–615.
Kirby, C. and Gregoriadis, G. (1984a). *In* "Liposome Technology" (G. Gregoriadis, ed.) Vol. I, pp. 19–28. CRC Press, Boca Raton.

Kirby, C. and Gregoriadis, G. (1984b). *In* "Liposome Technology" (G. Gregoriadis, ed.) Vol. II, pp. 69–82. CRC Press, Boca Raton.
Kirby, C. and Gregoriadis, G. (1984c). *J. Microencap.* **1**, 33–45.
Kirby, C., Clarke, J. and Gregoriadis, G. (1980a). *FEBS Lett.* **111**, 324–328.
Kirby, C., Clarke, J. and Gregoriadis, G. (1980b). *Biochem. J.* **186**, 591–598.
Krupp, L., Chobanian, A. V. and Brecher, I. P. (1976). *Biochem. Biophys. Res. Commun.* **72**, 1251–1258.
Mayhew, E. and Rustum, Y. (1983). *Biol. Cell.* **47**, 81–86.
Morell, A. G., Gregoriadis, G., Scheinberg, I. H., Hickman, J. and Ashwell, G. (1971). *J. Biol. Chem.* **246**, 1461–1467.
Patel, H. M., Tuzel, N. S. and Ryman, B. E. (1984). *Biochim. Biophys. Acta* **761**, 142–151.
Poste, G. (1983). *Biol. Cell* **47**, 19–38.
Proffitt, R. T., Williams, L. E., Presant, C. A., Tin, G. W., Uliana, J. A., Gamble, R. C. and Baldeschwielar, J. D. (1983). *Science* **220**, 502–505.
Ryman, B. E. and Tyrrell, D. A. (1980). *Essays Biochem.* **16**, 49–98.
Scherphof, G., Roerdink, F., Waite, M. and Parks, I. (1978). *Biochim. Biophys. Acta* **542**, 296–307.
Senior, J. and Gregoriadis, G. (1982a). *Life Sci.* **30**, 2123–2136.
Senior, J. and Gregoriadis, G. (1982b). *FEBS Lett.* **145**, 109–114
Senior, J. and Gregoriadis, G. (1984). *In* "Liposome Technology" (G. Gregoriadis, ed.) Vol. III, pp. 263–282. CRC Press, Boca Raton.
Senior, J., Gregoriadis, G. and Mitropoulos, K. (1983). *Biochim. Biophys. Acta* **760**, 111–118.
Senior, J., Crawley, J. C. W. and Gregoriadis, G. (1985). *Biochim. Biophys. Acta* **839,** 1–8.
Spanjer, H. H. and Scherphof, G. (1983). *Biochim. Biophys. Acta* **734**, 40–47.
Szoka, F. and Mayhew, E. (1983). *Biochem. Biophys. Res. Commun.* **110**, 140–146.
Teradaira, R., Kolb-Bachhofen, V., Schlepper-Schafer, J. and Kolb, H. (1983). *Biochim. Biophys. Acta* **759**, 306–310.
Toonen, P. A. H. M. and Crommelin, D. J. A. (1983). *Weekblad Scient. Edn* **5**, 269–280.
van Oss, C. J., Gillman, C. F., Bronson, P. M. and Border, J. R. (1974). *Immunol. Commun.* **3**, 321–328.
Wolff, B. and Gregoriadis, G. (1984). *Biochim. Biophys. Acta* **802**, 259–273.

9

Liposomes as Carriers for Gene Transfer in vivo

C. Nicolau

I. INTRODUCTION

Liposomes have already been used for *in vitro* gene transfer in eukaryotic cells in culture (Wong *et al.*, 1980). However, the efficiency of this procedure does not exceed that of other methods, such as calcium phosphate precipitation or treatment with DEAE-dextran (Fraley *et al.*, 1981; Schäfer-Ridder *et al.*, 1982; see also Chapter 12). Although liposomes may provide an attractive alternative with cells that are refractory to gene transfer with other methods, the greatest potentiality for liposome-mediated gene transfer seems to lie in its *in vivo* applications, in particular in adult animals.

Intravenous injection to rats of a recombinant plasmid containing the rat preproinsulin I gene encapsulated in large liposomes has indeed led to the transient expression of this gene in the liver and spleen of the recipient animals (Nicolau *et al.*, 1983a). A significant fraction of the expressed hormone was in its physiologically active form, as demonstrated by its effect on the blood glucose level of the inoculated animals.

I will present in the following pages some of the more significant experimental features of this work. This work has been already reviewed so that the more salient facts will be presented here (Cudd and Nicolau, 1984; Nicolau *et al.*, 1985).

II. LIPOSOME PREPARATION AND DNA ENCAPSULATION

Liposomes consisting of egg yolk phosphatidylcholine (Sigma, purified according to Singleton *et al.* (1965), ox brain phosphatidylserine (Sigma) and cholesterol (Sigma) [4:1:5 (mol/mol)] were prepared by reversed-phase

Microinjection and Organelle Transplantation Techniques

ISBN: 0-12-164722-6
ISBN: 0-12-164723-4 Pbk

evaporation (Szoka and Papahadjopoulos, 1978). Some preparations of liposomes included a 1:6 molar ratio of dihydro-LacCer (Sigma) to phospholipids (PL). Briefly, 60 μmol of lipids dissolved in 4.5 ml of freshly distilled ether was vortexed with 1.5 ml of phosphate-buffered saline containing 90 μg of DNA (including trace amounts of nick-translated ^{32}P DNA). The ether was removed under reduced pressure in a rotary evaporator and the liposomes were diluted to 4.5 ml with phosphate-buffered saline. Liposomes were stored at 4°C under nitrogen and were used within 1 week.

The percentage of encapsulation of the DNA was determined by treating an aliquot (200 μl) of the liposome suspensions with DNase I in the presence of 5 mM $MgCl_2$ at 37°C, followed by filtration on a Sepharose 4B column and monitoring the ^{32}P radioactivity in the excluded and retarded fractions.

The non-encapsulated DNA with a relative molecular mass greater than 30000 must be degraded in smaller fragments in order to be retained by the Sepharose 4B column. In order to recuperate the non-encapsulated DNA a centrifugation method of separation has been employed.

Liposomes (PC:PS:Chol in the molar ratios 4:1:5) at 80 μmol lipids/ml containing 4 mg/ml of the p(gRI 9.4) plasmid were prepared. This plasmid consists of the insertion of 9.4 kb of rat chromosomal DNA containing the rat preproinsulin I gene at the EcoRI site of the *Escherichia coli* pBR322 plasmid.

The percentage of DNA encapsulation is determined on a Sepharose 4B microcolumn [a Pasteur pipette of 2 ml of volume is filled with Sepharose 4B (Pharmacia) equilibrated with phosphate buffered saline (PBS) pH 7.4: 4 μmol of lipids are deposed on this column. 200 μl fractions are collected and subsequently counted for ^{32}P in a liquid scintillation counter]. The encapsulation efficiency is determined as the percentage of DNA molecules entrapped in the liposomes. Knowing this percentage and the lipid concentration one can calculate the capture efficiency of the liposome preparation as aqueous volume in litres per mole of lipids.

The recovery of the non-encapsulated DNA was achieved as follows: the liposome preparation is centrifuged for 30 min at 100000 $\times$ g and the ^{32}P radioactivity of the nick-translated DNA is counted in the sediment and the supernatant. In a typical preparation (ADN concentration = 1000 μg/ml; lipid concentration = 80 μmol/ml; PBS volume = 100 μl; ratio ether:PBS = 3:1) the encapsulation efficiency is 26% (6.5 l/mol of lipids). After centrifugation (30 min at 100000 $\times$ g) the percentage of radioactivity in the liposome sediment is 25%, so that 15% of the total DNA (1000 μg/ml) is recuperated.

An important aspect of the DNA encapsulation in liposome is the type of mechanical agitation. We find that even 15 s of mild sonication (10 kHz)

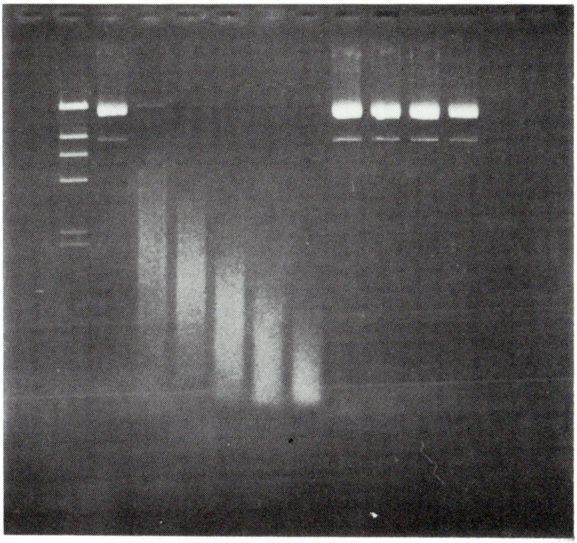

Fig. 1. Electrophoresis of an ADN subjected to sonication or vortexing. λ, size marker of λ-Phage DNA cut by Hind III, fragments size in kilobases (kb); 1, pRINS plasmid; 2, sonicated 15 s; 3, sonicated 30 s; 4, sonicated 1 min; 5, sonicated 2 min; 6, sonicated 4 min; 7, vortexing 1 min; 8, vortexing 3 min; 9, vortexing 5 min; 10, vortexing 8 min.

degrades most of the DNA (rel. mol. mass > 500000), whereas vortexing even for 8 min is without influence. Figure 1 shows electrophoresis in an agarose gel of liposomes preparations containing the pRINSg plasmid subjected to sonication or vortexing for different periods of time (Nicolau *et al.*, 1985).

Vortexing for various lengths of time influences the encapsulation efficiency of the prepared liposomes. For an agitation time of 30 s, the aqueous volume encapsulated by the liposomes is 5.5 l/mol of lipids; after 4 min of vortexing this volume is 7.2 l/mol lipid. Longer times of vortexing seem to reduce somewhat the encapsulated aqueous volume.

III. LIPOSOME DISTRIBUTION *IN VIVO*

To determine the location of the large PC/PS/Chol liposomes in the rat organism, liposomes encapsulating ^{111}In-labelled bleomycin were prepared. One millilitre aliquots were used for intravenous injection. Controls were injected with free ^{111}In-labelled bleomycin and free $^{111}InCl_3$.

Visualization of the organ distribution of liposome-encapsulated ^{111}In-labelled bleomycin was obtained by external γ-camera imaging. Anaesthetized rats (sodium pentobarbital at 40 mg/kg intraperitoneal) intubated via the jugular vein were placed on a Nuclear Chicago γ-camera equipped with a high-resolution 140 keV parallel collimator and a Simis 3 data system (Informatek, Birmingham, AL). Animals were injected with 20 μCi of ^{111}In-labelled bleomycin, $^{111}InCl_3$ (Commissariat à l'Energie Atomique, France; 4 mCi/ml), or liposome-entrapped ^{111}In-labelled bleomycin, in a volume adjusted to 1.5 ml with isotonic saline: 10-s dynamic scans were carried out continuously for 20 min using the 173 keV photopeak of ^{111}In. From the resultant images, the localization of radioactivity was determined for the areas of interest—the head (circulating blood), liver, spleen, kidneys and bladder. For the liposome-entrapped ^{111}In-labelled bleomycin injected rats, 10-min static scans were carried out 6 h after injection to estimate the remaining spleen and liver activity (Nicolau *et al.*, 1983a).

The images obtained show that, between the injection time and 20 min later, a rapid and intensive uptake by the liver of liposome-entrapped ^{111}In-labelled bleomycin occurred. A weak urinary elimination was also observed. By 6 h after injection the liposome organ distribution had changed only slightly. The radioactivity in the bladder is probably due to destruction of the liposomes in the liver and concomitant release of the label.

Six hours after injection, the rats were killed and the organs were individually visualized with the γ-camera. To check whether the liposomes were entirely responsible for the observed organ distribution of bleomycin, a similar experiment was carried out with free ^{111}In-labelled bleomycin and with $^{111}InCl_3$. The latter was used to determine the pattern of distribution of the free ion, which could have resulted from dissociation of ^{111}In-labelled bleomycin.

With these controls, the distribution pattern differed strongly from that observed with the liposome-encapsulated label. For ^{111}In-labelled bleomycin 2 min after injection, bleomycin was already present in liver and in urine. The urinary excretion was particularly strong 5 min after injection, and 20 min after injection practically all of the radioactivity was found in the urinary bladder. The absence of kidney radioactivity corresponds to the asymptotic phase of plasmatic clearance. The $^{111}InCl_3$ distribution differed from that of ^{111}In-labelled bleomycin in that urinary excretion was faster and more significant. Not even a transient liver uptake was observed (Nicolau *et al.*, 1983a).

The organ activities were measured individually 20 min after injection and the results are shown in Table I. The kinetics of organ uptake and of urinary excretion of the radioactivity are shown in Fig. 2. The kinetics of uptake and excretion were completely different for liposome-encapsulated ^{111}In-labelled bleomycin, free ^{111}In-labelled bleomycin and $^{111}InCl_3$. Three animals were used for each compound studied.

Table I. Percentage of ^{111}In radioactivity in various organs of the rat 20 min after intravenous injection (Nicolau *et al.*, 1983a).

Sample	Liver	Kidneys	Bladder
Liposome-encapsulated ^{111}In-labelled bleomycin	42 ± 4	< 5	15 ± 4
Free ^{111}In-labelled bleomycin*	10 ± 5	7 ± 5	82 ± 4
$^{111}InCl_3$	0	< 5	95 ± 4

Results represent mean ± s.d. of three measurements on four animals. For values lower than 5%, the statistical analysis does not allow the calculation of a standard deviation with any real significance.

* Liposome-free ^{111}In-labelled bleomycin tends to accumulate to some extent (10–15% of the administered dose) in the rat (as in the human liver). The level of accumulation is well below that of the liposome-encapsulated drug.

IV. EXPRESSION OF THE INSULIN GENE IN LIVER AND SPLEEN

The liposome-encapsulated p(gRI 9.4) plasmid, expressing rat preproinsulin I, was injected to non-fasting wistar male rats (300–350 g). At the same time controls were inoculated with liposome-encapsulated *E. coli* pBR322 plasmid, free p(gRI 9.4) plasmid, empty liposomes and a group of control rats received no inoculation at all. Glycaemia and blood insulin were measured at 0, 6, 10, 12 and 18 h after inoculation. In each experiment three rats were killed at 6 and 18 h after inoculation and liver and spleen insulin were assayed (Nicolau *et al.*, 1983a). The results are shown in Table II.

Table II shows that injection of the liposome-encapsulated insulin gene had a significant effect on the glycaemia and insulin levels of the animals so treated. Glycaemia in the treated animals showed a significant decrease 6 h after injection that correlated quite well with the increase in the insulin blood level in these animals. At the same time, 6 h after injection the insulin found in the liver and spleen was twice the amount in control animals. An interesting feature is the relatively short time of increased insulin synthesis observed with the treated animals. Glycaemia began to increase 10 h after injection and 12 h after injection it was higher than the control values, whereas the blood insulin decreased to less than the control values. The liver and spleen insulin values returned almost to normal by 18 h, after injection. Whatever control materials were injected — free insulin gene, empty liposomes, or liposome-entrapped pBR322 — the glycaemia and insulin values remained relatively stable over an 18 h period, as did those for untreated animals.

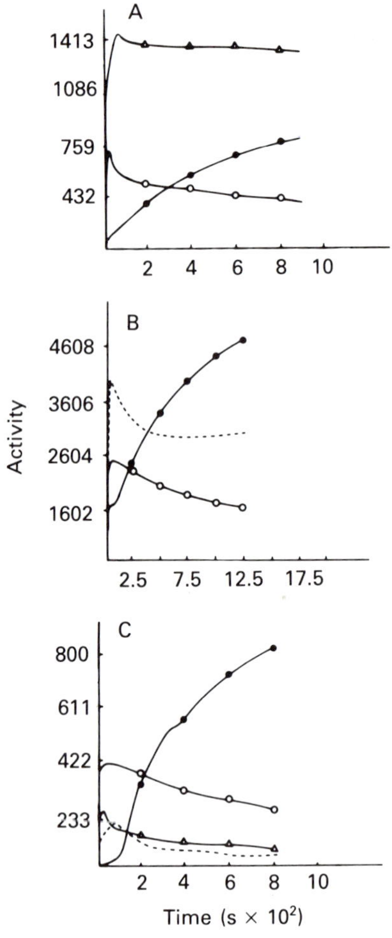

Fig. 2. Kinetics of organ uptake of ^{111}In after intravenous injection to rats in 1 ml of phosphate-buffered saline (pH 7.3). (A) Liposome-encapsulated ^{111}In-labelled bleomycin. (B) Free ^{111}In-labelled bleomycin. (C) $^{111}InCl_3$. △, liver; ●, urine; ○, blood; . . ., kidney. Results represent whole-body determination corrected for background radioactivity (Nicolau *et al.*, 1985).

The DNA segment encoding rat preproinsulin I that was used in this study contains, in addition to the insulin coding and intervening sequences, several kilobases of flanking sequences on each side of the gene (Cordell *et al.*, 1979). This suggests that regulatory signals are also included within the insulin plasmid and that the gene might be functional when transferred *in vivo* after its entrapment in liposomes. The observed organ distribution of the liposomes allowed us to assay the potentially expressed insulin in the

Table II. Glycaemia and blood, liver, and spleen insulin in control animals and in rats injected intravenously with the liposome-encapsulated insulin gene (Nicolau *et al.*, 1983a)

Group	n	Glycaemia, mg of glucose/100 ml of blood					Insulin: Blood, μU/ml					Insulin: Liver, μU/g of tissue			Insulin: Spleen, μU/g of tissue		
		0 h	6 h	10 h	12 h	18 h	0 h	6 h	10 h	12 h	18 h	0 h	6 h	18 h	0 h	6 h	18 h
Empty liposomes	4	110 ± 2	105 ± 2	118 ± 2	112 ± 2	110 ± 2	38 ± 6	40 ± 5	32 ± 8	42 ± 7	43 ± 8	85 ± 13	87 ± 15	84 ± 12	118 ± 15	112 = 20	127 ± 20
Free insulin gene	4	106 ± 2	109 ± 2	N.D.	104 ± 2	N.D.	41 ± 5	45 ± 5	N.D.	51 ± 7	N.D.	N.D.*	N.D.*	N.D.*	N.D.*	N.D.*	N.D.*
Liposome-encapsulated pBR322	4	115 ± 3	113 ± 3	N.D.	107 ± 7	N.D.	45 ± 5	36 ± 5	N.D.	46 ± 7	N.D.	89 ± 12	82 ± 13	82 ± 14	125 ± 20	121 = 18	123 ± 20
Not injected	4	103 ± 2	107 ± 2	116 ± 2	110 ± 2	103 ± 2	40 ± 6	43 ± 5	45 ± 6	50 ± 5	45 ± 7	N.D.*	N.D.*	N.D.*	N.D.*	N.D.*	N.D.*
Liposome encapsulated insulin gene	10	108 ± 3	72 ± 6	86 ± 5	129 ± 6	138 ± 9	41 ± 6	61 ± 8	42 ± 6	24 ± 6	30 ± 5	82 ± 10	205 ± 22	105 ± 15	115 ± 18	242 = 20	143 ± 20

For each animal, two determinations of each value were carried out and the s.d. was calculated for the mean value per animal μU, microunit(s).

* Because little variation of the glycaemia and insulin levels was observed during 18 h with these controls, the liver and spleen insulin levels were not assayed.

incorporating cells. Indeed, quite enhanced amounts of insulin were found in the livers and spleens of the treated rats whereas those of the controls did not change. Statistical evaluation of the significance of the results presented in Table II was not possible because, although 16 control animals were used, the numbers of animals per control group were too low for such evaluation (for instance, by Student's test). Nonetheless, the differences observed in the blood glucose and insulin levels 6 h after inoculation between controls on the one hand and treated animals on the other seem sufficiently clear that statistical tests, in this case, were not absolutely necessary. The insulin normally found in the liver and spleen of control animals is the blood pancreatic insulin that is bound on the insulin receptors present on these cells (Freychet *et al.*, 1971; Kahn and Roth, 1975).

These observations suggest that insulin is expressed in liver and spleen for a relatively short time (up to 10 h). The reason might be either the ejection of the gene by the host cells or a quenching of this gene (Nicolau *et al.*, 1983a). We are aware that Kupffer cells and splenic macrophages may not be the ideal host cells for insulin synthesis induced by uptake of exogenous DNA.

V. TARGETING OF LIPOSOME-MEDIATED GENE TRANSFER TO NON-PHAGOCYTIC CELLS

A. Liver

Hepatic uptake of large phospholipid-cholesterol liposomes after intravenous administration amounts to 40–60% of the injected dose and has been shown to be accounted for mainly by the Kupffer cells, to a minor extent by hepatocytes, and hardly at all by endothelial cells (Roerdink *et al.*, 1981; Spanjer and Scherphof, 1983). Because of the observed expression of the insulin gene *in vivo* and its transient character (Nicolau *et al.*, 1983a), an analysis of the intercellular location of the transported gene seemed necessary. Therefore we have isolated hepatocytes, Kupffer cells and endothelial cells from rat liver after intravenous injection of the liposome-entrapped rat preproinsulin I gene and assayed them for the presence of the exogenous DNA by Southern blot analysis (Soriano *et al.*, 1983).

Incorporation of a glycolipid with a terminal non-reducing β-galactose residue into the liposome bilayer has been reported to increase the fraction of the vesicles associating *in vivo* with hepatocytes, probably as a consequence of the interaction of the β-galactose residue with the galactose-specific lectin of the hepatocytes (Ghosh *et al.*, 1982). Because Kupffer cells, the major targets of intravenously injected liposomes, may not qualify very well for the lasting expression of an exogenous gene, we extended our experiments to lactosylceramide (LacCer)-containing liposomes, in an attempt to increase gene uptake by hepatocytes (Soriano *et al.*, 1983; Nicolau *et al.*, 1983b, 1984).

Liposomes encapsulating the p(gRI 9.4) plasmid were prepared by reversed-phase evaporation and checked for their entrapment efficiency by DNase I treatment followed by filtration on Sepharose 4B. Vesicles consisting only of PL and cholesterol (PL liposomes) or also containing LacCer (LC liposomes) encapsulated 13.4 and 16.3% of the aqueous volume, with an entrapped volume of 6.7 and 8.1 l/mol of PL, respectively. Electron micrographs of negatively stained liposomes showed the presence in both preparations of mostly unilamellar and oligolamellar vesicles with a size range of 0.1–1 μm (Soriano *et al.*, 1983).

Wistar rats were injected intravenously with 1 ml (13 μmol of total lipids or about 3 μg of encapsulated DNA) of both liposome preparations. As a control, rats were injected with 20 μg of the free rat insulin plasmid DNA. Four hours after liposome administration, livers were perfused and Kupffer cells, endothelial cells and hepatocytes were isolated (Soriano *et al.*, 1983). DNA was extracted from the three cell fractions, fractionated on agarose gels following digestion with Pst I, and subjected to Southern blot analysis (Figs 3–5). Because p(gRI 9.4), the liposome entrapped rat insulin plasmid, contains a repeated sequence that does not allow it to be used as a hybridization probe, a subclone designated p007, lacking the repeated sequence, was constructed and used as the hybridization probe (Bell *et al.*, 1980). The plasmid vector pBR322 was also used as a probe, thereby eliminating the background hybridization due to the endogenous rat insulin genes present in all liver cells.

By using p007 as a probe, injection of the free plasmid DNA does not result in any hybridization bands in addition to those found in normal rat liver DNA. Two hybridization bands, 5.2 and 3.0 kb, corresponding to the endogenous rat insulin I and II gene sequences, respectively, and expected to hybridize with the p007 probe, can be detected, particularly on long exposures of the autoradiograms (Fig. 5). The hybridization signal observed with the rat insulin I gene segment is the stronger of the two because the flanking sequences present in the probe originate from this gene. An additional 8 kb hybridizing fragment is also observed on long exposures (Fig. 5) and is thought to be due to some homology with the insulin flanking sequences present in p007, because it is not observed when using insulin cDNA probes. With PL liposomes, three bands of 8.7, 2.1 and 1.1 kb, expected from Pst I cleavage of p(gRI 9.4) and homologous to p007 sequences, can also be detected. These bands were in all cases absent in the controls. The bands are most intense in the Kupffer cell DNA fraction

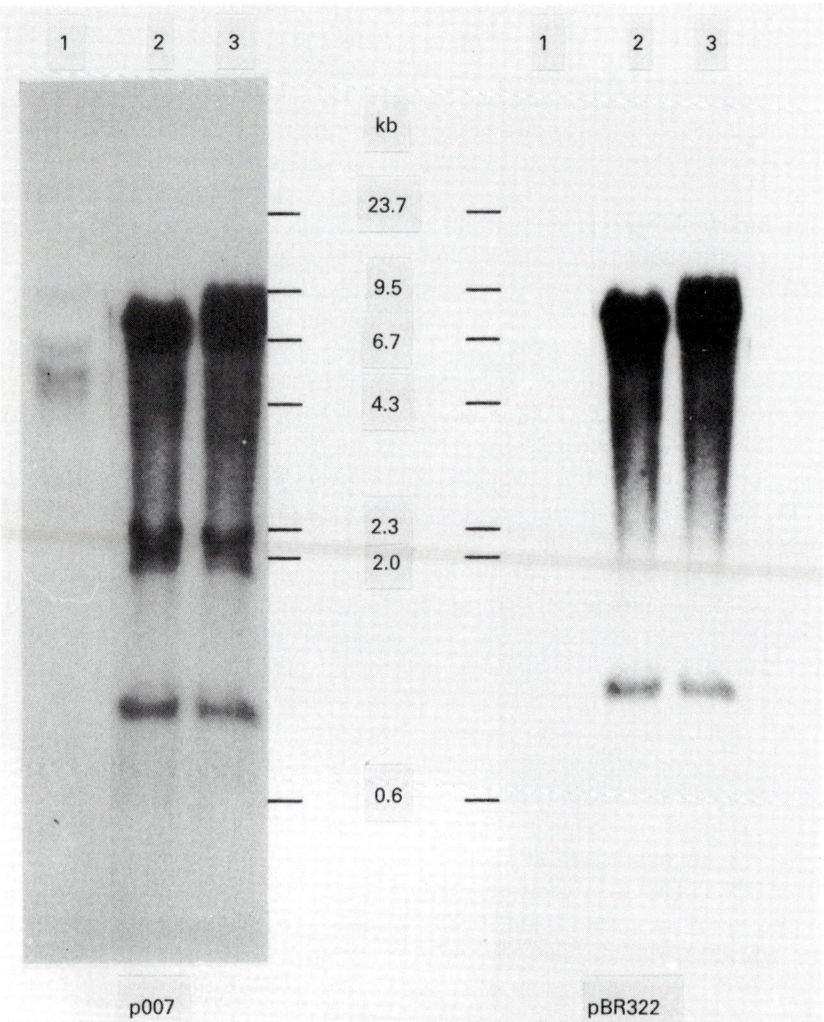

Fig. 3. Detection of the exogenous plasmid DNA in Kupffer cells. Twenty micrograms of Kupffer cell DNA from rats injected with 20 μg of free p(gRI 9.4) plasmid (lane 1), 3 μg of PL liposome-entrapped plasmid (lane 2), and 3 μg of LacCer liposome-entrapped plasmid (lane 3) was digested with Pst I, fractionated through 0.6% agarose gels, transferred to nitrocellulose filters, and hybridized with p007 or pBR322. Autoradiography was for 24 h. Hind III fragments of λ DNA were used as relative molecular mass markers and their lengths are indicated in kb (Soriano *et al.*, 1983).

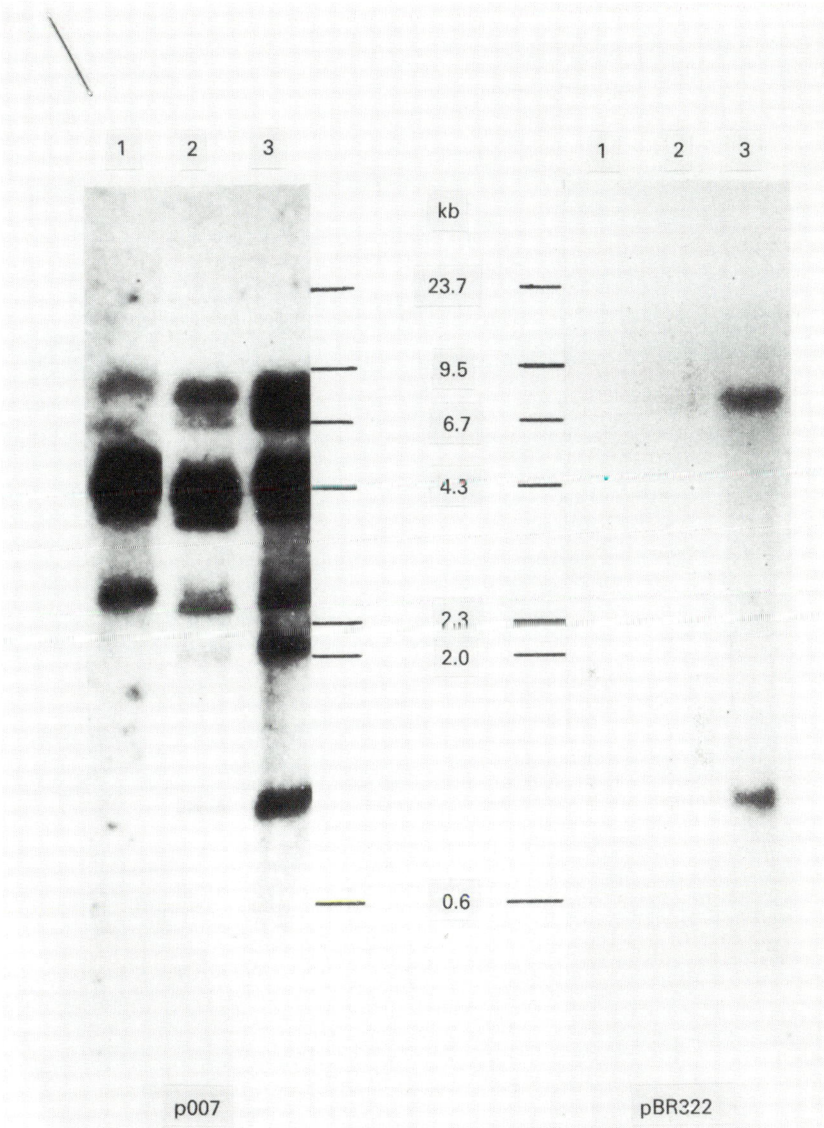

Fig. 4. Detection of the exogenous plasmid DNA in endothelial cells. The experimental procedure was as described in the legend to Fig. 1, except that 20 μg of endothelial cell DNA was used here. Autoradiography was for 24 h (Soriano *et al.*, 1983).

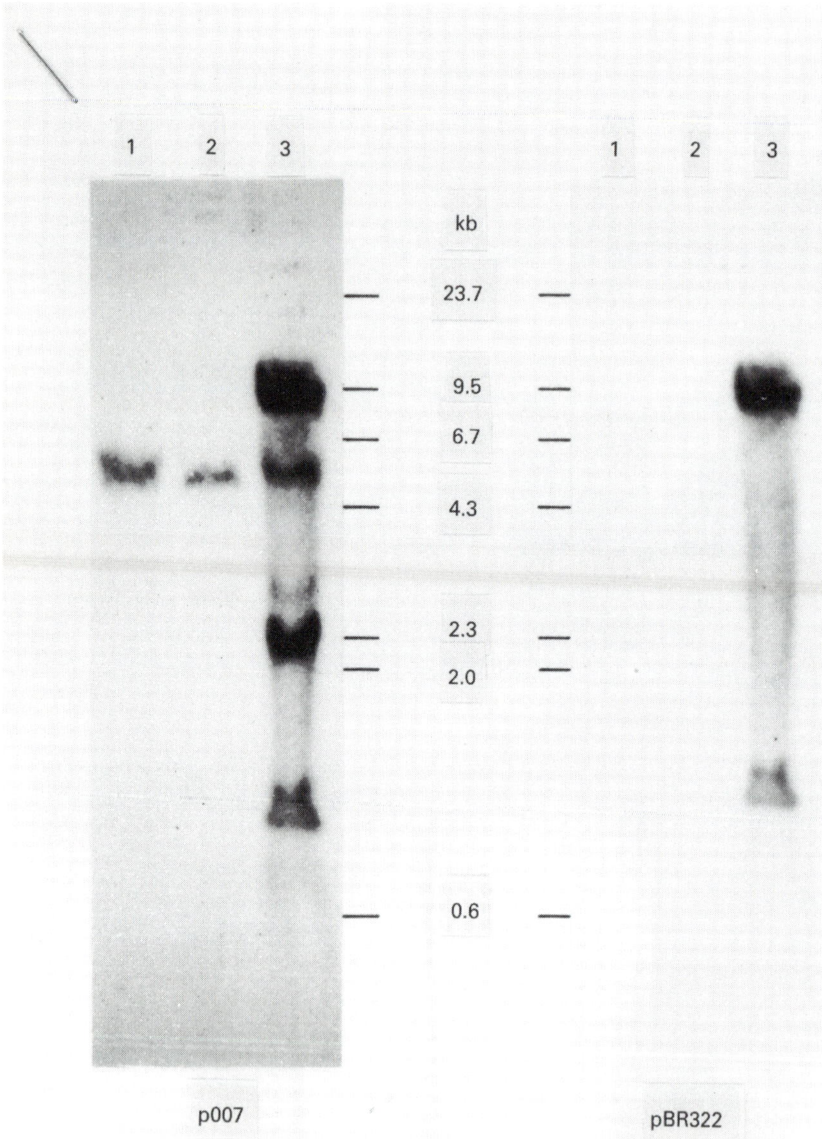

Fig. 5. Detection of the exogenous plasmid DNA in hepatocytes. The experimental procedure was as described in the legend to Fig. 1, except that 20 μg of hepatocyte DNA was used here. Autoradiography was for 12 days (Soriano *et al.*, 1983).

(Fig. 3, lane 2) and are much weaker in both endothelial cell (only visible on long exposures) and hepatocyte DNA fractions (Figs 4 and 5, lanes 2). Inclusion of LC within the lipid bilayer of the vesicles does not seem to have a great effect on the amount of exogenous DNA found in the Kupffer cells (Figs 4 and 5, lanes 2), although quantification of the hybridization data (see below and Table III) does reveal a small increase in this case. However, in both the endothelial cells and the hepatocytes, when LC liposomes are used a considerably larger amount of the plasmid is found in these cells than with PL liposomes (Figs 4 and 5, lanes 3). This effect is most marked in the endothelial cells. In all cases, a hybridization smear accompanied the presence of the plasmid bands and was accordingly found to be the strongest when the plasmid bands were the most intense.

By using pBR322 as a probe, the expected similar pattern of hybridization is observed, with the exception that there is no background hybridization (Figs 3–5, lanes 1) and that only two plasmid bands, 8.7 and 1.1 kb, are hybridized by the probe.

Quantification of the hybridization data was performed by scanning the autoradiograms of the Pst I-digested DNA samples with a microdensitometer. The results of this analysis are shown in Table III. The results presented further strengthen our previous observation on the expression of exogenous genes in adult animals (Nicolau *et al.*, 1983a). They demonstrate the feasibility of gene targeting to specific cells directly *in vivo*, within the limits the liposomes can reach, and thus further extend the application of gene transfer to eukaryotic cells.

Southern blot analysis shows that, with PL-cholesterol vesicles, the exogenous DNA is found in all liver cell fractions but in markedly different amounts. We have attempted to quantify the hybridization results by scanning the autoradiograms with a microdensitometer (Table III).

Table III. Distribution of the exogenous plasmid DNA among liver cell types 4 h after liposome administration (Soriano *et al.*, 1983).

	Plasmid copies, no. per cell		% of plasmid	
Cell type	PL liposomes	LC liposomes	PL liposomes	LC liposomes
Kupffer	12	16	>82	31
Endothelial	<0.2	8	<4	50
Hepatocytes	<0.2	1	<14	19

* Determined by assuming that the rat liver consists of 7% Kupffer cells, 23% endothelial cells and 70% hepatocytes.

Although the values we obtain are approximate values, they provide nonetheless an indication of the intrahepatic distribution of the liposome-entrapped plasmid. By using this method of quantification, it appears that with PL-cholesterol vesicles, Kupffer cells, although a minority in the liver cell population, are the major target of intravenously injected liposomes. This conclusion is in line with previous observations when labels other than DNA were used (Roerdink *et al.*, 1981; Spanjer and Scherphof, 1983).

Inclusion of LacCer in the lipid bilayer of the vesicles results in a significant change of the distribution pattern of the exogenous gene among the liver cells. Whereas with Kupffer cells only a minor increase in the amount of plasmid can be detected, a large increase is observed with both the endothelial cells and the hepatocytes. Quantification of the hybridization signals shows that, by using the "targeted" liposomes, all three cell fractions now become major targets.

The detection of the gene in the hepatocytes indicates that a fraction of the liposomes gained access to the liver parenchyma. For that to be possible, the liposomes must have crossed the endothelial lining of the sinusoid through the open fenestrations in these cells; indeed, there is a considerable overlap between the size range of the liposomes used (0.1–1.0 μm) and that of the fenestrations (0.1–0.3 μm; Nicolau *et al.*, 1983b).

The presence of a β-galactosyl receptor on the surface of hepatocytes is well documented (Ashwell and Morell, 1974). Wall *et al.* (1980) have shown that hepatocytes are the principal liver cells involved in the elimination of galactose-terminated glycoproteins from the blood circulation. The demonstrated function of the hepatocyte β-galactose-specific receptor in endocytosis might explain why liposomes exposing terminal non-reducing β-galactose residues are taken up much more readily than the non-glycosylated liposomes.

A galactose receptor similar to the one on hepatocytes has recently been reported on Kupffer cells (Kolb-Bachhofen *et al.*, 1982). This might account for the small increase observed in the amount of gene taken up by these cells when using the targeted liposomes. However, the very strong increase in uptake found in the endothelial cells is surprising because there is no galactose-specific receptor on these cells (Hubbard *et al.*, 1979). The liver endothelial cells have an endocytic activity (Simon, 1981). Nonetheless, despite the use of the same liposome concentrations, the very different efficiency of uptake of DNA entrapped in PL liposomes as compared to LC liposomes by the endothelial cells might point to uptake mechanisms other than straightforward endocytosis of the injected vesicles.

Concerning the intracellular localization of the exogenous plasmid DNA, it is possible to rule out any significant binding of DNA-loaded liposomes to the cell plasma membrane; the treatment used to separate the three types of liver cells, including density-gradient centrifugations and repeated washings, would indeed remove most liposomes. Moreover, the enzymatic treatment used to prepare the cell fractions (collagenase or pronase) would remove any adsorbed liposomes, because Pagano and Takeichi (1977) have shown that treatment of the cells with trypsin releases any adsorbed liposomes, suggesting a role for cell surface proteins. Lastly, should the cell separation procedure fail to remove all liposomes, it seems unlikely that such a significant fraction of them would be bound to the plasma membrane; indeed, we detect by Southern blotting up to 4 molecules of DNA per liver cell on average (Table III). This may be calculated as 6% of the injected dose (75 molecules of DNA per cell), assuming that the liver of a 220 g rat consists of 1400×10^6 cells and knowing that 50% of the liposomes are taken up by the liver (Nicolau *et al.*, 1983a).

Hepatocytes are secretory cells, having the enzymes required for the processing of prepolypeptides to polypeptides. This suggests that hepatocytes might qualify for the expression of liposome-transported insulin genes. The redistribution of the transported plasmid DNA among the liver cells, when changing from untargeted PL liposomes to targeted glycolipid-containing liposomes, leads to an uptake of 20% of all of the DNA recovered in the hepatocytes. This may prove to be significant for future work aimed at expression of the insulin gene in the liver in the physiologically active form of hormone.

B. Flow cytofluorometric studies of liposome targeting to hepatocytes

The results presented above showed, strictly speaking, that liposomal DNA associated with liver cells and that insertion of lactosylceramide in the liposome bilayer enhanced this association with hepatocytes and endothelial cells (Nicolau *et al.*, 1983a). In order to prove that the transfer of encapsulated material to the target cells is indeed enhanced, we used liposomes containing carboxyfluorescein and injected the animals intravenously. One hour later the animals had their livers perfused and then excised and the hepatocytes were separated (Grosse *et al.*, 1984). These cells were then analysed in a fluorescence-activated cell sorter analyser (FACS) for fluorescence. Carboxyfluorescein, a fluorescent dye which is self-quenched at high concentrations (Weinstein *et al.*, 1977), was entrapped in these liposomes. The internalization of the liposomes by the cells results in the release into the cytoplasm and dequenching of encapsulated carboxyfluorescein, causing an increase in the intensity of the cell-associated fluorescence.

Using this technique we demonstrate the influence of lactosylceramide in the liposome bilayer on the uptake of liposomes by hepatocytes after intravenous injection in mice.

(1) Liposome preparation

Liposomes encapsulating carboxyfluorescein were prepared by reverse-phase evaporation (Szoka and Papahadjopoulos, 1978). Briefly, 21 μmol of egg yolk PC (Sigma, purified according to Singleton *et al.*, 1965), ox brain phosphatidylserine (Sigma) and cholesterol (Sigma) were dissolved in 0.75 ml freshly distilled diethyl ether at a ratio of 4:1:5 mol/mol. The purity of the phospholipids was checked by thin-layer chromatography (TLC) in two solvent systems and they showed a single spot. The purity of the lactosylceramide (Sigma) was also checked by TLC. Liposome compositions are: PC:PS:cholesterol:lactosylceramide (4:1:5:0.5). Several mixtures of them were also used where the fraction of lactosylceamide liposomes varied from 25–100%. Carboxyfluorescein (Eastman), a mixture of isomers 5 and 6, was purified according to Leserman and Barbet (1982). Hydrophobic impurities were removed from carboxyfluorescein by adsorption chromatography on an LH-20 (Pharmacia) column (Leserman and Barbet, 1982).

Two hundred millimoles of carboxyfluorescein in 0.25 ml of phosphate-buffered saline (pH 7.4) were added to the diethyl ether solution of lipids and the mixture was sonicated. The diethyl ether was removed in a rotary evaporator under reduced pressure. Unencapsulated carboxyfluorescein was separated by repeated centrifugations at $100000 \times g$ and washing or by filtration on a Sepharose 4B column. Mixtures of liposome preparations were made which contained different percentages of lactosylceramide liposomes: 0%, 25%, 50%, 75% and 100%. The liposomes (fluorescence-quenched) were stored at 4°C under argon and used the same day.

The carboxyfluorescein content of the liposomes was determined by measuring the absorbance at 493 nm of a diluted liposome suspension in the presence of 1% Triton X-100. The size of the vesicle thus obtained was measured on a number of electron micrographs. Three hundred and fifty liposomes were analysed for each preparation. The average diameter of the liposomes was 260 nm, with sizes ranging from 50–500 nm. Addition of lactosylceramide changes neither the average size of the liposome nor their size distribution. Confirmation of the average diameter (260 nm) is also obtained from the fact that, as the spectroscopic assay shows, the encapsulated volume in our liposomes is 6 l/mol of phospholipid. This value corresponds to a liposome diameter of approximately 200 nm (Wilschut, 1982).

In order to see whether the phospholipid and lactosylceramide liposomes were subject to osmotic lysis, the variation of concentration-quenching of the encapsulated carboxyfluorescein was measured spectrofluorometrically over 48 h. During this time the quenching coefficient changed from 91% to 89% for both liposome preparations. Carboxyfluorescein was excited at 493 nm and the fluorescence emission was measured at 520 nm. A double-beam spectrofluorometer Fica MK-II was used.

The hepatocytes were isolated according to Klaunig *et al.* (1981). The animals were pre-perfused through the hepatic portal vein with 10 ml of pre-perfusion buffer [142 mM NaCl/6.7 mM KCl/10 mM Hepes (pH 7.4)] containing 0.04% EGTA, and then with 20 ml of EGTA-free pre-perfusion buffer. The liver was subsequently perfused with 35 ml of collagenase in buffer [120 mM NaCl/6.7 mM KCl/5 mM $CaCl_2$, $2H_2O$/5.5 mM glucose/20 mM Hepes (pH 7.5) and 0.05% collagenase (Boehringer)].

After perfusion the liver was excised and the cells sedimented at $1 \times g$ in Krebs buffer [120 mM NaCl/4.7 mM KCl/0.95 mM KH_2PO_4/1.2 mM $MgSO_4$, $7H_2O$/2.5 mM $CaCl_2$, $2H_2O$/5.5 mM glucose/10 mM Hepes (pH 7.4)]. The cells were filtered through nylon gauze (250, 100, 60 μm) and the filtrate containing mostly single cells was freed from contaminating non-parenchymal cells by repeated low-speed centrifugations (500 rpm). Viability of the cells, as assessed by their capacity to exclude Trypan blue, was 70–80%.

(2) Flow-cytofluorimetric analysis

Analysis of 5000 hepatocytes (after exclusion of the dead cells by light-scattering measurement in the cytofluorimeter) yields the results shown in Fig. 6a–c. The control hepatocytes, from animals inoculated with 200 mM of free, non-encapsulated carboxyfluorescein, show a weak non-specific fluorescence. This histogram is identical with that of hepatocytes isolated from uninoculated animals, indicating that free carboxyfluorescein injected intravenously is not taken up by hepatocytes 1 h after injection. When the animals have been injected with phospholipid liposomes containing carboxyfluorescein, the fluorescence emission shows a significant intensity enhancement (Fig. 6b). The intravenous inoculation with liposomes containing lactosylceramide further increases both the fluorescence intensity of the cells as well as the number of the strongly fluorescing cells (Fig. 6c), which is in qualitative agreement with the spectrofluorometric results. In Fig. 6a it is possible to distinguish three fluorescent populations. In the controls — i.e. hepatocytes from animals injected with free carboxyfluorescein — population 1 is very weakly fluorescent. This population shows the same weak intrinsic fluorescence in all hepatocyte preparations investigated, but the number of cells constituting it decreases from controls to lactosylceramide cells. Population 2 increases steadily from control cells to the lactosylceramide cells both in fluorescence intensity and in number of cells. The same holds for population 3. Remembering that the fluorescence scale is a logarithmic one, the increase in fluorescence intensity between control cells and lactosylceramide cells of population 3 is very significant. The mean

(a) Control spleen cells

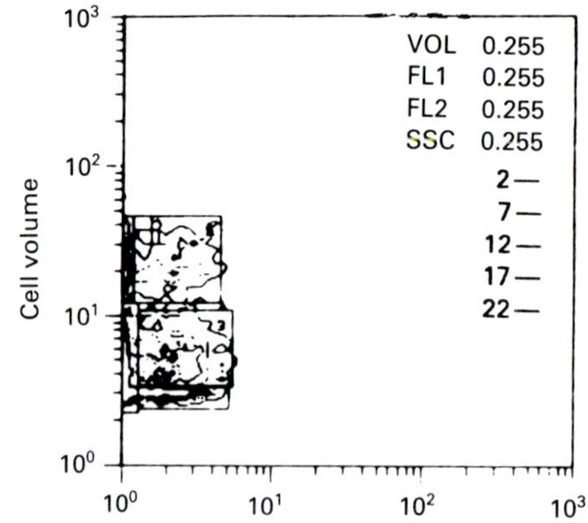

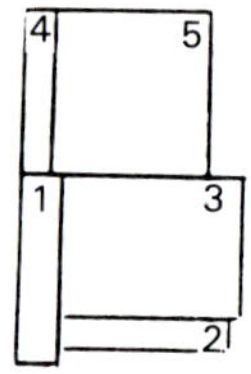

	% of cells in population	I_F
1	50.88	1.02
2	7.7	2.29
3	23.8	2.47
4	6.5	1.02
5	10.08	2.34

(b) Spleen cells PL-liposomes injected

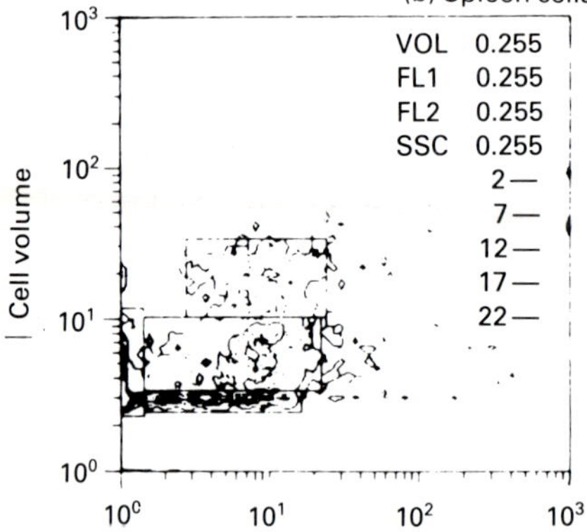

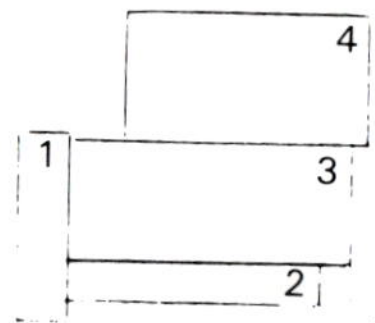

	% of cells in population	I_F
1	18.58	1.04
2	13.58	5.12
3	41.46	7.37
4	16.38	10.08

(c) Spleen cells C-liposomes injected

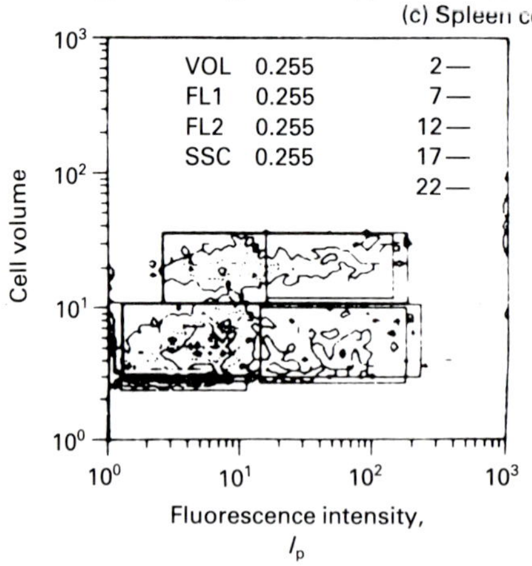

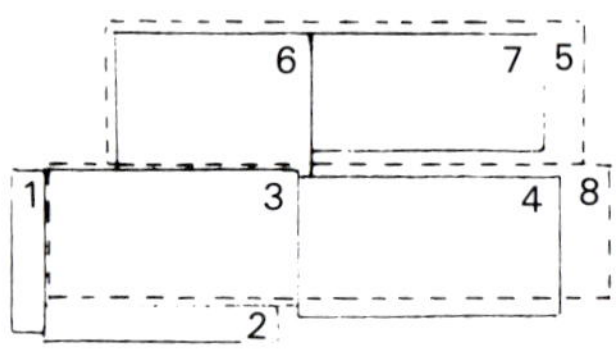

	% of cells in population	I_F
1	20.04	1.02
2	12.76	3.86
3	34.38	5.25
4	8.64	54.04
5	18.60	23.57
6	12.20	8.11
7	6.50	44.05
8	52.54	13.86

fluorescence intensity of this population goes from 5.16 for 41.6% of the phospholipid-treated cells to 8.36 for 47% of the lactosylceramide-treated cells.

When mixtures of phospholipid and lactosylceramide liposomes loaded with carboxyfluorescein were injected, the hepatocyte-associated fluorescence increased with the proportion of lactosylceramide liposomes (phospholipid liposomes only, 5.9; 25% lactosylceramide liposomes, 6.7; 50% lactosylceramide liposomes, 7.1; lactosylceramide liposomes only, 7.4. Values are the number of fluorescent cells ($\times 10^{-3}$). The results presented show that, upon insertion of lactosylceramide in the lipid bilayer of liposomes consisting of phospholipids and cholesterol, an increase both in association and uptake of these liposomes by hepatocyte cells is observed.

The increase of carboxyfluorescein fluorescence as a result of dilution-dequenching through the release of the dye from small liposomes (d = 30 nm) in the cell cytoplasm has been successfully used for the cytofluorimetric study of the uptake of targeted liposomes by cells *in vitro* (Truneh *et al.*, 1983). As these authors have indicated, once internalized, carboxy fluorescein is charge-neutralized by protonation in a low pH environment, rendering it membrane permeable and thus free to diffuse out into the cytoplasm (Truneh *et al.*, 1983).

Liposomes which have high cholesterol to LC or to phospholipid ratios have high stabilities and the release of carboxyfluorescein in the blood plasma is very low 150 min after intravenous inoculation (Kirby *et al.*, 1980). The observation of stronger fluorescence intensities in hepatocytes which have interacted with lactosylceramide liposomes suggests that not only do more cells take up liposomes upon lactosylceramide insertion in the bilayer, but each cell takes up a larger number of liposomes. The existence of the galactose-specific lectin on the hepatocyte plasma membrane (Ashwell and Morell, 1974) could possibly explain the increased interaction of the lactosylceramide-containing liposomes with the hepatocytes.

Fig. 6. Cytofluorimetric measurements of the uptake of carboxyfluorescein by hepatocytes. (a) Two-parameter analysis of control cells. On the ordinate is the cell volume; on the abcissa is the fluorescence intensity. Hepatocytes were separated by collagenase perfusion 1 h after intravenous injection of 200 mM carboxyfluorescein in phosphate-buffered saline into a mouse. The cells were not fixed. 5000 cells were analysed. I_F, fluorescence intensity. (b) Two-parameter analysis of hepatocytes separated from a mouse injected intravenously with PC/PS/cholesterol liposomes containing 200 mM of encapsulated carboxyfluorescein. The cells were isolated as described and were not fixed. 5000 cells were analysed. Lipid concentration, 8 μmol/mouse. (c) Two-parameter analysis of hepatocytes separated from a mouse injected intravenously with PC/PS/cholesterol/lactosylceramide liposomes containing 200 mM of encapsulated carboxyfluorescein. The cells were isolated as described and not fixed. 5000 cells were analysed. Lipid concentration 8 μmol/mouse. (Grosse *et al.*, 1984.)

This observation is in agreement with that of Spanjer and Scherphof (1983), who showed that lactosylceramide insertion in the liposome bilayer significantly enhances the uptake of small (sonication) liposomes by parenchymal cells, after intracardiac injection. They used [^{3}H] inulin as an aqueous marker. Using a much more sensitive detection procedure, namely Southern blot assay of the rat preproinsulin I gene transported by liposomes to the liver cells after intravenous injections, Soriano *et al.* (1983) showed that lactosylceramide liposomes (average diameter 260 nm) transferred 5 times as many gene copies to hepatocytes as did phospholipid liposomes. The sensitivity of this detection method is much higher than that of the [^{3}H] inulin counting, since as few as one gene copy per cell can be detected.

It appears that lactosylceramide insertion in the liposomes results not only in a higher degree of association of the liposomes with the hepatocytes, but also in an enhanced uptake of the liposomes by these cells (Grosse *et al.*, 1984).

VI. CONCLUSIONS

The data presented indicate that liposomes injected intravenously can be used successfully to transfer genetic material to cells within the reach of the liposomes. In the case of the rat preproinsulin I gene transient expression of this gene has been observed.

By inserting glycolipids in the liposome bilayer, it is possible to target the DNA-carrying liposomes to specific, non-phagocytosing cells of the liver and the spleen, provided that their sizes allow them to pass through the fenestrations of the endothelial cell lining. The terminal carbohydrate of the glycolipid seems to be recognized by surface sugar receptors (lectin) on hepatocytes; this leads to both an enhanced association of these liposomes with the hepatocytes and to increased uptake of the encapsulated material by the cells, as shown both by molecular hybridization assays and flow cytofluorimetry.

Further studies should be carried out in an attempt to construct DNA vectors for insulin expression with lasting expression and glucose regulation.

REFERENCES

Ashwell, G. and Morell, A. G. (1974). *Adv. Enzymol.* **41**, 99–128.

Bell, G. I., Pictet, R. and Rutter, W. J. (1980). *Nucl. Acids Res.* **8**, 4091–4109.

Cordell, B., Bell, G., Tischer, E., De Noto, F. M., Ulbrich, A., Pictet, R., Rutter, W. J. and Goodman, H. M. (1979). *Cell* **18**, 533–543.

Cudd, A. and Nicolau, C. (1984). *In* "Liposome Technology", (G. Gregoriadis, ed.) Vol. II, pp. 207–233. CRC Press, Boca Raton.
Fraley, R., Straubinger, R. M., Rule, G., Springer, E. L. and Papahadjopoulos, D. (1981). *Biochemistry* **20**, 6978–6987.
Freychet, P., Roth, J. and Neville, D. M. (1971). *Proc. Natl. Acad. Sci. USA* **68**, 1833–1837.
Ghosh, P., Das, P. K. and Bacchawat, B. K. (1982). *Arch. Biochem. Biophys.* **213**, 266–270.
Grosse, E., Kiéda, C. and Nicolau, C. (1984). *Biochim. Biophys. Acta* **805**, 354–361.
Hubbard, A. L., Wilson, G., Ashwell, G. and Stukenbrok, H. (1979). *J. Cell. Biol.* **83**, 47–64.
Kahn, C. R. and Roth, J. (1975). *Am. J. Clin. Pathol.* **63**, 656–668.
Kirby, C., Clarke, J. and Gregoriadis, G. (1980). *Biochem. J.* **186**, 591–598.
Klaunig, J. E., Goldblatt, P. J., Hinton, D. E., Lipsky, D. E., Chacko, M. M. and Trumpf, B. F. (1981). *In Vitro* **17**, 913–925.
Kolb-Bachhofen, V., Schlepper-Schäfer, J., Vogell, W. and Kolb, H. (1982). *Cell* **29**, 859–866.
Leserman, L. and Barbet, J. (1982). *In* "Liposome Technology", (L. Leserman and J. Barbet, eds) pp. 135–136. Les Editions INSERM, Paris.
Nicolau, C., Lepape, A., Soriano, P., Fargette, F. and Juhel, M. J. (1983a). *Proc. Natl. Acad. Sci. USA* **80**, 1068–1072.
Nicolau, C., Soriano, P., Lepape, A., Londos-Gagliardi, D., Legrand, A. and Grosse, E. (1983b). *Biol. Cell.* **47**, 121–131.
Nicolau, C., Legrand, A. and Soriano, P. (1984). *In* Ciba Foundation Symposium No. 103, "Cell Fusion", pp. 254–267. Pitman, London.
Nicolau, C., Legrand, A. and Grosse, E. (1985). *Methods Enzymol.*, in press.
Pagano, R. E. and Takeichi, M. (1977). *J. Cell. Biol.* **74**, 531–546.
Roerdink, F., Dijkstra, J., Hartman, G., Bolscher, G. and Scherphof, G. (1981). *Biochim. Biophys. Acta* **677**, 79–89.
Schäfer-Ridder, M., Wang, Y. and Hofschneider, P. H. (1982). *Science* **215**, 166–168.
Simon, G. T. (1981). *In* "The Reticuloendothelial System" (L. Carr and W. T. Daems, eds) pp. 481–482. Plenum Press, New York.
Singleton, W. S., Gray, M. S., Brown, M. L. and White, J. L. (1965). *J. Am. Oil Chem.* **42**, 53–61.
Soriano, P., Dijkstra, J., Legrand, A., Spanjer, H., Londos-Gagliardi, D., Roerdink, F., Scherphof, G. and Nicolau, C. (1983). *Proc. Natl. Acad. Sci. USA* **80**, 7128–7131.
Spanjer, H. H. and Scherphof, G. (1983). *Biochim. Biophys. Acta* **734**, 40–47.
Szoka, F., Jr and Papahadjopoulos, D. (1978). *Proc. Natl. Acad. Sci. USA* **75**, 4194–4198.
Truneh, A., Mishal, Z., Barbet, J., Machy, P. and Leserman, L. (1983). *Biochem. J.* **214**, 189–194.
Wall, A. D., Wilson, G. and Hubbard, A. L. (1980). *Cell* **21**, 79–93.
Weinstein, J. N., Yoshikami, S., Henkart, P., Blumenthal, R. and Hagins, W. A. (1977). *Science* **195**, 489–492.
Wilschut, J. (1982). *In* "Liposome Technology" (L. Leserman and J. Barbet, eds) pp. 9–24. Les Editions INSERM, Paris.
Wong, T. K., Nicolau, C. and Hofschneider, P. H. (1980). *Gene* **10**, 87–94.

10

Fusion-Mediated Microinjection of Macromolecules into Living Cultured Cells by "Targeted" Sendai Virus Envelopes

A. Loyter, A. G. Gitman, N. Chejanovsky and O. Nussbaum

I. INTRODUCTION

Infection of cells by enveloped animal viruses, belong to the paramyxovirus group, comprises two steps (Poste and Pasternak, 1978):

(a) Binding of virus particles to specific cell surface receptors, mainly sialic acid residues of glycoproteins and glycolipids (Poste and Pasternak, 1978). In the case of viruses of the paramyxovirus group, particularly Sendai virus particles, a specific viral envelope polypeptide, the haemagglutinin/neuraminidase (HN) glycoprotein, mediates binding between the virus particles and the cell surface sialic acid residues. Inactivation of the viral HN glycoprotein, either by proteolytic digestion (Sugawara *et al.*, 1982) or by reduction of its intramolecular S–S bonds with a reducing agent such as dithiothreitol (DTT) (Ozawa *et al.*, 1979), produces virus particles which are not able to attach to the appropriate cell receptors.

(b) Fusion of the viral envelope with the plasma membrane of the recipient cell with the concomitant injection of the viral nucleocapsid (Poste and Pasternak, 1978). The fusion process is mediated by a second viral envelope glycoprotein, the F (fusion) protein (Poste and Pasternak, 1978). The mechanism by which the F protein promotes fusion between the viral envelope and the cell plasma membrane is still obscure. Evidently, the virus–cell binding and the virus–cell fusion activities of Sendai virus particles are located in its envelope.

Microinjection and Organelle Transplantation Techniques

ISBN: 0-12-164722-6
ISBN: 0-12-164723-4 Pbk

In theory, an ideal vehicle for the efficient delivery of macromolecules directly to the cytoplasm of high numbers of living cells should be a membranous vesicle that will resemble membrane-enclosed viruses or, more specifically, the envelope of Sendai virus. Any molecule which can be enclosed within such a vesicle will be protected from digestion by any hydrolytic enzyme present during the delivery or fusion processes. Furthermore, such vesicles, like intact virus particles, should attach efficiently to specific receptors on the cell surface and then fuse with their plasma membranes.

Indeed, reconstituted viral envelopes which are vesicles containing the viral envelope phospholipids and the HN and F polypeptides, are able to promote cell agglutination, lysis and cell–cell fusion.

Trapping of macromolecules within Sendai virus envelopes has been achieved in two ways: (1) sonication of the virus particles in the presence of the macromolecules to be trapped (Uchida *et al.*, 1980); and (2) reconstitution of virus envelopes in a solution containing the soluble macromolecules (Uchida *et al.*, 1980; Loyter and Volsky, 1982; Loyter *et al.*, 1983). In this chapter we shall summarize and review work in which loaded, reconstituted Sendai virus envelopes (RSVE) have been used for the microinjection of molecules into living cells.

II. RECONSTITUTION OF FUSOGENIC SENDAI VIRUS ENVELOPES

Incubation of intact Sendai virus particles with non-ionic detergents such as Triton X-100 (Volsky and Loyter, 1978; Vainstein *et al.*, 1984) or Nonidet P-40 (Uchida *et al.*, 1980), results in complete solubilization of the viral envelope. The detergent-solubilized fraction contains both the viral phospholipid and the two envelope glycoprotein, namely the HN and F polypeptides, whose presence is essential for the promotion of virus–cell fusion (Poste and Pasternak, 1978; Loyter and Volsky, 1982). Removal of the detergent leads to the formation of empty, reconstructed Sendai virus envelopes (RSVE), which resemble the envelopes of intact Sendai virus particles but are devoid of the viral nucleocapsid (Volsky and Loyter, 1978; Loyter *et al.*, 1983; Vainstein *et al.*, 1984). Thus, it appears that RSVE are composed of relatively well-characterized and impermeable membranes, completely enclosing an aqueous space in which macromolecules can be trapped. Indeed, it has been shown that when soluble macromolecules or membrane components are present in the viral detergent-solubilized fraction, they are trapped within or inserted inside the membranes of the vesicles formed after removal of the detergent (Uchida *et al.*, 1980; Loyter and Volsky, 1982; Loyter *et al.*, 1983). Incubation of such loaded RSVE with cultured living cells at 37°C leads to fusion-mediated microinjection of the trapped material or transfer of the membrane components into the recipient cells (Loyter and Volsky, 1982; Loyter *et al.*, 1983; see also Chapter 12). RSVE, similar to resealed vesicles made of pure phospholipid molecules (liposomes) (Juliano *et al.*, 1983), have been used in the past few years as a biological carrier for the introduction of otherwise impermeable molecules into living cells. However, the use of RSVE as a biological carrier suffers from the following disadvantages:

(a) The RSVE obtained by the methods used during the past few years form a heterogeneous population of relatively small vesicles that are not as fusogenic as the intact Sendai virus (Volsky and Loyter, 1978; Loyter and Volsky, 1982). Moreover, since by the existing methods the detergent is removed from the mixture of the viral glycoproteins and phospholipids through a process of dialysis (Volsky and Loyter, 1978; Uchida *et al.*, 1980), it is practically impossible to trap molecules of low relative molecular mass within the vesicles formed after removal of the detergent.

(b) Both Sendai virus particles and RSVE interact and fuse with a wide variety of cells in culture because most of the cultured cells contain either sialoglycoproteins or sialoglycolipids as an integral part of their membrane (Gahmberg, 1977). Obviously, this makes the RSVE a very non-specific vehicle that will inject its content into almost any cell it encounters. If the only function of the Sendai virus HN glycoprotein were to bring the viral envelope into close contact with the recipient cell plasma membrane by binding to sialic acid residues and then allow their mutual fusion, it is conceivable that other molecules with similar binding activities would be able to substitute for the viral HN glycoprotein. An ideal fusogenic biological vehicle would be a vesicle containing the Sendai virus fusion factor and, instead of the viral HN glycoprotein, a specific binding molecule which would permit its interaction only with cells containing receptors for this molecule.

(c) The process of virus–cell and RSVE–cell fusion suffers from a lack of quantitative assay systems that would allow a better distinction between RSVE penetrating by endocytosis or via fusion with the plasma membrane.

Binding of virus particles to recipient cell membranes can be followed by the use of radiolabelled virus particles. However, many of the adsorbed virus particles fail to fuse with the membranes to which they are attached. The currently used methods for studying virus–cell fusion are semi-quantitative and indirect, based either on microscopic observations (Homma *et al.*, 1976) or lytic processes induced by enveloped viruses (Maeda *et al.*, 1977b).

In the present summary we describe attempts and experiments to overcome the above disadvantages.

(1) A new method for reconstituting highly fusogenic Sendai virus envelopes was developed in our laboratory recently (Vainstein *et al.*, 1984). As opposed to previously described techniques, in our new method the

detergent Triton X-100 is removed by direct addition of SM-2 Bio-beads to the detergent-solubilized mixture of the viral phospholipids and glycoproteins, therefore avoiding the long dialysis step. The vesicles obtained by this method resemble in their composition, size and features (Vainstein *et al.*, 1984) envelopes of intact Sendai virus particles. This method also allows the enclosure of low as well as high relative molecular mass material within the reconstituted viral envelopes.

(2) The fluorescent molecule *N*-4-nitro-benzo-2-oxa-1,3-diazole-phosphatidyl-ethanolamine (N-NBD-PE) has been inserted into Sendai virus envelopes, resulting in self-quenching. Incubation of fluorescent RSVE with biological membranes resulted in fluorescence dequenching. No change in the fluorescence value was observed when non-fusogenic RSVE were incubated with recipient cell membranes, showing that fluorescence dequenching can be used for a quantitative estimation of virus–membrane fusion (Chejanovsky and Loyter, 1985).

(3) A few methods for the construction of Sendai virus envelopes, bearing specific binding proteins such as antibodies or polypeptide hormones, have been developed recently in our laboratory (Gitman and Loyter, 1984; Gitman *et al.*, 1985). Anti-human erythrocyte antibodies (anti-HE-Ab) were inserted into the viral envelopes by the use of cross-linking reagents: succinimidyl-4-(*p*-maleimido-phenyl)butyrate (SMPB) and *N*-succinimidyl-3-(2-pyridyldithio)-propionate (SPDP). In addition, anti-HE-Ab or insulin molecules were covalently attached to the viral envelope glycoproteins. Our experiments clearly demonstrate that such "targeted" RSVE could interact and fuse with human erythrocytes (HE) or cultured cells from which the native viral receptors have been removed by treatment with neuraminidase (Gitman and Loyter, 1984; Gitman *et al.*, 1985). In addition, we have shown (Chejanovsky *et al.*, 1985) that specific hybrid antibody molecules can also be used for affinity targeting of RSVE to human erythrocytes devoid of virus receptors. Hybrid antibody molecules were obtained by chemical coupling of F(ab′) fragments obtained from anti-Sendai virus antibodies (anti-SV-Ab) to F(ab′) fragments obtained from anti-human erythrocyte antibodies (anti-HE-Ab). These hybrid antibodies were able to mediate binding and fusion of RSVE to desialized human erythrocytes (Chejanovsky *et al.*, 1985).

III. A NEW METHOD FOR THE RECONSTITUTION OF SENDAI VIRUS ENVELOPES: FUSION-MEDIATED INJECTION OF SV_{40}-DNA USING DNA-LOADED RECONSTITUTED SENDAI VIRUS ENVELOPES

Fusogenic vesicles can be prepared after solubilization of intact Sendai virus particles with a non-ionic detergent such as Triton X-100 (Volsky and

Loyter, 1978). However, removal of the detergent was previously performed by a long dialysis step (Volsky and Loyter, 1978; Uchida *et al.*, 1980). The use of dialysis as one of the steps in the reconstitution process prevented the trapping of molecules of low relative molecular mass because the dialysis tubings used are permeable to molecules with a relative molecular mass less than 14000 (Volsky and Loyter, 1978). In addition, the long dialysis process required (72 to 96 h) may cause inactivation of molecules of a certain biological activity such as enzymes or specific antibodies.

Recently (Vainstein *et al.*, 1984) we have developed a new method for the reconstitution of highly fusogenic vesicles made of Sendai virus envelopes. In this method we have avoided the long dialysis period by the addition of SM-2 Bio-beads directly to extremely small volumes of detergent-solubilized viral glycoproteins and phospholipids. Removal of the detergent leads to the formation of fusogenic vesicles which resemble intact virus particles much more than those prepared by previous methods, both in their appearance and activity (Vainstein *et al.*, 1984).

The results in Table I show that the amount of Triton X-100 remaining in the RSVE prepared by the new method of direct addition of SM-2 Bio-beads is very low, only about 0.005% (w/v), thus giving a molar ratio of Triton X-100 to envelope phospholipids of 0.02:0.03 (Vainstein *et al.*, 1984). Based on an average relative molecular mass of the viral glycoproteins of about

Table I. Preparation and trapping efficiencies of Sendai virus envelopes reconstituted by the "dialysis method" or by direct addition of SM-2 Bio-beads.

Method of removing Triton X-100 for RSVE reconstitution	Triton X-100 in RSVE (%, in w/v)	Trapping efficiency (% of total added)	
		^{32}P-DNA	$Na_3{}^{32}PO_4$
Dialysis in Spectraphor tubing	0.020	2–4	0
Direct addition of SM-2 Bio-beads	0.005	7–8	1

Sendai virus particles were dissolved by Triton X-100 essentially as described earlier (Volsky and Loyter, 1978; Vainstein *et al.*, 1984). After shaking for 1 h at 20°C, the detergent soluble material was removed by centrifugation (100000 × g for 60 min). Triton X-100 was removed either by dialysis in Spectraphor tubing (Volsky and Loyter, 1978) or by the direct addition of SM-2 Bio-beads (Vainstein *et al.*, 1984). The turbid suspension obtained (containing reconstituted viral envelopes) was centrifuged at 100000 × *g* for 1 h. The pellet was then suspended in 100 μl of Solution A (160 mM NaCl and 20 mM Tricine-HCl, pH 7.4). The amount of Triton X-100 in the different preparations was determined by the use of [^{3}H]Triton X-100. Trapping of macromolecules (DNA) was performed as follows: [^{3}H]labelled pBR322 (Vainstein *et al.*, 1983) or $Na_3{}^{32}PO_4$ (Vainstein *et al.*, 1984) were added to the detergent soluble fraction obtained after centrifugation of the detergent insoluble viral components. After removal of the detergent and obtaining RSVE, externally adsorbed DNA was hydrolysed by pancreatic DNase I (Loyter *et al.*, 1983; Vainstein *et al.*, 1984). At the end of the incubation period, the RSVE were collected by centrifugation, and radioactivity associated with the viral envelopes was estimated by scintillation counter following their solubilization with picofluor (Packard).

60000 (Poste and Pasternak, 1978), the calculated molar ratio of Triton to viral glycoproteins is 2:3. This is significantly lower than the amount of detergent (Triton X-100) left in RSVE prepared by the previously described methods (Loyter and Volsky, 1982). Table I also shows that macromolecules such as DNA can be enclosed within the RSVE prepared by direct addition of SM-2 Bio-beads, with an efficiency slightly higher than that obtained with the previously described methods. Furthermore, the new technique allows, for the first time, the trapping of molecules of low relative molecular mass such as $Na_3{}^{32}PO_4$ within the reconstituted viral envelopes. It is therefore obvious that the resealed fusogenic envelopes may be of great potential as a vehicle for transferring DNA molecules into living cells. This is so because the DNA molecules are protected from hydrolysis by serum or cell-secreted nucleases.

The results in Table II demonstrate that RSVE can serve as a carrier for the introduction of biologically active SV40 DNA into permissive cells. Fusion of SV40 DNA-loaded RSVE with CV1 cells induced the synthesis of SV40 T antigen in the recipient cells. SV40 DNA molecules were trapped within RSVE as described in Table I and elsewhere (Loyter *et al.*, 1983).

The best results were obtained with RSVE reconstituted by the direct addition of SM-2 Bio-beads (Table II). These DNA-loaded viral envelopes induced the synthesis of T antigen in 55% of the cells, as compared to synthesis in 20% of the cells when RSVE, prepared by the previous method (long dialysis step), were used. Our results (Loyter *et al.*, 1983; Vainstein *et al.*, 1983) clearly indicate that the induction of SV40 T antigen in CV1 cells and in other cell lines is due to fusion-mediated microinjection of the DNA and not to entry of DNA by other routes. In control or untreated cells, synthesis of T antigen was observed in less than 0.2% of the cells (Loyter *et al.*, 1983).

In our laboratory (Vainstein *et al.*, 1983), loaded RSVE were used also to

Table II. Induction of SV40 T antigen in CV_1 cells by fusion-mediated injection of SV40 DNA.

Method of reconstitution of SV40 DNA in RSVE	T antigen positive cells (% of total)
Dialysis method	20
Direct addition of SM-2 Bio-beads	55

Fusion of DNA-loaded RSVE with monolayers of CV1, an African green monkey kidney cell line, was performed as described previously (Loyter *et al.*, 1983). After fusion-mediated injection of SV40 DNA, the cells on a coverslip were allowed to grow between 24 and 48 h. At the end of the growth period, the cells were dried and stained with rhodamine B-conjugated immunoglobulin G from hamster anti-SV40 serum as previously described (Graessmann *et al.*, 1976).

transfer the HSV-TK gene (*Herpes simplex* thymidine kinase gene) to LTK$^-$ cells with relatively high efficiency. This was found from experiments showing that about 0.08–0.1% of LTK$^-$ cells which were incubated with RSVE loaded with the plasmid PTK×1 were transformed to LTK$^+$ (Vainstein *et al.*, 1983; see also Chapter 12). The LTK$^+$ cells, after cultivation in HAT medium, showed an 8-fold increase in the activity of the enzyme thymidine kinase, as compared to the activity of the enzyme in control, untransformed cells (LTK$^-$ cells).

IV. THE USE OF FLUORESCENT PROBES FOR THE QUANTITATIVE ESTIMATION OF FUSION BETWEEN RSVE AND BIOLOGICAL MEMBRANES

For the construction of a highly fusogenic and efficient biological vehicle, a quantitative assay system to follow RSVE–cell fusion is necessary. Fluorescent molecules have recently been used to study fusion processes occurring between pure phospholipid liposomes. When the fluorescent molecules N-NBD-PE were inserted into phospholipid liposomes at relatively high concentrations, their fluorescence was reduced due to self-quenching (Shroit and Pagano, 1981). Dilution of the N-NBD-PE due to fusion processes led to fluorescence dequenching (Shroit and Pagano, 1981).

We have recently shown (Chejanovsky and Loyter, 1985) that fluorescent RSVE can be prepared, if the above fluorescent probe N-NBD-PE is added to the detergent solution of the Sendai virus phospholipids and glycoproteins. Removal of the detergent results in the formation of vesicles containing the viral phospholipids and the fluorescent molecules within the same membrane in a weight ratio of viral lipids to N-NBD-PE of 96:4.

The results in Table III show that incubation of fluorescent RSVE with human erythrocyte ghosts (HEG) or Friend erythroleukemic cells (FELC) yielded a significant increase in the fluorescence value. Such an increase in the fluorescence degree was not observed when non-fusogenic viral envelopes such as trypsinized or PMSF-treated RSVE were incubated at 37°C with HEG. The results in Table III also show that anti-viral antibodies which are known to inhibit fusion between the viral envelopes and biological membranes (Loyter and Volsky, 1982), inhibited the increase in fluorescence observed upon incubation of fluorescent RSVE and HEG as well. Our results (Table III) show, too, that very little fluorescence dequenching (about 6–7%) occurred when fluorescent RSVE were incubated at 37°C with glutaraldehyde-fixed HEG or FELC. RSVE are able to bind to and agglutinate glutaraldehyde-fixed cells and to promote lipid–lipid exchange, but are incapable of fusing with these cells (Maeda *et al.*, 1977a). Hence, based on our observations (Table III), it can be inferred that most of the dequenching observed upon interaction of RSVE with HEG is due to fusion between the viral envelopes and the erythrocyte membranes, and only very little (6–7%) of the total increase in the fluorescence value is contributed by lipid–lipid exchange.

Based on the above results, one can deduce that the dequenching observed in fluorescent RSVE can be used as a quantitative system to estimate, in a given system such as HEG or FELC, the number (or percentage) of RSVE which are fused with recipient cell membranes.

The results are given in Table IV, which show that incubation of relatively low amounts of fluorescent RSVE (0.5 μg) with relatively high amounts (200 μg) of HEG resulted in maximum dequenching in the fluorescence of the virus-associated NBD. This indicates that at a high HEG/RSVE ratio,

Table III. Fusion between RSVE and human erythrocyte ghosts or Friend erythroleukemic cells as monitored by fluorescence dequenching.

System	Fluorescence dequenching (%)
RSVE + HEG	98.4
RSVE + anti-RSVE-Ab + HEG	2.0
Tryps-RSVE + HEG	3.2
PMSF-RSVE + HEG	0
RSVE + glutaraldehyde-fixed HEG	6.6
RSVE + FELC	55
Tryps-RSVE + FELC	8
RSVE + glutaraldehyde-fixed FELC	<1

Fluorescent RSVE were prepared by the addition of 2.5–3 mg protein of detergent (Triton X-100)-solubilized Sendai viral phospholipids and glycoproteins to a thin layer of 170 μg of N-NBD-PE, to give a ratio of 94:6 viral lipids:N-NBD-PE (w/w) as described previously (Chejanovsky and Loyter, 1985). After this addition, the mixture was shaken and the detergent was removed, again as described previously (Vainstein *et al.*, 1984). Fluorescent RSVE were incubated with either 300 μg of human erythrocyte ghosts (HEG) or with about 1.5×10^6 cultured FELC for 2 min at room temperature (20°C) to allow binding of virions to the cell membranes. After determination of the fluorescence degree (zero time of incubation), the systems were incubated for 30 min at 37°C, after which the degree of fluorescence was again estimated. Total fluorescence dequenching was estimated by addition of Triton X-100 (0.1% final concentration) to the incubation system, as described (Chejanovsky and Loyter, 1985).

All fluorescence measurements were performed on a Perkin Elmer MPF-4 spectrofluorimeter or on a Spex computerized spectrofluorimeter. NBD fluorescence was measured at 473 nm excitation and 545 nm emission (Chejanovsky and Loyter, 1985). The dequenching degree (of the N-NBD-PE) was determined as described before (Schroit and Pagano, 1981; Chejanovsky and Loyter, 1985).

The fluorescent RSVE were treated with trypsin (Tryps-RSVE) or with PMSF (PMSF-RSVE) as previously described (Chejanovsky and Loyter, 1985). Fixation of HEG and FELC with glutaraldehyde (0.1%) as well as preparation of anti-Sendai virus antibodies (anti-RSVE-Ab) were as described previously (Chejanovsky and Loyter, 1985).

Table IV. Quantitative estimation of RSVE-HEG fusion by the use of fluorescent RSVE

System	Fluorescence dequenching (%)
Fusogenic RSVE	98
Fusogenic RSVE + non-fusogenic RSVE (1:1, w/w)	47
Fusogenic RSVE + non-fusogenic RSVE (1(4, w/w)	19

Fluorescent, active RSVE (2.5 μg) were incubated with 200 μg of HEG at 37°C, at the end of which increasing concentrations of trypsinized RSVE (non-fusogenic RSVE) were added, and the suspension was allowed to incubate for another 20 min at 37°C. At the end of the incubation period, the fluorescence degree was estimated as described on p. 186 and elsewhere (Chejanovsky and Loyter, 1985). All other experimental conditions were as described before (Chejanovsky and Loyter, 1985).

most of the RSVE in the population fused (92–93%) with the HEG membranes. It is thus expected that addition of increasing concentrations of non-fusogenic fluorescent RSVE to the system will result in a decrease in the percentage of dequenching observed after incubation at 37°C. Indeed, the results in Table IV show that at a 1:1 (w/w) ratio of fusogenic to non-fusogenic (trypsinized) RSVE, in which theoretically 50% of the RSVE in the population are expected to fuse, 47% of dequenching was observed at the end of the incubation period. At a ratio of 1:4 (w/w) of fusogenic to non-fusogenic RSVE, where 20% of the population are expected to fuse, 19% of dequenching was observed (Table IV). These results demonstrate that fluorescent RSVE can be used for a quantitative estimation of RSVE–membrane fusion. In addition, this method will allow us to follow the fusogenic properties of liposomes containing various amounts of the viral F or HN glycoproteins. This, in turn, may lead to the construction of highly fusogenic vesicles which will become an efficient vehicle for the introduction of macromolecules into the recipient cell cytoplasm.

V. TARGETING OF RSVE TO NEURAMIDASE-TREATED CELLS

During recent years, efforts have been made to couple specific antibodies or other ligands to phospholipid liposomes with the aim of constructing a specific "targeted" liposome. It appears that the most efficient method is to couple chemically IgG or F(ab) molecules to the amino groups of phospholipids via cross-linking reagents such as SPDP or SMPB (Martin *et al.*, 1982). Indeed, liposomes bearing specific antibodies interacted effectively with cells carrying the appropriate antigens (Martin *et al.*, 1982).

Construction of "targeted" RSVE is a more complicated process. Such a method should result in the neutralization of the virus binding protein, the HN glycoprotein, while preserving the virus fusogenic activity. Recently (Tomasi *et al.*, 1982) the cross-linking reagent SPDP has been used to couple chemically anti-human erythrocyte antibodies to the envelope glycoproteins of intact Sendai virus particles. Virus particles to which anti-human erythrocyte antibodies (anti-HE-Ab) were attached were able to agglutinate and bind to human erythrocytes (HE) from which the virus receptors were removed by treatment with neuraminidase (Tomasi *et al.*, 1982). However, fusion between Sendai virus particles and neuraminidase-treated HE, as monitored by virus-induced haemolysis, was very low. This may be due to the fact that the two viral polypeptides, the HN and F glycoproteins, were inactivated by the chemical modification (reduction with DTT) required for the coupling reaction.

Experiments in our laboratory (Nussbaum *et al.*, 1984) and in others (Heath *et al.*, 1983) indicated that the viral HN glycoprotein has a dual function in the virus–membrane fusion process; in addition to its function as a binding protein, it also plays a crucial role in the membrane fusion step. From these observations (Heath *et al.*, 1983; Nussbaum *et al.*, 1984), it became clear that in "targeted" RSVE the two viral envelope glycoproteins should remain active and intact. To achieve this goal, we have recently (Gitman and Loyter, 1984; Chejanovsky *et al.*, 1985; Gitman *et al.*, 1985) developed three different methods through which highly fusogenic "targeted" RSVE can be constructed (see scheme in Fig. 1):

(a) The cross-linking reagent SMPB was used to attach covalently anti-HE-A6 to the thiol-containing paraffin, dodecanethiol (Gitman and Loyter, 1984). The complex formed, dodecanethiol-MPB (maleimidophenylbutyrate) antibody was then added to a detergent solution containing the viral phospholipids and glycoproteins. Removal of the detergent led to the formation of vesicles containing intact, unmodified viral glycoproteins and the dedocanethiol–MPB antibody complex within the same membrane. The results in Table V show that RSVE bearing anti-HE-Ab were able to interact and fuse with neuraminidase-treated HE. Fusion is inferred from the ability of the "targeted" (bearing antibodies) RSVE to induce haemolysis of neuraminidase-treated HE. Induction of cell lysis by enveloped viruses, especially by Sendai virus particles, has been shown to reflect a virus–cell fusion process (Maeda *et al.*, 1977b). It is noteworthy that DTT-reduced RSVE-bearing anti-HE-Ab were able to agglutinate (bind to) desialized (neuraminidase-treated) HE, but failed to haemolyse them (Table V). Reduction of RSVE with DTT under the conditions used specifically inactivated the viral HN glycoprotein without affecting the viral fusion (F) polypeptide (Gitman and Loyter, 1984). Hence, these results confirm

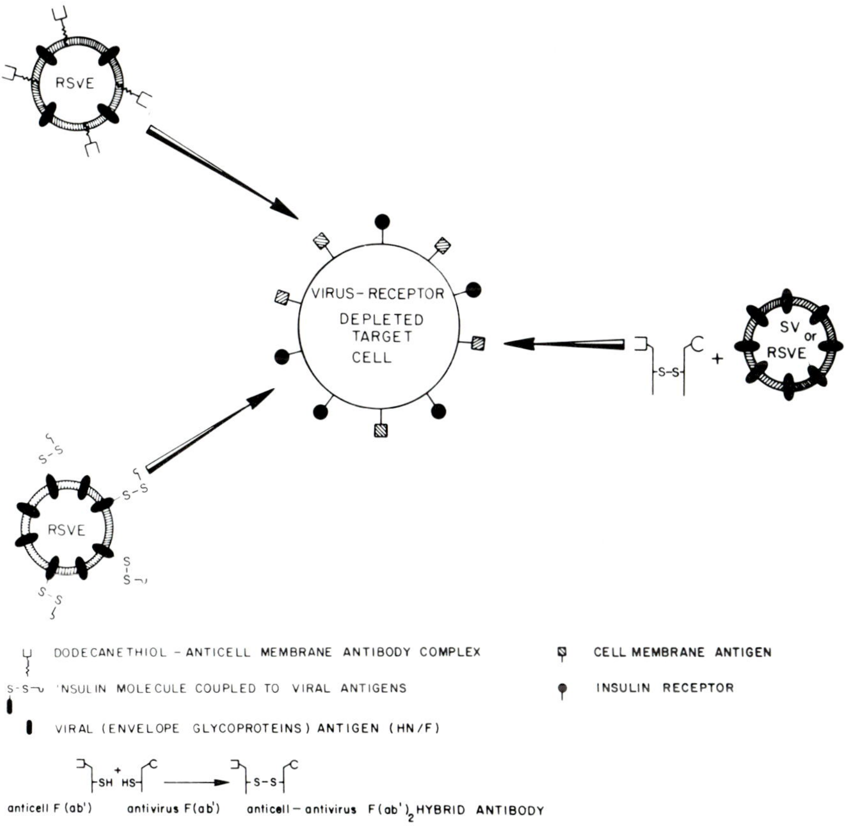

Fig. 1. Schematic illustration of the different methods used for the preparation of "targeted" RSVE.

previous observations indicating that the viral HN glycoprotein, besides mediating binding of the viral particles to cell membranes, also plays an active role in the fusion (haemolytic) process. The involvement of the viral fusion factor in the haemolysis obtained by "targeted" RSVE (RSVE-Ab) is evident from the results showing that PMSF greatly inhibited haemolysis but not agglutination of desialized human erythrocytes induced by RSVE-Ab (Table V) (see also Gitman and Loyter, 1984).

(b) A second method for the construction of highly fusogenic "targeted" RSVE is to couple proteins such as specific antibodies or polypeptide hormones to the viral envelope glycoproteins after they have been solubilized with Triton X-100 (Gitman *et al.*, 1985). Using this method, anti-HE-Ab or insulin molecules were covalently coupled to the viral HN

Table V. The ability of anti-human erythrocyte antibodies to mediate binding and fusion of RSVE to desialized human erythrocytes.

System	Agglutination of desialized human erythrocytes	Haemolysis of desialized human erythrocytes
(a) "Targeted" RSVE were constructed by the use of dodecanethiol to insert IgG into RSVE membranes		
RSVE	−	7
RSVE-Ab	+	63
DTT–RSVE-Ab	+	9
RSVE–human-IgG	−	6
RSVE-Ab + PMSF	+	16
(b) "Targeted" RSVE were constructed by coreconstitution of viral glycoproteins bearing antibodies with unmodified glycoproteins		
RSVE	−	5
RSVE-Ab	+	45
RSVE-Ab + F(ab) fragment	−	12
RSVE–human IgG	−	9
(c) Targeting of RSVE by the use of anti-SV–anti-HE $F(ab')_2$ preparation		
RSVE	−	11.0
RSVE + anti-SV–anti-HE	+	59.0
RSVE + anti-SV–anti-SV	−	3.5
RSVE + anti-HE–anti-HE	+*	7.5
RSVE + anti-SV–anti-SV + anti-HE–anti-HE	+*	3.8
RSVE + anti-SV–rabbit IgG	−	9.0

* Agglutination is due to the presence of anti-HE–anti-HE $F(ab')_2$ fragments.

(a) Anti-human erythrocyte antibody (anti-HE-Ab) was first coupled to dodecanethiol, using SMPB as a bifunctional cross-linking reagent, and then the IgG-MPB-dodecanethiol complex was inserted into RSVE as described before (Gitman and Loyter, 1984). Human IgG was inserted into RSVE by the same method. All other experimental conditions of reduction of RSVE with DTT or treatment with PMSF were as described earlier (Gitman and Loyter, 1984).

(b) Haemolytic RSVE bearing anti-HE-Ab (RSVE-Ab) were obtained by mixing detergent-solubilized, modified viral glycoproteins (viral glycoproteins with covalently attached anti-HE-Ab) with unmodified detergent-solubilized viral glycoproteins, as described previously (Gitman *et al.*, 1985). RSVE–human-IgG were likewise obtained, except that MPB–human-IgG was attached to the viral glycoproteins instead of anti-HE-Ab. F(ab) fragments of anti-HE-Ab were prepared as described previously (Gitman *et al.*, 1985).

(c) All the $F(ab')_2$ molecules were obtained after reoxidation of the appropriate F(ab'), as described before (Chejanovsky *et al.*, 1985).

Incubation with desialized HE and estimation of virus-induced agglutination and haemolysis were as previously described (Gitman and Loyter, 1984; Chejanovsky *et al.*, 1985).

and F polypeptides with SMPB as a cross-linking reagent. RSVE bearing covalently attached anti-HE-Ab or insulin molecules were able to bind to, but not to fuse with, virus receptor-depleted human erythrocytes or HTC (Gitman *et al.*, 1985). Only coreconstitution of Sendai virus glycoproteins, bearing attached anti-HE-Ab or insulin molecules, with intact untreated viral glycoproteins led to the formation of fusogenic "targeted" RSVE (Loyter *et al.*, 1984; Gitman *et al.*, 1985; see also scheme in Fig. 1), again indicating the requirement for both Sendai virus envelope glycoproteins for the fusion process. The results in Table V show that RSVE containing active viral glycoproteins and bearing anti-HE-Ab were able to agglutinate (bind to) and haemolyse (fuse with) neuraminidase-treated HE. Our results (Gitman *et al.*, 1985; and Table V) show that binding and fusion of RSVE-Ab with neuraminidase-treated HE was inhibited by the monovalent F(ab) fragments obtained from anti-HE-Ab. The specific requirement for anti-HE-Ab for allowing interaction of RSVE with neuraminidase-treated HE was also evident from these results (Gitman *et al.*, 1985; and Table V), showing that covalently attached human IgG (or BSA, not shown) did not substitute for covalently attached anti-HE-Ab. RSVE bearing human IgG neither bind to nor induce haemolysis of desialized HE (Table V).

(c) In order to avoid chemical modification or manipulation of the Sendai virus envelope, as was required in the methods summarized above (a and b), and yet be able to use molecules of specific binding properties for mediating the binding of virus particles to receptor-depleted cells, we studied in our laboratory (Chejanovsky *et al.*, 1985) the function of hybrid antibody molecules. Hybrid antibody molecules are $F(ab')_2$ molecules each of whose F(ab′) fragment possesses a different binding specificity (Nisonoff and Rivers, 1961; see scheme in Fig. 1). We constructed hybrid antibody molecules by coupling F(ab′) fragments obtained from anti-Sendai virus antibody (anti-SV-Ab) to F(Ab′) fragments obtained from anti-HE-Ab. These specific hybrid antibodies were formed after reoxidation of chemically reduced anti-SV-Ab and anti-HE-Ab $F(ab')_2$ fragments (Chejanovsky *et al.*, 1985; and scheme in Fig. 1). As a model system, the ability of such hybrid antibodies to mediate binding and fusion (virus-induced agglutination and haemolysis) to neuraminidase-treated HE was studied. The results in Table V(c) show that, similarly to the above two methods (a and b), RSVE "targeted" by the use of hybrid antibodies were also able to bind to (agglutinate) and fuse with (haemolyse) desialized human erythrocytes. Neither hybrid molecules obtained after reoxidation of a mixture containing anti-SV F(ab′) and F(ab′) of rabbit IgG nor $F(ab')_2$ fragments consisting of anti-SV-anti-SV or anti-HE-anti-HE or a mixture of the latter, could stimulate virus-induced agglutination or haemolysis in neuraminidase-treated HE (Table V).

VI. "TARGETED" SENDAI VIRUS ENVELOPES AS A BIOLOGICAL CARRIER

It has been mentioned above (see results in Table II) that loaded Sendai virus envelopes can serve as an efficient carrier for the microinjection of SV40 DNA into permissive cells such as African green monkey kidney cells. The results in Table VI show that loaded Sendai virus envelopes can also transfer their content into virus receptor-depleted cells, namely, cultured cells from which the virus receptors have been removed by treatment with neuraminidase. This can be achieved if specific antibodies (not shown) or insulin molecules (Table VI) are chemically coupled to the virus envelope glycoproteins, substituting for the virus binding protein (HN glycoprotein).

The results in Table VI confirm previous observations (Loyter *et al.*, 1983) and those in Table II, showing that RSVE serve as an efficient vehicle for transferring SV40 DNA, this time into HTC cells. SV40 T antigen appeared in 47% of the HTC incubated with loaded RSVE. However, synthesis of SV40 T antigen was not induced in desialized HTC (Table VI), indicating that the RSVE failed to fuse with and therefore transfer their content into these virus receptor-depleted cells. On the other hand, when the desialized HTC were incubated with insulin-bearing, loaded RSVE, SV40 T antigen appeared in 35% of the cells (Table VI). Addition of free insulin to this system completely avoided the appearance of the SV40 T antigen in the desialized HTC, clearly showing that binding and fusion of the "targeted" RSVE to the cells was mediated by the virus-associated insulin molecules. This can also be inferred from the results in Table VI showing that virus envelopes, to which BSA molecules had been chemically coupled, were able to transfer the SV40 DNA to non-treated cells but not to virus receptor-depleted cells, i.e. desialized HTC.

Similar observations were obtained when using RSVE loaded with fragment A of the plant toxin ricin (ricin A) (Oeltman and Health, 1979). Ricin is a potent toxin composed of two subunits, the B subunit whose function is to mediate binding of the whole toxin to cell surface receptors, and the A subunit which, after being transferred to the intracellular space, causes inhibition of protein synthesis and eventually cell death (Oeltman and Heath, 1979). Fragment A of the toxin, by itself — in the absence of the B subunit — is harmless, unless it is microinjected into the intracellular space of living cells (Oeltman *et al.*, 1979). Indeed, the results in Table VI show that very little, if any, inhibition of protein synthesis was caused by incubation of non-treated or desialized HTC with a solution containing free ricin A. Nevertheless, when ricin A was enclosed within Sendai virus envelopes and the resulting loaded RSVE were incubated with HTC, about 98% inhibition of protein synthesis was observed (Table VI). Only a 15%

Table VI. Fusion-mediated microinjection of SV40 DNA and ricin A by "targeted" RSVE.

System	T antigen positive cells in hepatoma tissue cultured cells (% of total)		Inhibition of protein synthesis in hepatoma tissue cultured cells (%)	
	Desialized	Non-treated	Desialized	Non-treated
(a) RSV loaded with SV40 DNA				
RSVE	0	47		
RSVE-Ins	35	41		
RSVE-BSA	0	43		
RSVE-Ins + free insulin	0	N.D.*		
(b) RSVE loaded with fragment A of ricin				
RSVE			15	98
RSVE-Ins			98	95
RSVE-BSA			17	99
RSVE-Ins + free insulin			5	N.D.
Ricin A			7	9
None			0	0

*N.D. = not determined.

Sendai virus was reconstituted and SV40 DNA or ricin A was enclosed within the RSVE, as described earlier for the enclosure of calf thymus DNA and IgG (Vainstein *et al.*, 1984). Insulin and BSA were covalently attached to the viral glycoproteins to prepare RSVE-Ins and RSVE-BSA, respectively, as described previously (Gitman *et al.*, 1985).

(a) For induction of the synthesis of SV40 T antigen, 10 μg protein of RSVE loaded with SV40 DNA were incubated for 30 min at 37°C with a monolayer containing 5×10^4 HTC. Appearance of T antigen was determined after 24–28 h of incubation as described before (Loyter *et al.*, 1983).

(b) A suspension containing 1×10^6 HTC was incubated with 10 μg protein of RSVE loaded with ricin A for 45 min at 37°C. After washing, the extent of protein synthesis was determined by estimating the incorporation of [^{3}H]-leucine into TCA insoluble material (Wasserman *et al.*, 1977). When used, free insulin (50 μg/ml) was added to the HTC cells 5 min prior to the addition of the RSVE.

inhibition of protein synthesis was obtained when the loaded RSVE were incubated with desialized HTC (Table VI).

Incubation of loaded RSVE, bearing chemically-coupled BSA, also caused very little inhibition of protein synthesis (17%) in desialized HTC, as compared to total inhibition of protein synthesis in non-treated cells (Table VI), again showing that the virus envelope did not fuse with virus receptor-depleted cells. However, conjugation of insulin molecules to the viral envelopes enabled them to interact with and to transfer their content into desialized cells. The results in Table VI indeed show that incubation of RSVE bearing insulin molecules with desialized HTC resulted in almost complete (98%) inhibition of protein synthesis. Free insulin molecules drastically inhibited the effect of the loaded RSVE, and very little inhibition of protein synthesis was observed when loaded RSVE bearing insulin molecules were incubated with desialized HTC in the presence of free insulin (Table VI). These results strengthen the view that the virus-attached insulin molecules mediated binding of the RSVE to the desialized HTC.

A. RSVE as a possible carrier for use *in vivo*

Phospholipid vesicles (liposomes) have been extensively used during the past few years as carrier to deliver specific drugs (Juliano *et al.*, 1983) and recently also DNA molecules (Soriano *et al.*, 1983) into the organs of whole animals. It has been well established that after intravenous injection most of the injected liposomes are taken up, probably by endocytic-like processes,

Table VII. The *in vivo* distribution of ^{125}I-RSVE in laboratory mice.

Organ	% of total ^{125}I injected: 10 min post-injection	90 min post-injection	180 min post-injection
Liver	50	45	15
Spleen	3	3	2
Lung	15	5	2
Blood circulation	25	8	8
Intestine	2	4	11
Others (kidney, pancreas, etc.)	2	2	4
Whole animal	100	67	42

^{125}I-RSVE was prepared from ^{125}I-Sendai virus (F particles) which were radiolabelled as previously described (Wolf *et al.*, 1980). ^{125}I-RSVE was injected intravenously at a dosage of 100 μg protein of ^{125}I-RSVE per mouse. Each value is the average obtained from 4–6 injected mice.

by the hepatocytes and the Kupffer cells of the injected animal (Roerdink *et al.*, 1981).

Theoretically, loaded RSVE may be used, similarly to liposomes, for the *in vivo* delivery of drugs and macromolecules. However, the use of RSVE *in vivo*, as opposed to their use in cell cultures, raises two major problems: (1) RSVE contain viral envelope glycoproteins (Loyter and Volsky, 1982) and their repeated injection would raise immunological response in the infected animal. Obviously this will nullify their continual injection into any particular animal. (2) Preparation of RSVE is a much more complex process than that of phospholipid liposomes, and their use as drug carriers would necessitate the growth and production of huge amounts of viruses.

The use of RSVE for the delivery of drugs and probably also macromolecules may have one important and crucial advantage over phospholipid liposomes. If RSVE will fuse with recipient cells *in vivo* as they do in cell cultures, their use as a biological carrier may be highly efficient and would necessitate low doses, and perhaps only one or two injections. No information as yet exists about the fusogenic properties and the fate of RSVE *in vivo*, after they have been injected into laboratory animals. In our laboratory we have recently injected ^{125}I-RSVE into mice and followed its distribution with time. The results in Table VII show that, as with liposomes, most of the injected RSVE accumulated in the liver a short time after injection. As can be seen in this table, about 50% of the radioactive material was found to be associated with the liver as soon as 10 min after injection, and 15% of the radioactive material was still found in the liver 3 h after injection of ^{125}I-RSVE. A relatively large percentage of the radioactive material was also found in the blood circulation. The results in Table VII show that approximately 10% of the radioactive material was found in the circulation 3 h after injection of ^{125}I-RSVE.

Currently, attempts are being made to study the fate of the injected RSVE, especially whether they fused with the liver cells. Electron microscopy and immunoprecipitation techniques are being used to reach this goal.

VII. CONCLUSIONS

RSVE have been shown to be able to transfer their content into cultured cells, thus serving as an efficient biological carrier. However, their use for the delivery of drugs and macromolecules *in vivo* is still questionable. Methods and techniques which have been developed during the past few years allow a quantitative estimation of the number of RSVE that are fused with recipient cells. Furthermore, specific antibodies and polypeptide hormones can be inserted into or chemically coupled to the viral envelopes without impairing the viral fusogenic activity. Such ligand-bearing RSVE can bind to and fuse with virus receptor-depleted cells. The illustration in Fig. 1 summarizes schematically the different methods developed in our laboratory for the preparation of "targeted" RSVE. It is possible that the binding of specific ligands to the viral envelopes will make them more useful as a drug delivery system *in vivo*.

ACKNOWLEDGEMENTS

This work was supported by grants from: International Genetic Sciences Partnership (IGSP), Stiftung Volkswagenwerk, National Council for Research and Development, Israel asnd GSF, Munich, Germany.

REFERENCES

Chejanovsky, N. and Loyter, A. (1985). *J. Biol. Chem.* **260**, 911–918.

Chejanovsky, N., Fridlender, B. and Loyter, A. (1985). *Biochim. Biophys. Acta* **812**, 353–361.

Gahmberg, C. G. (1977). *In* "Cell Surface Reviews" (G. Poste and G. L. Nicolson, eds) Vol. 3, pp. 370–421. Elsevier/North Holland, Amsterdam.

Gitman, A. G. and Loyter, A. (1984). *J. Biol. Chem.* **259**, 8913–8920.

Gitman, A. G., Kahane, I. and Loyter, A. (1985). *Biochemistry* **27**, 2762–2768.

Graessmann, A., Graessmann, M., Bobrik, R., Hoffmann, E., Lauppe, F. and Mueller, C. (1976). *FEBS Lett.* **61**, 81–85.

Heath, T. D., Martin, F. J. and Macher, B. A. (1983). *Exp. Cell Res.* **149**, 162–175.

Homma, M. K., Shimizu, K., Shimizu, Y. K. and Ishida, N. (1976). *Virology* **71**, 41–47.

Juliano, R. L., Lopez-Berenstein, G., Mehta, R., Hopfer, R., Mehta, K. and Kasi, L. (1983). *Biol. Cell.* **47**, 39–47.

Loyter, A. and Volsky, D. J. (1982). *In* "Cell Surface Reviews" (G. Poste and G. L. Nicolson, eds) Vol. 8, pp. 215–266. Elsevier/North Holland, Amsterdam.

Loyter, A., Vainstein, A., Graessmann, M. and Graessmann, A. (1983). *Exp. Cell Res.* **143**, 415–425.

Loyter, A., Tomasi, M., Gitman, A. G., Etinger, L. and Nussbaum, O. (1984). *In* "The use of specific antibodies to mediate fusion between sendai virus envelopes and living cells". CIBA Foundation, pp. 163–180. Pitman, London.

Maeda, T., Asano, A., Okada, Y. and Onishi, S. I. (1977a). *J. Virol.* **21**, 232–241.

Maeda, Y., Kim, J., Koseki, I., Mekada, E., Shiokawa, Y. and Okada, Y. (1977b). *Exp. Cell Res.* **108**, 95–106.

Martin, F. J., Papahadjopoulos, D. and Vail, W. J. (1982). *J. Biol. Chem.* **257**, 286–288.

Nisonoff, A. and Rivers, M. M. (1961). *Arch. Biochem. Biophys.* **93**, 460–462.

Nussbaum, O., Zakai, N. and Loyter, A. (1984). *Virology* **138**, 185–197.

Oeltman, F. K. and Heath, E. C. (1979). *J. Biol. Chem.* **254**, 1022–1028.

Ozawa, M., Asano, A. and Okada, Y. (1979). *Virology* **99**, 197–202.

Poste, G. and Pasternak, A. (1978). *In* "Membrane Fusion" (G. Poste and G. L. Nicolson, eds) pp. 305–317. Elsevier/North Holland, Amsterdam.

Roerdink, F., Dykatra, J., Hartman, G., Bolscher, B. and Scherphof, G. (1981). *Biochim. Biophys. Acta* **677**, 79–89.

Schroit, A. J. and Pagano, R. E. (1981). *Cell* **23**, 105–112.

Soriano, P., Dijkstra, J., Légrand, A., Spanjer, H., Gagliardi, D. L., Roerdink, F., Scherphof, G. and Nicolau, C. (1983). *Proc. Natl. Acad. Sci. USA* **80**, 7128–7131.

Sugawara, K. E., Tashiro, M. and Homma, M. (1982). *Virology* **117**, 444–455.

Tomasi, M., Gitman, A. G., Fridlender, B. and Loyter, A. (1982). *FEBS Lett.* **143**, 252–256.

Uchida, T., Yamaizumi, M., Mekada, E. and Okada, Y. (1980). *In* "Introduction of Macromolecules into Mammalian Cells" (Baserga, R., Croce, C. and Rovera, C., eds) pp. 169–185. Liss, New York.

Vainstein, A., Razin, A., Graessmann, A. and Loyter, A. (1983). *Methods Enzymol.* **101**, 492–512.

Vainstein, A., Hershkovitz, M., Israel, S., Rabin, S. and Loyter, A. (1984). *Biochim. Biophys. Acta* **773**, 181–188.

Volsky, D. J. and Loyter, A. (1978). *FEBS Lett.* **92**, 190–194.

Wasserman, M., Loyter, A. and Kulka, R. G. (1977). *J. Cell Sci.* **27**, 157–165.

Wolf, D., Kahana, I., Nir, S. and Loyter, A. (1980). *Exp. Cell Res.* **130**, 361–369.

11

Transformation of Mammalian Cells with DNA Using the Calcium Technique

R. D. McKinnon and F. L. Graham

I. INTRODUCTION

The introduction of exogenous DNA into mammalian cells has become an integral step in the analysis of gene structure, gene function, and the regulation of gene expression. Examining the biological properties of isolated genes usually requires an efficient process for delivery of genetic information into the nucleus of recipient cells and subsequent identification of cells that are expressing the foreign DNA. DNA transfer into mammalian cells can be achieved using several techniques, the suitability of which depends on the biological activity assayed and the type of DNA to be transferred. For transfection of nucleic acids into mammalian cells, we consider three basic types of biological activity to be assayed: infectivity of viral nucleic acid (DNA or RNA); transformation, that is heritable change in phenotype resulting from stable expression of the transferred DNA; and transient expression, assayed by detection of mRNA or proteins encoded by the transferred DNA.

One of the most frequently used methods for DNA transfer in mammalian cells is the DNA–calcium phosphate coprecipitation technique or calcium technique (Graham and van der Eb, 1973a). This technique is a simple and reproducible method for assaying all three types of biological activity mentioned above. For certain types of assays the calcium technique may be less efficient than, for example, the direct microinjection technique for transformation (Capecchi, 1980; see also Chapters 1, 2 and 12), electroporation (Potter *et al.*, 1984), the spheroplast fusion technique for transient expression (Schaffner, 1980; Sandri-Goldin *et al.*, 1981), or the DEAE-dextran mediated transfection technique for infectivity of small virus

Microinjection and Organelle Transplantation Techniques

ISBN: 0-12-164722-6
ISBN: 0-12-164723-4 Pbk

genomes (McCutchan and Pagano, 1968; Warden and Thorne, 1968). However, for most experimental protocols the calcium technique is quite suitable and is often the most straightforward and reliable assay for examining the biological activity of purified DNA.

The principle of this technique is to mix together DNA, sodium phosphate, and calcium chloride in concentrations which generate a coprecipitate of DNA and calcium phosphate. The resulting suspension is inoculated onto a cell monolayer and virtually all of the cells take up the DNA in a calcium ion-dependent process occurring over several hours at 37°C. Biological activity of transfected DNA can then be assayed as viral infectious units (for example by plaque assay), transient gene expression (assay for mRNA or protein production), or as a stable (heritable) transformation after selection for an altered phenotype. In this chapter we review the procedure for DNA transfer using the calcium technique with certain modifications which optimize expression in various assays, describe several systems for selection of transformed cells, and describe some of the more recent applications of this technique for the isolation and characterization of mammalian genes.

II. TRANSFORMATION PROTOCOL

The calcium technique was developed and originally optimized for the detection of infectivity of viral DNA (Graham and van der Eb, 1973a). Several parameters were found to have a pronounced effect on infectivity of adenovirus DNA, including the pH of the buffer in which viral DNA was diluted, the DNA and $CaCl_2$ concentrations during formation of the coprecipitate, and the length of time that cells were exposed to this precipitate (see Graham and van der Eb, 1973a). This technique is particularly suitable for assaying infectivity of viral DNA with intrinsically low activity such as that of adenovirus DNA, for assaying high relative molecular mass viral DNA such as herpes virus DNA (Graham *et al.*, 1973), or for assaying DNA preparations containing a mixture of infectious and non-infectious DNAs. Other techniques such as the DEAE-dextran method which function best at low DNA concentrations seem better suited for assaying infectivity of DNA from the smaller viruses such as the papova virus. A detailed description of the procedure for assaying infectivity of viral DNA using the calcium technique is given by Graham and Bacchetti (1983).

Although the calcium technique could be used to detect the morphological transformation of mammalian cells with viral DNA (Graham and van der Eb, 1973b; Graham *et al.*, 1974), the efficiency of this assay was low. Several groups subsequently demonstrated that herpes simplex viral DNA could be used to transfer the viral encoded thymidine kinase (TK) gene into TK^- recipient cells using the calcium technique (Bacchetti and Graham, 1977; Maitland and McDougall, 1977; Wigler *et al.*, 1977; Minson *et al.*, 1978). Once cloned TK genes became available it was possible to re-evaluate the parameters for optimal transformation of mammalian cells using TK transformation as an assay (Graham *et al.*, 1980). The following sections describe the assay for both morphological and biochemical transformation of mammalian cells, and we comment on a few of the key parameters which have been changed from those optimized for the assay of DNA infectivity.

A. Materials

Buffers required include 2X Hepes buffered saline (HeBS: 10 g/l *N*-2-Hydroxyethyl-piperazine-*N*′-2-ethanesulphonic acid, 16 g/l NaCl, 0.74 g/l KCl, 0.25 g/l $Na_2HPO_4 \cdot 2H_2O$, 2 g/l D-glucose, final pH 7.1) and 2.5 M $CaCl_2$. The HeBS is aliquoted into small glass bottles, sterilized by autoclaving and stored at 4°C. $CaCl_2$ stocks are prepared in water, sterilized by filtration, and stored at 4°C in plastic containers.

Carrier DNA is generally isolated from the cell type that is to be used as recipient of transforming DNA. For cultured cell lines, monolayers of cells growing in 150 mm × 15 mm dishes are rinsed once with phosphate-buffered saline without divalent cations, lysed, and digested at 37°C for 4–5 h with 2 ml per dish of 500 μg/ml pronase in 0.01 M Tris-HCl (pH 7.5), 0.001 M EDTA (TE-buffer) plus 0.4% SDS. Cell lysates are then collected from the dishes with a rubber policeman and gently extracted with phenol. After extensive dialysis against several changes of sterile 0.1 × SSC and then against TE-buffer (pH 7.5), the DNA is recovered aseptically from the dialysis bag and stored at 4°C in sterile plastic tubes. There is no need to remove RNA from these preparations. It is convenient to prepare large batches of carrier DNA so that one standardized preparation may be used for several assays.

Recipient cells are prepared from established cell lines one day prior to use by seeding cells in Petri dishes at the desired density (see Section II.C). Culture medium should not contain high concentrations of phosphate ions. While many cell lines are suitable recipients for exogenous DNA, the efficiency of transformation varies greatly between lines (Section II.C). This may, at least in some cases, be a result of differing sensitivities of various cell lines exposed to high concentrations of $CaCl_2$. For morphological transformation with viral DNA, we routinely use primary rodent kidney cells as recipients. The preparation of primary cultures is described in detail by van der Eb and Graham (1980).

B. Methods

The preparation of a DNA–calcium phosphate coprecipitate is carried out at room temperature under sterile conditions. The following protocol gives us optimal results for preparation of the coprecipitates and delivery to recipient cells:

(a) The desired concentration of transforming DNA is added to carrier DNA in 0.1 × TE-buffer (pH 8.1), then 2.5 M $CaCl_2$ is slowly added with gentle mixing to give a final concentration of 0.25 M $CaCl_2$. The final concentration of high relative molecular mass carrier DNA in this solution should be approximately 10 μg/ml, although the optimum must be determined empirically (see below).

(b) For preparation of precipitates the DNA–$CaCl_2$ is added slowly to an equal volume of 2 × HeBS while mixing constantly by bubbling air through a Pasteur pipette placed at the bottom of the tube. A visible precipitate should form within minutes.

(c) After sitting at room temperature for 15–30 min, the resulting precipitate is suspended by gentle mixing and then added to subconfluent cell monolayers (without removal of growth medium) at a volume ratio of transforming cocktail to medium of 1:10.

(d) Cells are exposed to the DNA–calcium phosphate coprecipitate in incubators at 37°C and the medium replaced with fresh growth medium after 4–20 h (depending on the recipient cells used). After a further 24–72 h, during which time the cells continue to divide and monolayers reach confluency, the medium is replaced with selective medium to allow for growth of transformed cells and to eliminate untransformed cells. A description of various selective regimens is given in Section III.

(e) The culture medium is replaced with fresh selective medium every 3–4 days, and transformed colonies are visible after 1–3 weeks, depending on the assay and the recipient cell type. For most selection systems (see Section III), cells are maintained in the original culture dishes during this period. For $G418^r$ (neo) transformants (Colbere-Garapin *et al.*, 1979; Southern and Berg, 1982), we find it generally necessary to passage transfected cells and reseed at a lower density in selective medium (growth-arrested cells are relatively resistant to G418). Once the background of untransformed recipient cells has been eliminated we routinely stain the dishes with 1% crystal violet in 30% formaldehyde to score for colonies.

C. Parameters for optimal efficiency

The above procedure is based largely on the original technique optimized for DNA infectivity, but it incorporates several modifications introduced for the transfer of a recombinant HSV TK gene into TK^- cells. If plasmid DNA is

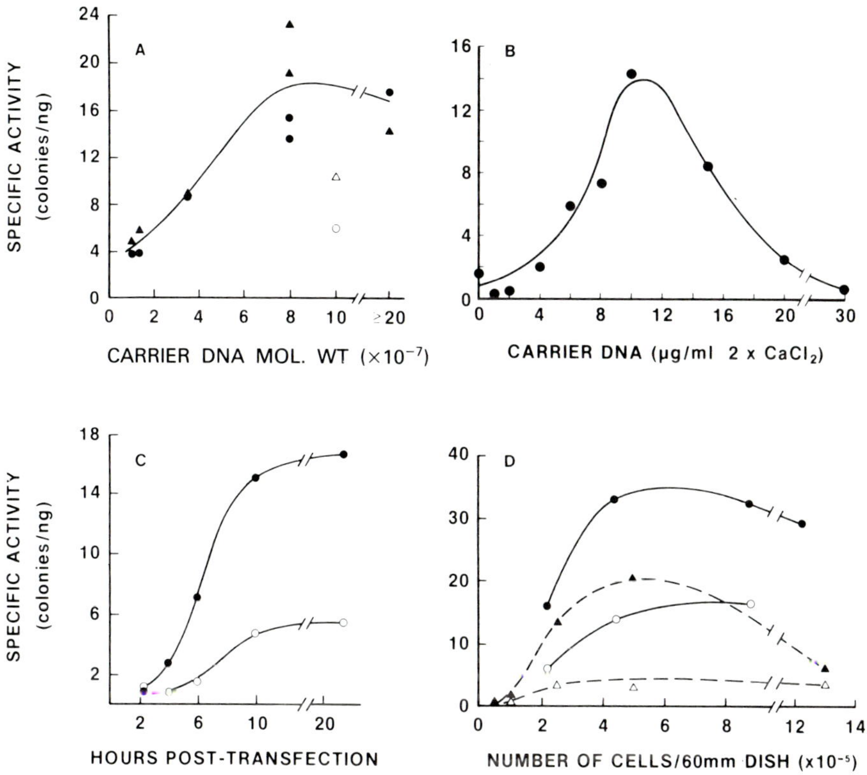

Fig. 1. Transformation of LTK$^-$APRT$^-$ cells with pTK1 plasmid DNA. Effect of (A) carrier DNA relative molecular mass, (B) carrier DNA concentration, (C) time of exposure of cells to the DNA coprecipitates, and (D) cell density. (A,B) cells were exposed to 10 ng plasmid DNA per dish. (C,D) cells were exposed to 10 ng (●) or 25 ng (○) of pTK1 DNA. In (D) cells were also treated with 20 ng (▲) or 50 ng (△) of linearized plasmid DNA (specific activity × 20). Reproduced from Graham *et al.* (1980) with permission.

used as the donor, the DNA is purified by alkaline extraction (Birnboim and Doly, 1979) followed by CsCl density gradient centrifugation, and then dialysis against TE-buffer. We use circular plasmid DNA for these assays, although we have not observed any difference in transformation efficiency between linearized and closed circular plasmid DNA (Graham *et al.*, 1980).

Maximum transformation efficiencies are usually obtained when the DNA–calcium phosphate precipitates are prepared using a concentration of approximately 10 μg/ml of high relative molecular mass carrier DNA (Graham *et al.*, 1980) as shown in Figs 1A and B. However, the optimum DNA concentration can vary among different carrier DNA preparations and should be determined empirically. Although we have not systematically examined the effect of relative molecular mass, it is likely that the size of the carrier DNA determines the optimum concentrations; the higher the carrier DNA relative molecular mass, the lower the concentration needed for optimal efficiency of transfection. Precipitates formed in the presence of a steady stream of air bubbles as first described by Wigler *et al.* (1979a) seem to be more active than precipitates formed by rapid mixing. In combination, these three factors — carrier DNA relative molecular mass, carrier DNA concentration, and method of precipitate formation — can have pronounced effects on the morphology of the resultant precipitate, the nature of which seems to be important for best results (Graham *et al.*, 1980). In general, higher efficiency of transformation is obtained with a rather coarse precipitate with a tendency to settle out of suspension within a few minutes.

The effect of the time of exposure of mouse L cell monolayers to the DNA precipitate is shown in Fig. 1C. The efficiency of transformation increases markedly with the length of time that the precipitate is left on the cells (Graham *et al.*, 1980; Corsaro and Pearson, 1981a). The limiting factor may be the sensitivity of various cell types to exposure to high concentrations of calcium ions. For cells sensitive to this procedure, we recommend leaving the DNA precipitate on for 3–4 h, but with TK^- mouse L cells and with primary rodent kidney fibroblasts we routinely leave precipitates on the cells for 15–20 h prior to the first medium change. Although successful transformation of many mammalian cell types has been described, including rodent, simian and human cells, the optimum parameters for transformation of a particular cell line by DNA-mediated gene transfer must be determined empirically.

Transformation efficiency is also affected by the density of the recipient culture, as shown in Fig. 1D for transformation of mouse TK^- cells using cloned HSV TK DNA. In general, best results are obtained if the recipient cells undergo 1–2 cell divisions after exposure to the DNA precipitate and before the cultures become confluent. In assays of HSV DNA infectivity (Graham *et al.*, 1973) it was found that removal of the culture medium was not necessary for efficient adsorption. Subsequent experiments have confirmed this for transformation assays. In addition, we find that a change of growth medium prior to application of the precipitate is unnecessary and in some instances can reduce the transformation efficiency (Graham *et al.*, 1980).

One of the most critical factors for efficient transformation is the cell type used as recipient for exogenous DNA (Graf *et al.*, 1979; Graham *et al.*, 1980; Peterson and McBride, 1980; Corsaro and Pearson, 1981b). In our experience the most efficient recipient cell line is LTA, a TK^-APRT^- line derived by R. Hughes and P. Plagemann (pers. commun.) from the LTK^- Clone 1D mouse cell line described by Kit *et al.* (1963). We routinely obtain transforming activity in the range of 10–20 colonies per ng plasmid DNA for transfer of HSV TK into LTA cells. Under optimal conditions we have obtained specific activities up to 100 colonies per ng plasmid DNA, and efficiencies of up to 1 transformant per 2–5 × 10^3 recipient cells.

We have not attempted to boost transforming activity by using either DMSO (Stow and Wilkie, 1976) or glycerol shocks (Frost and Williams, 1978). Corsaro and Pearson (1981a) have reported that a DMSO boost may be useful when other parameters such as length of exposure to the precipitate are suboptimal. Several other modifications have been employed to boost transforming efficiency for certain assays. Luthman and Magnusson (1983) have reported that chloroquine treatment can increase transformation efficiency by 6-fold, possibly by preventing nuclease degradation of transfected DNA. Similarly, Gorman and Howard (1983) reported that sodium butyrate enhances both transformation and transient expression of exogenous plasmid DNA, and Mak *et al.* (1985) found that cycloheximide treatment enhances adenovirus transformation 4- to 6-fold (although this effect seems to be adenovirus specific). Given the efficiency of transformation using the procedure described in Section II.B, we generally find it unnecessary to employ these boosts, although they may prove necessary under certain circumstances such as for the detection of single copy cellular genes (Section III).

III. TRANSFORMATION ASSAYS AND APPLICATIONS

Under optimal conditions only 0.1% of cells exposed to a DNA precipitate stably express a transformed phenotype (see also Chapter 12). While cells stably expressing exogenous DNA can be identified using techniques such as immunocytochemistry, the low efficiency of transformation generally necessitates selection for transformants under growth conditions that eliminate non-transformed cells. The two types of selection systems employed are morphological or oncogenic transformation and acquired drug resistance transformation, selecting for cells capable of forming colonies either under stringent growth conditions or in the presence of metabolic inhibitors. The selection schemes outlined below have allowed the detection of transforming activity of both viral genes and single copy cellular genes using DNA-mediated gene transfer.

A. Biochemical transformation

While cell lines such as galK$^-$ CHO cells (Thirion *et al.*, 1976) have been used to detect transformants of auxotrophic mammalian cells (Schumperli *et*

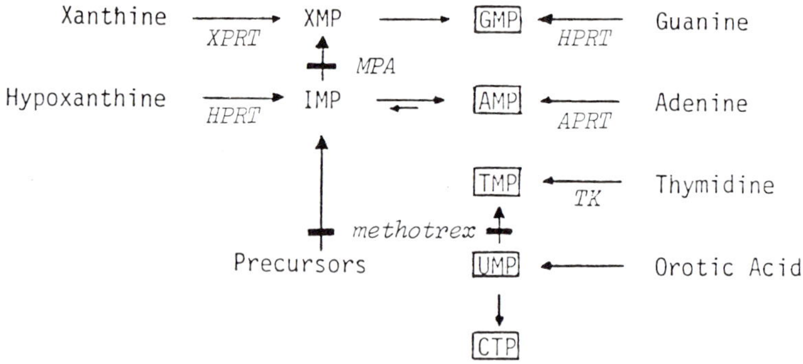

Fig. 2. Metabolic pathways involved in purine and pyrimidine synthesis and various inhibitors. Abbreviations are defined in the text.

al., 1982), the majority of selective systems employed to date use acquired resistance to metabolic inhibitors. A number of drug selection regimens have been developed for mammalian cell transformation. For example, detection of DNA-mediated gene transfer of several enzymes involved in purine and pyrimidine biosynthesis is based on the sensitivity of mammalian cells to methotrexate, as outlined in Fig. 2.

In *de novo* purine biosynthesis (Fig. 2) both GMP and AMP are formed from IMP. IMP is converted to AMP via adenylosuccinate and to XMP by IMP dehydrogenase. This latter enzyme is inhibited by mycophenolic acid (Franklin and Cook, 1969), while IMP synthesis is inhibited by aminopterin (Szybalski and Szybalski, 1962). The salvage pathway for free purines occurs by condensation with phosphoribosyl pyrophosphate (PRPP). Adenine is converted to AMP by adenine phosphoribosyltransferase (APRT) and hypoxanthine and guanine to IMP and GMP, respectively, by hypoxanthine phosphoribosyltransferase (HPRT). There is no mammalian enzyme comparable to the bacterial enzyme (XGPRT) that converts xanthine to XMP (Krenitsky *et al.*, 1969). In *de novo* pyrimidine biosynthesis both TMP and CTP are formed from orotic acid via UMP. As with IMP formation, synthesis of TMP from UMP via thymidylate synthetase is sensitive to methotrexate (MTX). The salvage pathway for TMP synthesis from thymidine requires thymidine kinase (TK).

Szybalski and Szybalski (1962) first described the use of the HAT (hypoxanthine, aminopterin and thymidine) selection system to identify $HPRT^+$ transformants of a human $HPRT^-$ cell line. HAT selection has been employed to detect transformation of $BUdR^r$ thymidine kinase-deficient (TK^-) cells to TK^+, initially using herpes simplex virus (Munyon *et al.*, 1971) and subsequently with viral DNA (Bacchetti and Graham, 1977; Maitland and McDougall, 1977; Wigler *et al.*, 1977; Minson *et al.*, 1978).

Wigler *et al.* (1978) further demonstrated transformation of TK^- cells with single-copy cellular genes. HAT selection has since been used to detect HPRT transformation using cellular DNA (Graf *et al.*, 1979; Willecke *et al.*, 1979; Lester *et al.*, 1980; Peterson and McBride, 1980). Other cellular genes detected by DNA-mediated gene transfer include APRT (Wigler *et al.*, 1979a; Lester *et al.*, 1980) dihydrofolate reductase (Lewis *et al.*, 1980; Wigler *et al.*, 1980) and a human DNA repair gene (Rubin *et al.*, 1983).

The use of dominant genetic markers for mammalian cell transformation eliminates the requirement for an enzyme-deficient cell line to detect transformants. For example, Simonsen and Levinson (1983) have isolated an altered dihydrofolate reductase (DHFR) gene from MTX^r murine cells which can be used as a dominant selectable marker in cells expressing normal levels of the wild-type enzyme. Similarly, Corsaro and Pearson (1981b) have reported transfer of ouabain resistance to mouse L cells using DNA from $ouabain^r$ cells, and Mulligan and Berg (1981) devised a selection system for transfer of the *Escherichia coli* xanthine–guanine phosphoribosyl transferase gene (gpt) to mammalian cells using aminopterin and micophenolic acid selection.

One of the most powerful dominant selective markers employed to date for transformation of eukaryotic cells is the gene coding for aminoglycoside 3′ phosphotransferase (neo) from the bacterial transposon Tn5, which renders bacteria resistant to the aminoglycoside antibiotics neomycin and kanamycin. This enzyme also confers resistance to geneticin (G-418), as first reported for yeast (Jimenez and Davies, 1980) and subsequently for higher eukaryotic cells (Colbere-Garapin *et al.*, 1981; Southern and Berg, 1982). A series of plasmid vectors have been developed that employ transcription regulatory signals from the simian virus SV40 for efficient expression of the bacterial genes neo and gpt in mammalian cells (see Subramani and Southern, 1983).

B. Morphological transformation

Oncogenic transformation of primary cells in simplified terminology can be described as a two-step process involving acquisition of infinite growth potential (immortalization) and deregulated proliferative capacity (neoplastic transformation). These two steps in transformation correspond to two complementation groups of oncogenes (Land *et al.*, 1983; Ruley, 1983) isolated from both viral and cellular genomes. The calcium technique has been used to identify oncogenes that are capable of inducing a morphological transformation of both primary mammalian cells and established (immortal) cell lines.

While it is possible to assay for transforming activity of DNA by injecting transfected cells or even pure DNA into an animal and then scoring for tumours, it is more common to assay transformation by scoring for morphologically identifiable colonies of transformed cells growing in culture. The selection system used in a morphological transformation assay depends on the type of cells employed and the DNA being assayed. For example, for primary cell transformation by adenovirus DNA, we generally select for transformed cells able to form colonies in medium containing low calcium ion concentrations and supplemented with minimal serum (Joklik's MEM plus 5% donor horse serum). Under these conditions the untransformed fibroblasts detach within 7 days and colonies of epitheloid transformants are visible by day 10. For established cell lines such as NIH3T3, selection of morphological transformants generally involves outgrowth of colonies of transformed cells against a background of growth-arrested fibroblasts. The identification of transformants thus does not require specialized selective medium and colonies can be distinguished on the basis of altered cellular morphology and altered growth properties.

C. Transfection with non-selectable genes

The above systems allow the isolation of mammalian cells expressing exogenous genes that confer a selectable phenotype. Mammalian cells expressing non-selectable exogenous DNA have also been isolated using several approaches. Wigler *et al.* (1979b) first demonstrated the cotransfer of unlinked genes. Subsequent work has demonstrated that cells isolated for expression of a selective marker are capable of expressing either linked or unlinked cotransferred non-selective markers (Huttner *et al.*, 1979; Mantei *et al.*, 1979; Wold *et al.*, 1979; Breathnach *et al.*, 1980; Lai *et al.*, 1980). In theory, mammalian cells can be isolated expressing any transfected gene using cotransfer of a selective marker to isolate transformants.

Fluorescence-activated cell sorting (FACS) has also been used to enrich for cells expressing a transfected cell surface antigen gene. This approach requires both specific antisera against the surface marker and a recipient cell line capable of expressing exogenous surface antigens. This has proven useful in the characterization of class I (Goodenow *et al.*, 1983) and class II (Malissen *et al.*, 1983; Rabourdin-Combe and Mach, 1983) genes of the major histocompatibility complex. Detection of surface antigens by a specific antibody has also been used in the screening of cells transformed by DNA determining a cell surface antigen associated with human chronic lymphocytic leukemia (Stanners *et al.*, 1981, 1983). As described below, the application of plasmid rescue approaches should make this a useful approach for cloning genes for other cell surface markers.

D. Plasmid rescue

Transformation of mammalian cells with DNA can also be used as an assay in order to isolate and clone genes. A particularly elegant application of this technology for the isolation of mammalian genes is the use of plasmid rescue to recover the transforming gene from transformed cells. This was pioneered for the chicken thymidine kinase gene (Perucho *et al.*, 1980), and has since proven useful in the rescue of several genes including the Chinese hamster APRT gene (Lowy *et al.*, 1980) and a human DNA repair gene (Westerveld *et al.*, 1984). This approach can also be applied to isolate junction sequences at integration sites of exogenous DNA in transformed cells. One limitation of plasmid rescue is the frequent generation of rearranged sequences (Kiessling *et al.*, 1984). However, this technique may prove useful for the isolation and characterization of any genes which express a distinguishing phenotype on transformed cells, and for the rescue of cellular DNA sequences adjacent to integration sites in mammalian chromosomes.

E. Transient expression assays

The low frequency of stable transformants in transfected cultures presumably reflects the frequency of successful integration of transcriptionally active genes into a cellular replicon. However, a high proportion of transfected cells (up to 25%) are at least transiently able to express exogenous DNA (Chu and Sharp, 1981). The calcium technique has been used in the absence of any selection to examine transient expression of exogenous DNA in mammalian cells.

One of the more recent applications of transient expression assays is as a test for transcription activity of recombinant DNA molecules. The system of choice for such an assay is usually the chloramphenicol acetyltransferase (CAT) enzyme (Gorman *et al.*, 1982). Mammalian cells that have taken up CAT express only limited resistance to chloramphenicol (Gorman *et al.*, 1982) and, therefore, may not be selectable. However, the level of CAT gene expression in transfected cells can be readily assayed enzymatically, facilitating the analysis of transcriptional activity and the relative strength of transcriptional promoters and enhancers (Gluzman and Shenk, 1983).

The levels of transient gene expression can be increased by providing exogenous DNA with a functional replication origin. Gluzman (1981) has developed an African green monkey kidney cell line (COS cells) which contains and expresses the SV40 large-T tumour antigen and will replicate episomal copies of exogenous plasmids containing the SV40 origin region. Thus this system allows amplification of exogenous templates for transient gene expression.

Shen *et al.* (1982) have described a transfection technique for cells growing in suspension which enhances both transient expression and transformation, although from our experience the value of this approach may depend on the recipient cell type used in this assay. For example, treatment of CHO TK^- cells in suspension appears to enhance transient expression of the HSV TK gene, but gives results similar to those obtained in monolayer with LTA (TK^-) mouse cells. Since the calcium technique as described in Section II.C is the most straightforward and reproducible method of transfecting cells, it is advisable to test its suitability for transient expression assays in a particular system prior to adopting more elaborate protocols.

IV. MECHANISM OF TRANSFORMATION

Although the mechanism whereby exogenous DNA is taken up by and expressed in mammalian cells is largely unknown, several studies have shed some light on some of the steps in cell transformation. Using fluorescent dye to monitor the fate of exogenous DNA, Loyter *et al.* (1982) showed that virtually all recipient cells in a culture take up calcium phosphate–DNA complexes, possibly by phagocytosis, although these complexes reach the nucleus in only a small percentage of transfected cells. Since 10–25% of cells can transiently express exogenous DNA, it is likely that DNA is released from these complexes in the cytoplasm and then migrates to the nucleus.

Subsequent to transfection the donor DNA molecules become linked to high relative molecular mass carrier DNA (Perucho *et al.*, 1980) in complexes termed "transgenomes" (Scangos and Ruddle, 1981). Although the carrier is not essential for efficient transformation using nuclear microinjection (Capecchi, 1980), transfection efficiency using the calcium technique in the absence of carrier DNA is reduced by one or more orders of magnitude for both viral DNA infectivity (Graham and van der Eb, 1973a) and transformation assays (Graham *et al.*, 1980). Carrier DNA may facilitate nuclear transport or alternatively may protect DNA from nuclease degradation. Within the nucleus these transgenome complexes may be amplified (Reyes *et al.*, 1982), as has been reported for episomal copies of plasmid DNA introduced in absence of carrier DNA (Spandidos *et al.*, 1982). The increased frequency of unstable transformants in the presence of carrier DNA further suggests that carrier DNA may provide replication origins or transcription regulatory signals (Scangos and Ruddle, 1981).

Evidence from several laboratories suggests that in the nucleus at least a fraction of exogenous DNA becomes transcriptionally competent. Transient expression of exogenous DNA can be increased by the presence of an enhancer sequence. The interesting correlation between transient levels of gene expression and efficiency of stable transformation (Gorman and

Howard, 1983; Lang *et al.*, 1983; Weeks and Jones, 1983; Berg and Anderson, 1984) suggests that enhancer sequences facilitate the organization of a transcriptionally active chromatin structure for both episomal and integrated forms of exogenous DNA. Alternatively, enhanced transient expression may allow cells to survive the initial stages of selection (Gorman and Howard, 1983), or sequences such as promoters and enhancers that facilitate transcription may also affect accessibility to enzymes catalysing integration.

While both TK (Jolly *et al.*, 1983; Lang *et al.*, 1983) and neo (F. Yoshimura, pers. commun.) constructs that lack enhancer sequences transform less efficiently than constructs with enhancers, both give rise to drug-resistant cell lines expressing comparable levels of these mRNAs. Thus there is no apparent relationship between transient levels of gene expression and the level of expression of the selected marker in stably transformed cells. It is possible that drug-resistant cells transformed with constructs lacking an enhancer sequence have integrated the exogenous DNA into an environment near a cellular enhancer, facilitating the efficient expression of the marker gene.

The integration of transgenomes into a cellular chromosome apparently is the limiting factor in stable transformation (Scangos and Ruddle, 1981). Integration does not proceed by homologous recombination (Steele *et al.*, 1984), although mammalian cells can catalyse homologous recombination of exogenous DNA (see Lin *et al.*, 1984). This is in marked contrast to transformation in yeast (Hinnen *et al.*, 1978). The failure of transfected DNA to integrate by homologous recombination is a general phenomenon associated with all presently available methods of DNA delivery to mammalian cells. It is thus impossible to study the expression of transfected DNA in the context of its normal locus in the recipient cell chromosome. The failure of exogenous genes to insert at the site of an endogenous copy may limit the usefulness of DNA-mediated gene transfer for so-called "gene therapy" as well as for the study of control of gene expression, since DNA which has integrated randomly may not be subject to the same developmental controls as the normal copy. A major goal of DNA-mediated gene transfer into mammalian cells therefore should not only be to enhance efficiencies of transformation, but also to develop methods for achieving homologous recombination.

ACKNOWLEDGEMENTS

Supported by the Medical Research Council and the National Cancer Institute of Canada. RMcK is a Research Fellow and FLG a Research Associate of the National Cancer Institute of Canada.

REFERENCES

Bacchetti, S. and Graham, F. L. (1977). *Proc. Natl. Acad. Sci. USA* **74**, 1590–1594.

Berg, P. E. and Anderson, W. F. (1984). *Mol. Cell. Biol.* **4**, 368–370.

Birnboim, H. C. and Doly, J. (1979). *Nucl. Acids Res.* **7**, 1513–1523.

Breathnach, R., Manter, N. and Chambon, P. (1980). *Proc. Natl. Acad. Sci. USA* **77**, 740–744.

Capecchi, M. (1980). *Cell* **22**, 479–488.

Chu, G. and Sharp, P. A. (1981). *Gene* **13**, 197–202.

Colbere-Garapin, F., Horodniceanu, F., Kourilsky, P. and Garapin, A.-C. (1979). *J. Mol.Biol.* **150**, 1–14.

Corsaro, C. M. and Pearson, M. L. (1981a). *Somat. Cell Genet.* **7**, 603–616.

Corsaro, C. M. and Pearson, M. L. (1981b). *Somat. Cell Genet.* **7**, 617–630.

Franklin, T. J. and Cook, J. M. (1969). *Biochem. J.* **113**, 515–524.

Frost, E. and Williams, J. (1978). *Virology* **91**, 39–50.

Gluzman, Y. (1981). *Cell* **23**, 175–182.

Gluzman, Y. and Shenk, T., eds (1983). *In* "Communications in Molecular Biology". Cold Spring Harbor Laboratory, Cold Spring Harbor.

Goodenow, R. S., Stroynowski, I., McMillan, M., Nicholson, M., Eakle, K., Sher, B. T., Davidson, N. and Hood, L. (1983). *Nature* **301**, 388–394.

Gorman, C. M., Moffat, L. F. and Howard, B. H. (1982). *Mol. Cell. Biol.* **2**, 1044–1051.

Gorman, C. M. and Howard, B. H.L (1983). *Nucl. Acids Res.* **11**, 7631–7648.

Graf, L. H., Jr., Urlaub, G. and Chasin, L. A. (1979). *Somat. Cell Genet.* **5**, 1031–1044.

Graham, F. L. and Bacchetti, S. (1983). *In* "Techniques in the Life Sciences" B5, Nucleic Acid Biochemistry (R. A. Flavell, ed.) pp. 1–14. Elsevier, Ireland.

Graham, F. L. and van der Eb, A. J. (1973a). *Virology* **52**, 456–467.

Graham, F. L. and van der Eb, A. J. (1973b). *Virology* **54**, 536–539.

Graham, F. L., Veldhuisen, G. and Wilke, N. M. (1973). *Nature New Biol.* **245**, 265–266.

Graham, F. L., van der Eb, A. J. and Heijnecker, H. L. (1974). *Nature* **251**, 687–691.

Graham, F. L., Bacchetti, S., McKinnon, R. D., Stanners, C., Cordell, B. and Goodman, H. M. (1980). *In* "Introduction of Macromolecules into Viable Mammalian cells". Alan Liss, New York. pp. 3–25.

Hinnen, A., Hicks, J. B. and Fink, G. R. (1978). *Proc. Natl. Acad. Sci. USA* **75**, 1929–1933.

Huttner, K. M., Scangos, G. and Ruddle, F. H. (1979). *Proc. Natl. Acad. Sci. USA* **76**, 5820–5824.

Jimenez, A. and Davies, J. (1980). *Nature* **287**, 869–871.

Jolly, D. J., Esty, A. C., Subramani, L., Friedmann, T. and Verma, I. M. (1983). *Nucl. Acids Res.* **11**, 1855–1872.

Kiessling, U., Platzer, M. and Strauss, M. (1984). *Mol. Gen. Genet.* **193**, 513–519.

Kit, S., Dubbs, D., Peikarski, L. and Hsu, T. (1963). *Exp. Cell Res.* **31**, 297–312.

Krenitsky, T. A., Papaioannou, R. and Elion, G. B. (1969). *J. Biol. Chem.* **244**, 1263–1270.

Lai, E. C., Woo, S. L. C., Bordelon-Riser, M. E., Fraser, T. H. and O'Malley, B. W. (1980). *Proc. Natl. Acad. Sci. USA* **77**, 244–248.

Land, H., Parada, L. F. and Weinberg, R. A. (1983). *Nature* **304**, 596–602.

Lang, J. C., Wilkie, N. M. and Spandidos, D. A. (1983). *J. Gen. Virol.* **64**, 2679–2696.
Lester, S. C., LeVan, S. K., Steglich, C. and DeMars, R. (1980). *Somat. Cell Genet.* **6**, 241–259.
Lewis, W. H., Srinivasan, P. R., Stokes, N. and Siminovitch, L. (1980). *Somat. Cell Genet.* **6**, 333–348.
Lin, F.-L., Sperle, K. and Sternberg, N. (1984). *Mol. Cell. Biol.* **4**, 1020–1034.
Lowy, I., Pellicer, A., Jackson, J. F., Sim, G.-K., Silverstein, S. and Axel, R. (1980). *Cell* **22**, 817–823.
Loyter, A., Scangos, G. A. and Ruddle, F. H. (1982). *Proc. Natl. Acad. Sci. USA* **79**, 422–426.
Luthman, H. and Magnusson, G. (1983). *Nucl. Acids Res.* **11**, 1295–1308.
Malissen, B., Steinmetz, M., McMillan, M., Peirres, M. and Hood, L. (1983). *Nature* **305**, 440–443.
Maitland, H. and McDougall, J. (1977). *Cell* **11**, 233–241.
Mak, I., Lai Fatt, R. and Mak, S. (1986). *Can. J. Biochem. and Cell Biology,* in press.
Mantei, N., Boll, W., and Weissmann, C. (1979). *Nature* **281**, 40–46.
McCutchan, J. H. and Pagano, J. S. (1968). *J. Natl. Cancer Inst.* **41**, 351–357.
Minson, A. C., Wildy, P., Buchan, A. and Darby, G. (1978). *Cell* **13**, 581–587.
Mulligan, R. C. and Berg, P. (1981). *Proc. Natl. Acad. Sci. USA* **78**, 2072–2076.
Munyon, W., Kraiselburd, E., Davis, D. and Mann, J. (1971). *J. Virol.* **7**, 813–820.
Perucho, M., Hanahan, D. and Wigler, M. (1980). *Cell* **22**, 309–317.
Perucho, M., Hanahan, D., Lipsich, L. and Wigler, M. (1980). *Nature* **285**, 207–210.
Peterson, J. L. and McBride, O. W. (1980). *Proc. Natl. Acad. Sci. USA* **77**, 1583–1587.
Potter, H., Weir, L. and Leder, P. (1984). *Proc. Natl. Acad. Sci. USA* **81**, 7161–7165.
Rabourdin-Combe, C. and Mach, B. (1983). *Nature* **303**, 670–674.
Reyes, G. R., Mclane, M. W. and Hayward, G. S. (1982). *J. Gen. Virol.* **60**, 209–224.
Rubin, J. S., Joynes, A. L., Bernstein, A. and Whitmore, G. F. (1983). *Nature* **306**, 206–208.
Ruley, H. E. (1983). *Nature* **304**, 602–606.
Sandri-Goldin, R. M., Goldin, A. L., Levine, M. and Glorioso, J. C. (1981). *Mol. Cell Biol.* **1**, 743–752.
Scangos, G. and Ruddle, F. H. (1981). *Gene* **14**, 1–10.
Schaffner, W. (1980). *Proc. Natl. Acad. Sci. USA* **77**, 2163–2167.
Schumperli, D., Howard, B. H. and Rosenberg, M. (1982). *Proc. Natl. Acad. Sci. USA* **79**, 257–261.
Shen, Y.-M., Hirschhorn, R. R., Mercer, W. E., Surmacz, E., Tsutsui, Y., Soprano, K. J. and Baserga, R. (1982). *Mol. Cell. Biol.* **2**, 1145–1154.
Simonsen, C. C. and Levinson, A. D. (1983). *Proc. Natl. Acad. Sci. USA* **80**, 2495–2499.
Southern, P. J. and Berg, P. (1982). *J. Mol. Appl. Genet.* **1**, 327–341.
Spandidos, D. A., Harrison, P. R. and Paul, J. (1982). *Exp. Cell Res.* **141**, 149–158.
Stanners, C. P., Lam, T., Chamberlin, J. W., Stewart, S. S. and Price, B. B. (1981). *Cell* **27**, 211–221.
Stanners, C. P., Chamberlin, J. W. and Price, B. B. (1983). *In* "Oncogenes and Retroviruses: Evaluation of Basic Findings and Clinical Potential", pp. 173–183. Alan Liss, New York.
Steele, R. E., Bakken, A. H. and Reeder, R. H. (1984). *Mol. Cell. Biol.* **4**, 576–582.

Stow, N. and Wilkie, N. (1976). *J. Gen. Virol.* **33**, 447–458.
Subramani, S. and Southern, P. J. (1983). *Anal. Biochem.* **135**, 1–15.
Szybalski, E. H. and Szybalski, W. (1962). *Proc. Natl. Acad. Sci. USA* **48**, 2026–2034.
Thirion, J.-P., Banville, D. and Noel, H. (1976). *Genetics* **83**, 137–147.
van der Eb, A. J. and Graham, F. L. (1980). *Methods Enzymol.* **65**, 826–839.
Warden, D. and Thorne, H. V. (1968). *J. Gen. Virol.* **3**, 371–377.
Weeks, D. L. and Jones, N. C. (1983). *Mol. Cell. Biol.* **3**, 1222–1234.
Westerveld, A., Hoeijmakers, J. H. J., van Duin, M., de Wit, J., Odijk, H., Pastink, A., Wood, R. D. and Bootsma, D. (1984). *Nature* **310**, 425–429.
Wigler, M., Silverstein, S., Lee, L. S., Pellicer, A., Cheng, Y. C. and Axel, R. (1977). *Cell* **11**, 223–232.
Wigler, M., Pellicer, A., Silverstein, S. and Axel, R. (1978). *Cell* **11**, 725–731.
Wigler, M., Pellicer, A., Silverstein, S., Axel, R., Urlaub, G. and Chasin, L. (1979a). *Proc. Natl. Acad. Sci. USA* **76**, 1373–1376.
Wigler, M., Sweet, R., Sim, G.-K., Wold, B., Pellicer, A., Lacy, E., Maniatis, T., Silverstein, S. and Axel, R. (1979b). *Cell* **16**, 777–785.
Wigler, M., Perucho, M., Kurtz, D., Dana, S., Pellicer, A., Axel, R. and Silverstein, S. (1980). *Proc. Natl. Acad. Sci. USA* **77**, 3567–3570.
Willecke, K., Klomfass, M., Mierau, R. and Doehmer, J. (1979). *Mol. Gen. Genet.* **170**, 179–185.
Wold, B., Wigler, M., Lacy, E., Maniatis, T., Silverstein, S. and Axel, R. (1979). *Proc. Natl. Acad. Sci. USA* **76**, 5684–5688.

12

The Somatic Cell as a Test Tube: Comparison Between Various Transfer Techniques

J. E. Celis

I. INTRODUCTION

Several techniques to introduce macromolecules into somatic cells have been developed during the last decade (for references see Poste *et al.*, 1976; Graham, 1977; Schlegel and Rechsteiner, 1978; Graessmann *et al.*, 1979b, 1980a; Kulka and Loyter, 1979; Baserga *et al.*, 1980; Celis *et al.*, 1980a; Furusawa, 1980; Gregoriadis and Allison, 1980; Paraf and Nicolau, 1981; Gregoriadis *et al.*, 1982; Rechsteiner, 1982; Nicolau *et al.*, 1983a; Wu *et al.*, 1983; Evered and Whelan, 1984; Celis, 1984b; see also previous chapters in this book). These techniques which aim at using the somatic cell as a living test tube, can be divided into three types depending on the way the macromolecules are delivered to the recipient cells.

(1) Direct microinjection

(a) Microinjection with glass capillaries. Graessmann, 1968; Graessmann and Graessman, 1971; Diacumakos, 1973; Stacey and Allfrey, 1976; Celis, 1977, Capecchi, 1980.

(2) Vehicle-mediated transfer

(a) Erythrocytes. Furusawa *et al.* (1974, 1976); Loyter *et al.* (1975); Schlegel and Rechsteiner (1975); Kaltoft and Celis (1978); Krieger *et al.* (1978); Schlegel and Mercer (1980); Uchida *et al.* (1980); Rechsteiner (1982); Brown *et al.* (1985).

The work in the author's laboratory was supported by grants from Euratom, the Danish Medical and Natural Science Research Councils, the Danish Cancer Foundation, NOVO, and the Aarhus University Research Fund.

Microinjection and Organelle Transplantation Techniques

ISBN: 0-12-164722-6
ISBN: 0-12-164723-4 Pbk

(b) Liposomes. Gregoriadis and Buckland (1973); Papahadjopoulos *et al.* (1974a,b, 1980a,b); Pagano *et al.* (1974); Poste *et al.* (1976); Pagano and Weinstein (1978); Fraley *et al.* (1979, 1980); Gregoriadis (1980); Poste (1980); Wong *et al.* (1980); Nicolau and Sene (1982); Nicolau *et al.* (1983a).

(c) Reconstituted Sendai virus envelopes. Uchida *et al.* (1977, 1980); Volsky *et al.* (1979); Loyter and Volsky (1979, 1982); Vainstain *et al.* (1983, 1984); Beigel and Loyter (1983); Loyter *et al.* (1983, 1984).

(3) Transfer aided by facilitators

(a) Calcium phosphate. Graham and van der Eb (1973); Wigler *et al.* (1978); Graham *et al.* (1980); Lewis *et al.* (1980); Graham and Baccheti (1983).

(b) DEAE-dextran. Pagano and Vaheri (1965); Vaheri and Pagano (1965); McCutchan and Pagano (1968); Warden and Thorne (1968); Graham (1977).

(c) Polyethylene glycol/sucrose shock. Chu and Sharpe (1981); Shen *et al.* (1982).

(d) Osmotic lysis of pinosomes. Okada and Rechsteiner (1982).

To date, a wide range of macromolecules (DNA, drugs, lipids, proteins, RNA, small molecules) as well as organelles (chromosomes, nuclei, membrane fragments) and virus particles have been introduced or transplanted into somatic cells by using these techniques (Table I; see also previous chapters in this book). It is becoming increasingly clear, however, that there are limitations inherent in each one of these methods and that certain biological problems are best approached using a particular technique.

The purpose of this chapter is to present a comparative evaluation of the various transfer techniques. Since the method of direct microinjection has brought us closer to the final goal of using the somatic cell as a test tube I have chosen to centre this chapter on this technique. A brief description of the other transfer techniques is given to facilitate comparison.

II. DIRECT MICROINJECTION

A. Microinjection of somatic cells with glass capillaries

The technique of microinjection of somatic cells with glass capillaries was developed originally by Graessmann (1968) and Diacumakos (1973; see also

Table I. Some characteristics of various transfer techniques.*

Technique	Macromolecules or organelles transferred	Recipient somatic cells	Site of delivery	Main lines of research in which these techniques have been used
Direct microinjection				
Microinjection with glass capillaries	DNAs, RNAs, proteins, small molecules, cell organelles, virus particles	All types, no restriction	Cytoplasm or nucleus	Gene structure, function and regulation of gene expression; transit of proteins across the nuclear envelope; studies of the cytoskeleton; translation of mRNAs.
Vehicle-mediated transfer				
Erythrocytes	Proteins, RNAs, only limited information on DNAs	All types, no restriction	Cytoplasm†	Degradation and turn-over of proteins. Nuclear localization of proteins. Identification and mutant selection.
Liposomes	DNAs, RNAs, proteins, lipids	All types, no restriction‡	Cytoplasm	*In vitro* delivery of macromolecules. Gene transfer and delivery of drugs into living organisms.
Reconstituted Sendai virus envelopes	DNAs, RNAs, proteins, membrane receptors	Restricted to cells	Cytoplasm having Sendai virus receptors	Degradation and turn-over of membrane proteins. Gene transfer.
Suborganelle vesicle transplantation	Mitochondria, mitochondrial-outer membrane	Apparently no restriction	Cytoplasm	Degradation and turn-over of membrane proteins
Transfer aided by facilitators				
Calcium phosphate	DNAs	Restricted to special cell types	Cytoplasm	Gene structure, function and regulation of gene expression
DEAE-dextran	DNAs	Restricted to special cell types	Cytoplasm	Gene function and regulation of gene expression
Polyethylene glycol/sucrose shock	DNAs	Restricted to special cell types	Cytoplasm	Gene function and regulation of gene expression

* Modified from Graessmann and Graessmann (1984).
† Nuclear transfer can be achieved by fusing loaded erythrocytes with mitotic cells.
‡ There is restriction for transfer into living organisms.

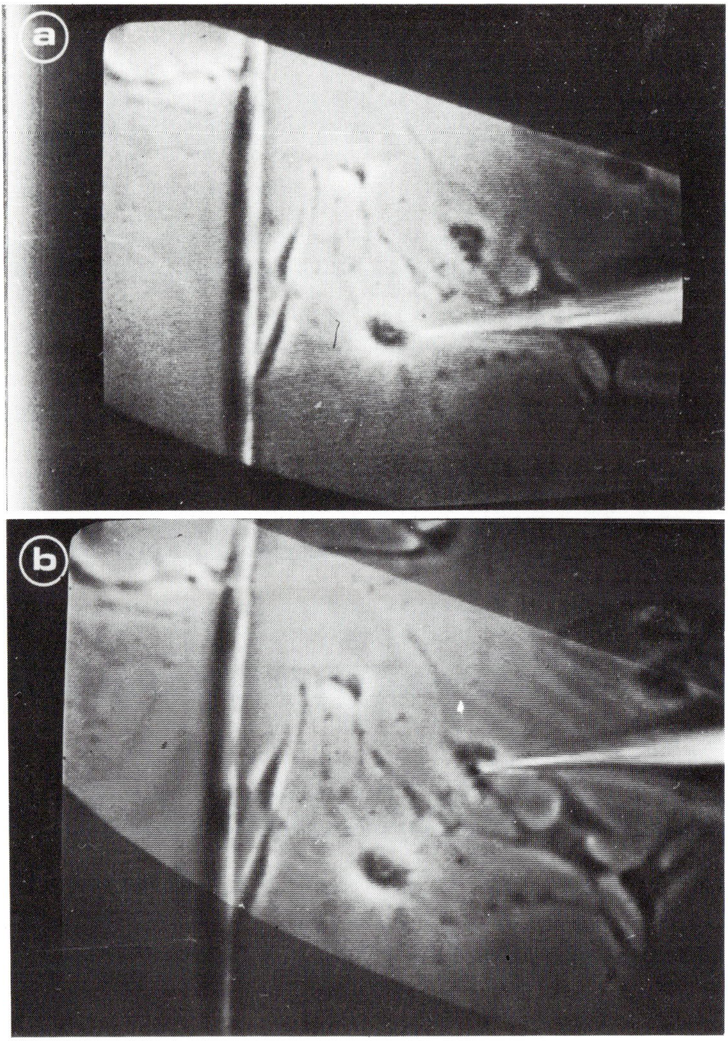

Fig. 1. Micrograph from a television monitor showing (a) cytoplasmic and (b) nuclear injections (from Celis *et al.*, 1980b). The glass coverslip (144 or 9 mm^2) with the attached cells is placed in a 5 cm Petri dish containing 8 ml of warm medium minus serum or Hank's buffered solution. The cells are viewed under phase contrast (×180). Once the cells are focused the tip of the glass capillary is lowered until it is in the same focal plane as the cells. To inject the cell, we position the tip of the glass capillary so that it lies just outside the cell. It is necessary just to touch the cells in order to penetrate them. The glass capillary is connected to a 50 ml glass syringe, to assist the injection of liquid. Injection is assessed visually. Once a cell has been injected, the glass capillary is raised and moved closer to the next cell to be injected. The procedure is simple and about 100 cells can be injected in 15 min. Various microinjection set-ups are currently available and these are described in articles by Graessmann (1968; see also other chapters concerned with direct microinjection), Diacumakos (1973), Celis (1977), Yamamoto and Furusawa (1978), Stacey (1981), Ansorge (1982), Graessmann and Graessmann (1983a) and Timm *et al.* (1983).

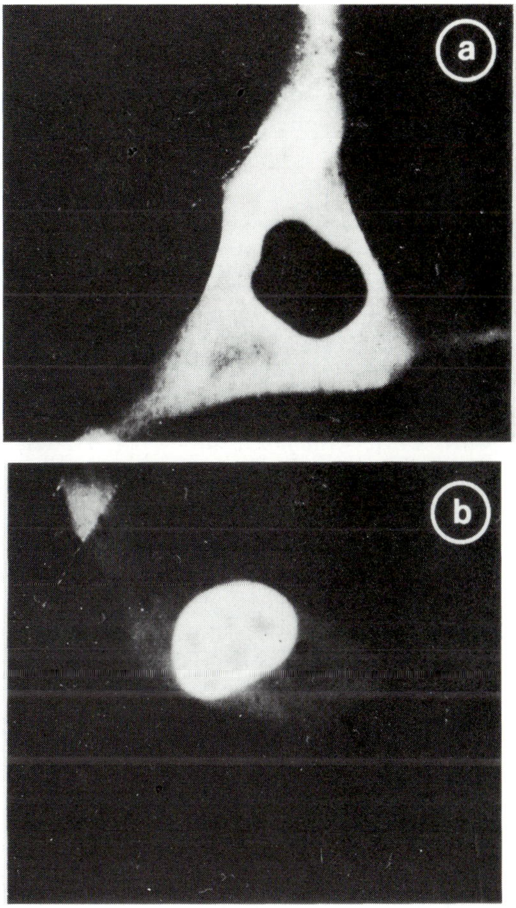

Fig. 2. Direct microinjection of FITC-BSA (16 O.D. 490/ml) into (a) the cytoplasm and (b) the nucleus of mouse 3T3 cells.

previous chapters concerned with direct microinjection). The technique is based on the use of small glass capillaries (0.5–1 μm diameter at the tip) which allow the direct transfer of macromolecules into recipient somatic cells grown on a solid support or artificially bound to a substrate (Graessmann *et al.*, 1980c; see also Fig. 1). This technique has no cell-type restriction and the macromolecules can be delivered either into the cytoplasm (Figs 1a and 2a) or the nucleus (Figs 1b and 2b) of the recipient cells.

To assess the possibilities of direct microinjection and to allow a comparison with other transfer methods (see also Tables I and II), it is necessary to weight the advantages and disadvantages of this technique (see also Chapters 1 and 2). The main advantages can be summarized as follows:

(1) A wide variety of recipient cultured somatic cells (primary or secondary cultures) can be used. Even cells that grow in suspension can be microinjected if bound to a substrate by a suitable linker [concanavalin A, poly(L-lysine) or phytohaemagglutinin; Graessmann *et al.*, 1980c].

(2) Only a small amount of sample is required; usually about 1–2 μl is sufficient.

(3) Injected cells can be easily identified by using marked glass slides.

(4) The average number of molecules injected per cell can be estimated. About 5×10^{-11}–10^{-10} ml can be injected per cell without any significant effect on cell viability (Stacey and Allfrey, 1976; Celis, 1977; Graessmann and Graessmann, 1983a,b).

(5) There is no apparent limitation on the size or type of macromolecules that can be injected. To date DNA (for references see Graessmann *et al.*, 1976, 1978, 1979b, 1981; Mueller *et al.*, 1978; Anderson *et al.*, 1980; Capecchi, 1980; Kopchick *et al.*, 1981; Pugatsch and Stacey, 1982; Timm *et al.*, 1983; Graessmann and Graessmann, 1983a,b, 1984; Izant and Weintraub, 1984; Kopchick and Stacey, 1985; see also Chapters 1 and 2), RNA (for references see Graessmann and Graessmann, 1971, 1976, 1982; Graessmann *et al.*, 1974; Stacey and Allfrey, 1976; Celis, 1977, 1984a; Stacey *et al.*, 1977; Liu *et al.*, 1979; Bravo and Celis, 1980; Celis *et al.*, 1980b,c; Huez *et al.*, 1980; Stacey, 1980a,b; Franke *et al.*, 1984), proteins (for references see Stacey and Allfrey, 1977, 1984; Tjian *et al.*, 1978; Feramisco, 1979; Kreis *et al.*, 1979; Graessmann *et al.*, 1980b; Wehland and Weber, 1980; Klimkowsky, 1981; Lin and Feramisco, 1981; Glacy, 1983; Mercer *et al.*, 1983, 1984; Einck *et al.*, 1984; Feramisco *et al.*, 1984; Stacey and Kung, 1984; Mulcahy *et al.*, 1985; see also Chapter 3), small molecules, organelles and virus particles have been introduced into the cytoplasm or the nucleus of a wide range of cultured somatic cells. DNA species are efficiently expressed following microinjection (Table II; nearly 100% for transient expression) and stable TK^+ transformants have been obtained with frequencies of 0.1–0.2% of the intranuclearly injected cells (Table II; Capecchi, 1980). mRNA species (Table II; for references see Celis, 1984a) and complementary RNAs (Graessmann and Graessmann, 1976, 1982) are readily translated and suppressor tRNA species have been shown to correct nonsense mutations (Hudziak *et al.*, 1982; see also Chapter 16). Microinjected proteins have been shown to find their cellular localization and to exhibit biological activity. Often, however, injected proteins are misplaced, a fact that is worrisome.

(6) The biological effect of the injected molecules can be analysed in a natural environment. Assays can be performed in single cells if autoradiographic, immunofluorescent or histochemical tests are available. At the protein synthesis level the effect can be assessed in 10–50 injected cells if improved [^{35}S]-methionine labelling techniques (Bravo *et al.*, 1981; Celis

Table II. Comparison between the various transfer techniques (from Celis, 1984a,b).

Technique	DNA: Thymidine kinase gene: Cells expressing thymidine kinase (%)	DNA: Thymidine kinase gene: TK$^+$ colonies (%)	DNA: SV40 genes: Number of molecules of SV40 DNA required for plaque formation	DNA: SV40 genes: Cells expressing T antigen (%)	Proteins (average number of molecules injected per cell): Serum albumin	Proteins (average number of molecules injected per cell): IgG	mRNA (average number of molecules injected per cell): Protamine mRNA	mRNA (average number of molecules injected per cell): Globin mRNA
Direct microinjection								
Microinjection with glass capillaries	50–100[a]	0.1–0.2[b]	1[f]	100[g]	2.4×10^{7j}		$(3–6) \times 10^{5m}$	2.9×10^{4c}
Vehicle-mediated transfer								
Erythrocytes		0.005–0.001[7c]			2.7×10^{6k}	$(2–5) \times 10^{5l}$	$(1.2–2.4) \times 10^{4n}$	
Liposomes	10[a]	0.02[a]	10^{6f}					1×10^{4p}
Reconstituted Sendai virus envelopes		0.08–0.1[d]	5×10^{5f}	1–20[h]		$(1–4) \times 10^{4l}$		
Transfer aided by facilitators								
Calcium phosphate	3[a]	0.05[a]	10^{6f}	5–10[i]				
DEAE-dextran	0.1–1[a]	<0.0001[a]						
Polyethylene glycol sucrose shock		≈0.03[e]		70[e]				

[a] From Schäfer-Ridder *et al*. (1982). [b] Capecchi (1980). [c] Iino *et al*. (1983). Correspond to the highest value reported.
[d] Vainstain *et al*. (1983). Correspond to the highest value reported. [e] Shen *et al*. (1982). Correspond to the highest value reported.
[f] From Graessmann and Graessmann (1984). [g] Graessmann *et al*. (1976). [h] Loyter *et al*. (1983).
[i] Rassoulzadegan *et al*. (1982). [j] These data have been calculated assuming injection of 10^{-7} μl of a 1.7 mg/ml solution of bovine serum albumin.
[k] Wassermann *et al*. (1976). [l] Cited in Loyter and Volsky (1982)
[m] These data have been calculated assuming injection of 10^{-7} μl of a 1 mg/ml solution of protamine mRNA.
[n] Boogard and Dixon (1983b).
[o] These data have been calculated assuming injection of 10^{-7} μl of a 0.1 mg/ml solution of globin mRNA.
[p] Ostro *et al*. (1980).

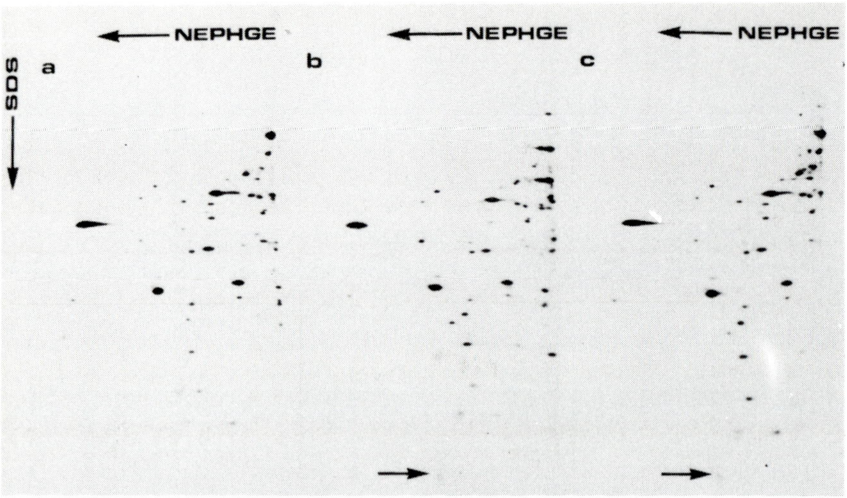

Fig. 3. Two-dimensional gel electrophoresis (NEPHGE) of [^{35}S]-methionine labelled polypeptides from 3T3 injected with globin mRNA. (a) 100 control cells; (b) 100 control cells plus globin synthesized *in vitro*; and (c) 100 cells injected with total globin mRNA (0.5 mg/ml). The arrows indicate the position of globin. From Bravo and Celis, 1980.

and Bravo, 1981) are used in combination with polyacrylamide gel electrophoresis (Bravo and Celis, 1980; Celis *et al.*, 1980b; Graessmann and Graessmann, 1982) (see Fig. 3).

The main disadvantages of the technique can be summarized as follows.

(1) The number of cells that can be injected is limited. An experienced researcher can inject a maximum of about 1000 cells/h. Thus, the technique cannot be used to study biological or biochemical processes that require a much higher number of cells. This disadvantage can be partially overcome by microinjecting multinucleated giant cells produced by polyethylene glycol-induced fusion of cultured cells (Graessmann *et al.*, 1979a). These cells, however, are not viable.

(2) The technique cannot be used to deliver macromolecules into cells of living organisms or to implant components into the membrane of cultured somatic cells.

(3) There is a damaging effect produced by the introduction of the glass capillary and by the pressure exerted by the injected fluid. The extent of the damage cannot be estimated at present.

The main areas of research in which this technique has uniquely contributed to an advance in knowledge are listed in Table I.

III. VEHICLE-MEDIATED TRANSFER

A. Erythrocyte-mediated transfer

The erythrocyte-mediated transfer is based on the fusion of red blood cells, preloaded with macromolecules, together with somatic cells by using inactivated Sendai virus (Furusawa *et al.*, 1974; Loyter *et al.*, 1975; Schlegel and Rechsteiner, 1975) or polyethylene glycol (Kaltoft and Celis, 1978; Krieger *et al.*, 1978; Brown *et al.*, 1985; see also Chapter 5) as fusogenic agents. First, the macromolecules are trapped within the erythrocyte ghost during hypo-osmotic haemolysis (step 1, Fig. 4), and secondly the resealed vesicles are fused with the recipient cell (step 2, Fig. 4; usually a 100-fold excess of erythrocytes over cultured cells are used; see also Schlegel and Rechsteiner, 1978; Rechsteiner, 1982). Sendai virus is recommended as fusogen for cells

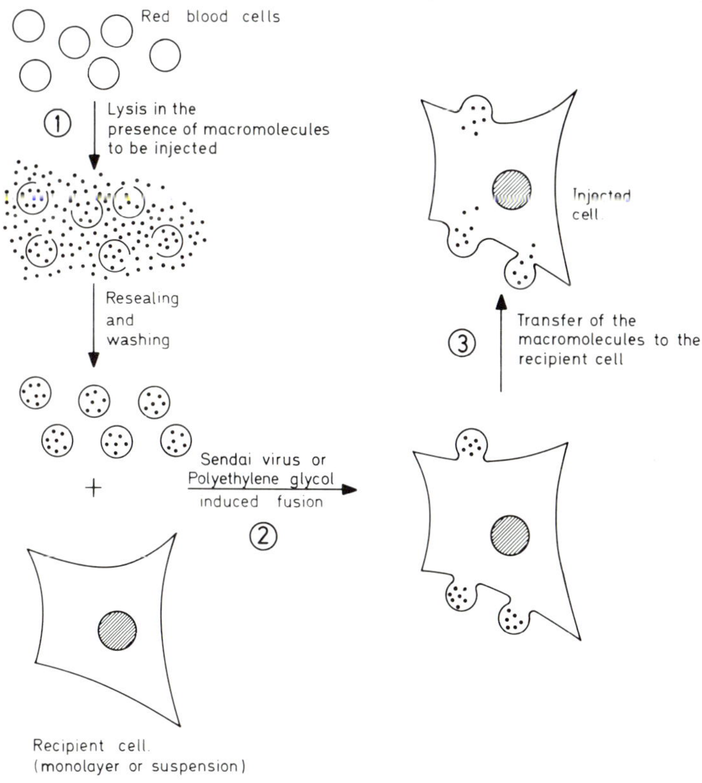

Fig. 4. Schematic representation of the erythrocyte-mediated transfer. (1) Erythrocyte loading; (2) fusion of loaded erythrocytes with recipient cells; and (3) transfer of macromolecules to the recipient cells. Modified from Celis (1977).

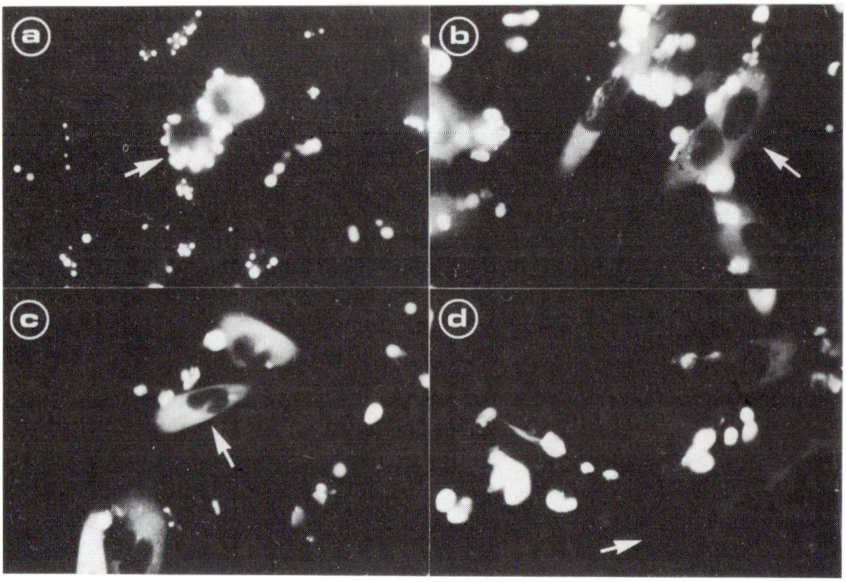

Fig. 5. Fusion of CHO cells with human erythrocytes loaded with FITC-BSA (16 O.D. 490/ml). (a) 10 min after fusion; (b), (c) and (d) 30 min after fusion. From Kaltoft and Celis, 1978.

in suspension while PEG is more suitable for monolayers. The average number of erythrocytes fusing with recipient cells is about 5 in polyethylene glycol-induced fusions as compared with 1–3 for Sendai virus fusions. Recently, Schlegel and Mercer (1980) have improved the efficiency of microinjection by combining the use of polyethylene glycol (fusogenic agent; 44%) and the lectin phytohaemagglutinin (50–75 μg/ml). Under these conditions 70–75% of the quiescent fibroblasts could be injected with a viability of 80–95%. Various procedures to improve the efficiency of transfer both in suspensions as well as in monolayers are discussed in Chapter 5. Protocols have also been developed for antibody-directed targeting of ghosts to cell surface antigens (Godfrey *et al.*, 1981, 1983). For example, avidin-coupled erythrocytes have been successfully fused to mouse lymphocytes labelled with biotin anti-mouse immunoglobulins (Godfrey *et al.*, 1983).

By this technique, macromolecules are introduced into the cytoplasm of the recipient cultured cells. For those macromolecules that do not usually cross the nuclear membrane, access to the nucleus can be achieved by using cells in mitosis (Schlegel, 1984). Proteins (for references see Loyter *et al.*, 1975; Schlegel and Rechsteiner, 1975, 1978; Wassermann *et al.*, 1976; Rechsteiner and Kuehl, 1979; Yamaizumi *et al.*, 1979; Zavortink *et al.*, 1979; Antman and Livingston, 1980; Wille and Willecke, 1980; Bigelow *et al.*,

1981; Chin *et al.*, 1982; Ohara *et al.*, 1982; Rechsteiner, 1982; Bennett *et al.*, 1983; Boney *et al.*, 1983; McGarry *et al.*, 1983; Vogt *et al.*, 1983; Osawa *et al.*, 1984; Jacobsen and Wojciezyn, 1984; Rechsteiner *et al.*, 1984; Schlegel, 1984; Yoshimori *et al.*, 1984) and RNA (Kaltoft *et al.*, 1976; Schlegel *et al.*, 1976, 1978; Anderson *et al.*, 1977; Capecchi *et al.*, 1977; Boogard and Dixon, 1983a,b) have been transferred into somatic cells by using this technique but the average number of molecules injected per cell is about 10 times lower than that achieved by the direct microinjection (Table II; calculations are based on the injection of bovine serum albumin; compare also Figs 2a and 4b and c). There are a few reports concerning transfer of DNA (Iino *et al.*, 1983; Wiberg *et al.*, 1983), but this requires special loading conditions. For example, in the protocol described by Wiberg *et al.* (1983) both the presence of EDTA and repeated freeze–thawings of the ghosts during loading are required to trap DNA (see also Chapter 6). The reported efficiency of transformation (TK^+ transformants) is, however, significantly lower than that achieved by the direct microinjection approach, by the reconstituted Sendai virus envelope method or by the calcium phosphate technique (Table II).

The main advantage of this technique over the direct microinjection is that a large number of cells (10^7–10^8) can be injected simultaneously. The main disadvantages are the cotransfer of residual erythrocyte components and the need for a fusogenic agent. Various applications of this technique are listed in Table I.

B. Liposome-mediated transfer

In this technique, the macromolecules are first trapped within phospholipid vesicles (liposomes) before delivery to the recipient cells (Gregoriadis and Buckland, 1973; Pagano *et al.*, 1974; Papahadjopoulos *et al.*, 1974a,b, 1980a,b; Poste *et al.*, 1976; Pagano and Weinstein, 1978; Fraley *et al.*, 1979, 1980; Gregoriadis, 1980; Poste, 1980; Wong *et al.*, 1980; Nicolau and Sene, 1982; Nicolau *et al.*, 1983a; Straubinger *et al.*, 1985). Fusogenic agents such as polyethylene glycol are often not used in liposome-mediated transfer. Various types of vesicles have been described (for references see Straubinger and Papahadjopoulos, 1983; see also Chapter 7), but of these the large unilamellar vesicles are the best suited for transfer as they exhibit a relatively high ratio of internal aqueous space per unit lipid and because they have a higher delivery ratio. The mechanism by which the content of the vesicles is transferred to cells is still unknown, although endocytosis seems to be an important pathway of uptake (for references see Finkelstein and Weissmann, 1978; Straubinger *et al.*, 1983). Fusion of liposomes with plasma membrane is now believed to be a rare event (Pagano and Takeuchi, 1977;

Szoka *et al.*, 1981). Liposomes containing colloidal gold have been shown to be bound to coated pits, intracellular coated and uncoated vesicles and secondary lysosomes, including dense bodies (Straubinger *et al.*, 1983). These observations emphasize the topographical difficulties encountered with DNA in gene transfer experiments and may account for the low efficiency of transformation achieved with this technique as compared with direct nuclear microinjection (see below). Efforts are now being devoted to devise experimental conditions which may promote the escape of encapsulated molecules from the endocytic pathway (Straubinger *et al.*, 1983, 1985; see also Chapter 7).

Liposomes have been used to introduce proteins (Gregoriadis and Buckland, 1973; Gad *et al.*, 1979; Eytan and Eytan, 1980; Uchida *et al.*, 1984; Straubinger *et al.*, 1985), DNA (Fraley *et al.*, 1980, 1981; Papahadjopoulos *et al.*, 1980a,b; Nicolau and Sene, 1982; Schäffer-Ridder *et al.*, 1982), RNA (Dimitriadis, 1978; Ostro *et al.*, 1978, 1980; Wilson *et al.*, 1979), lipids (Martin and McDonald, 1976; Struck and Pagano, 1980), metaphase chromosomes (Mukherjee *et al.*, 1978) and small molecules (for references see Papahadjopoulos, 1979; Nicolau and Gersonde, 1979; Gersonde and Nicolau, 1979; Machy and Leserman, 1984) into a variety of cultured cells (no cell restriction). This technique, however, is less efficient than the direct microinjection for the injection of RNA (Table II) or proteins. Likewise, the efficiency of the liposome-mediated gene transfer, and expression, does not exceed that of more conventional methods (Table II). The technique, however, has the advantage that it can be used with cells that are refractory to transformation by the calcium phosphate technique.

From the above observations it would seem that future applications of this technique will rest mainly on the possibility of delivering drugs (for references see Gregoriadis *et al.*, 1982; Gregoriadis, 1983, 1984) and genetic material (for references see Nicolau *et al.*, 1982, 1983a,b; see also Chapter 9) into cells of living organisms. Techniques are now being developed to improve the specificity of delivery of liposomes by coupling specific antibodies to their surface (targeted liposomes) (for references see Barbet *et al.*, 1981; Heath *et al.*, 1981, 1983; Martin *et al.*, 1981; Martin and Papahadjopoulos, 1982; Huang *et al.*, 1983; Bragman *et al.*, 1983; Machy and Leserman, 1984).

C. Reconstituted Sendai virus envelopes

In this technique the macromolecules to be injected or transplanted are first trapped within the viral envelopes or incorporated into the vesicle membrane during their reconstitution (Fig. 6). Fusion of the loaded reconstituted Sendai virus envelopes (RSVE) with the plasma membrane of recipient cells

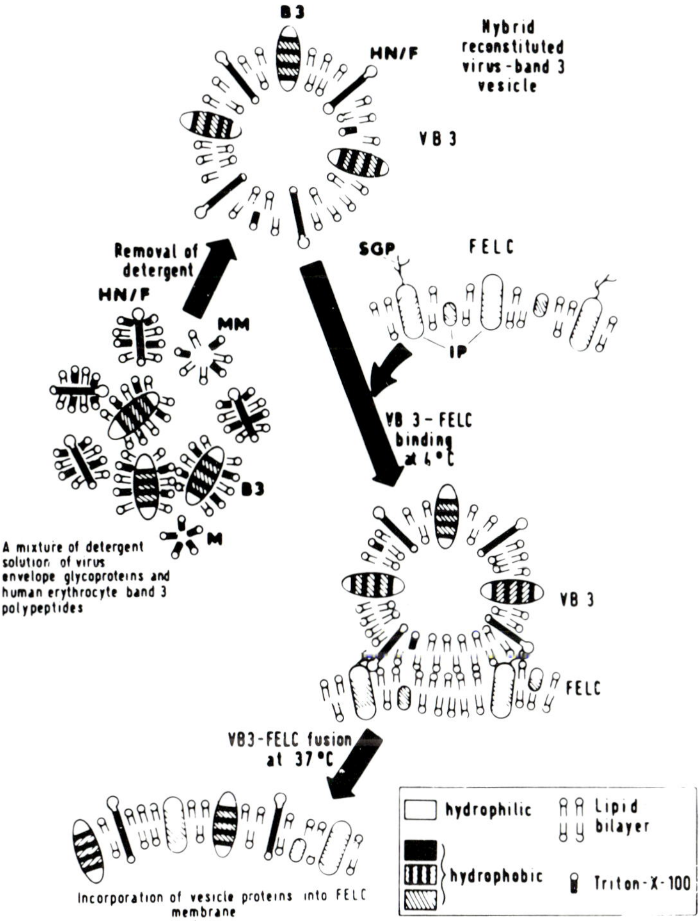

Fig. 6. Schematic representation of the method for using reconstituted Sendai virus envelopes for implantation of membrane protein band 3 into living animal cells. Isolated band 3 is first mixed with a detergent solution of viral envelopes and upon removal of the detergent by codialysis, vesicles containing band 3 are formed (VB3). Next, the hybrid vesicles are bound to the recipient cells by incubation at 4°C. Finally, integration takes place following incubation at 37°C. HN/F, agglutinin-neuraminidase or fusion glycoprotein of Sendai virus envelopes; B3, human erythrocyte band 3 polypeptide; FELC, Friend erythroleukaemic cells; M, detergent micelle; MM, mixed membrane phospholipid/detergent micelle; SGP, sialoglycoprotein; IP, integral membrane protein. From Loyter *et al.* (1980).

is then promoted by the presence of the virus F protein (fusion factor) in the reconstituted vesicles (Fig. 6) (for references see Uchida *et al.*, 1977, 1980; Volsky and Loyter, 1978; Loyter and Volsky, 1979, 1982; Volsky *et al.*, 1979; Beigel and Loyter, 1983; Loyter *et al.*, 1983, 1984; Vainstain *et al.*, 1983, 1984; see also Chapter 10). This technique is restricted to cells having receptors for Sendai virus, although efforts are currently being made to couple anti-cell membrane antibodies to the viral envelopes so as to extend its use to receptor-depleted cells (Loyter *et al.*, 1984; Chejanovsky *et al.*, 1985). A method for the preparation of highly fusogenic target RSVE has recently been published by Gitman *et al.* (1985; see also Chapter 10). Reconstituted Sendai virus envelopes have been used to transfer proteins (Loyter and Volsky, 1979, 1982; Uchida *et al.*, 1980) and DNA (Loyter *et al.*, 1983; Vainstain *et al.*, 1983) into cultured cells as well as to transplant membrane proteins (Volsky *et al.*, 1979, 1980; Loyter and Volsky, 1982; Beigel and Loyter, 1983; Loyter *et al.*, 1984). This technique does not present any significant advantage over the direct microinjection technique for the injection of proteins (Table II; immunoglobulin G), or RNA, but it may be of value for gene-transfer studies (Table II) for cells that cannot be transfected by using the calcium phosphate technique. Also it is possible that, in the future, this technique may be of use to deliver macromolecules (especially DNA) into cells of living organisms. Various applications of this technique are listed in Table I.

Recently, Evans and Mayer (1983) described a technique, polyethylene glycol-induced sub-organelle vesicle transplantation, which can also be used to study the degradation of proteins after transplantation of organelles into appropriate target cells. Specifically, this method offers new possibilities for studying the degradation of intracellular proteins that function in defined extracytosolic sites. So far, this technique has been used to study the degradative fate of transplanted total mitochondrial proteins and mitochondrial outer membrane proteins (Evans and Mayer, 1983, 1984; Russell and Mayer, 1983; Mayer *et al.*, 1984; see also Chapter 13).

IV. TRANSFER AIDED BY FACILITATORS

A. Calcium phosphate technique

This technique, which was originally developed to determine the infectivity of viral DNA (Graham and van der Eb, 1973; see also Chapter 11 and references therein) is now widely used to assay the transforming activity of viral DNA (for references see Graham, 1977; Graham and Baccheti, 1983) as well as of DNA extracted from eukaryotic cells (for references see Wigler *et al.*, 1978; Willecke *et al.*, 1979; Graham *et al.*, 1980; Lewis *et al.*, 1980; Rubin *et al.*, 1983). The technique requires the incubation of the recipient cells with coprecipitates of DNA and calcium phosphate. The precipitate binds to the cells and is then taken up via an endocytotic-like process (Loyter *et al.*, 1982). Intracellularly, the DNA molecules have been shown to be trapped in phagocytic vacuoles and secondary lysosomes (Loyter *et al.*, 1983), but very little is known as to how they gain access to the nucleus and become integrated in the host genome. There is evidence that the donor DNA molecules become linked to high molecular mass carrier DNA (Perucho *et al.*, 1980) forming complexes termed "transgenomes" (Scangos and Ruddle, 1981; see also Chapter 11). The technique necessitates the use of specific cell lines such as mouse L cells and NIH3T3 cells.

To date, this technique has proved invaluable in studies of gene transfer in cultured somatic cells, and it is increasingly being used to transfect genomic clones into target cells. The percentage of stably transformed TK^+ cells obtained with this technique is comparable with that obtained by microinjection, but many more cells can be transfected at a time. Furthermore, transfection of DNA isolated from neoplastic cells into non-neoplastic recipient cells has provided a unique approach for the study of the genetic control of cancer (for references see Cooper, 1982).

B. DEAE-dextran

In this method, the DNA is added to the cultured cells in the presence of the polycation DEAE-dextran (Pagano and Vaheri, 1965; Vaheri and Pagano, 1965; McCutchan and Pagano, 1968; Warden and Thorne, 1968; Graham, 1977). The efficiency of transformation (TK^+; Table II) achieved with this technique is considerably lower than that obtained with other methods currently used for gene transfer (Table II).

C. Polyethylene glycol/sucrose shock

This technique is essentially a modification of the procedure of Chu and Sharpe (1981) to transfect cells in suspension. Briefly, after transfection the cells are plated and after 4 h they are shocked for 2–4 min with a 60–70% concentration of polyethylene glycol in sucrose (Shen *et al.*, 1982). The optimum concentration of polyethylene glycol must be worked out for each individual cell line. This procedure gives excellent results in terms of transient gene expression (phenotypic expression; Table II) and represents a reasonable alternative to direct microinjection in those cases in which transfer of genes to a large number of cells is required. The percentage of stably transformed cells (TK^+; Table II) obtained with this technique is low.

D. Osmotic lysis of pinosomes

This technique, which was developed by Okada and Rechsteiner (1982), has been used mainly to introduce proteins (horseradish peroxidase and ricin antibodies) and Dextran 70000 into the cytoplasm of mouse L929 cells. In short, cells are first incubated in the presence of 0.5 M sucrose/10% polyethylene glycol 1000 and the macromolecules to be injected, followed by a short incubation in hypo-osmotic medium. Under these conditions, the pinocytic vesicles formed during the sucrose treatment release their content as a result of the osmotic lysis.

The technique can be used for large-scale transfer of proteins into cultured mammalian cells and the efficiency of transfer has been shown to be similar to that achieved by the erythrocyte-mediated transfer (Okada and Rechsteiner, 1982). By the technique of osmotic lysis of pinosomes, however, it may be possible to transfer larger macromolecules. The technique requires the use of cultured cells exhibiting a high rate of fluid-phase pinocytosis (Steinman *et al.*, 1974; Okada and Rechsteiner, 1982).

V. CONCLUSION

In general, the various transfer techniques described here as well as in previous chapters have opened the possibilities of studying complex biological phenomena that are not amenable to experimentation with conventional systems *in vitro*. The technique of direct microinjection of cultured somatic cells with glass capillaries is perhaps the most versatile of the transfer techniques, and, despite its disadvantages, it has brought us closer to the final goal of using the somatic cell as a test tube.

The applications of the various transfer techniques in basic research are numerous and evident (see text and Table I). In medicine, techniques such as liposome-mediated transfer and Sendai virus reconstituted envelopes may provide a realistic basis for important applications in areas such as gene transfer (genetic engineering *in vivo*) and delivery of drugs to specific cell types in living organisms.

Note added in proof

Recently, Doxsey *et al.* (Doxey, S. J., Sambrook, J., Helenius, A. and White, J. 1985: *J. Cell Biol.* **101**, 19–27) have used a modification of the erythrocyte-mediated transfer technique to inject 1.4×10^7 IgG molecules into the cytoplasm of Cvl cells. The technique uses loaded erythrocytes as delivery vesicles and for attachment and membrane fusion it exploits the activities of influenza virus haemagglutinin expressed on the surface of the recipient cells. Extensive membrane fusion is triggered by mildly acidic pH.

REFERENCES

Anderson, W. F., Deisseroth, A., Nienhuis, A. W., Gopalakrishnan, T. V., Huang, A. and Krueger, L. (1977). *Natl. Cancer Inst. Monogr.* **48**, 65–73.

Anderson, W. F., Killos, L., Sanders-Haigh, L., Kretschmer, P. J. and Diacumakos, E. G. (1980). *Proc. Natl. Acad. Sci. USA* **77**, 5399–5403.
Ansorge, W. (1982). *Exp. Cell Res.* **140**, 31–37.
Antman, K. H. and Livingston, D. M. (1980). *Cell* **19**, 627–635.
Barbet, J., Machy, P. and Leserman, L. D. (1981). *J. Supramol. Struct. Cell. Biochem.* **16**, 243–258.
Baserga, R., Croce, C. and Rovera, G. eds (1980). "Introduction of Macromolecules into Viable Mammalian Cells". Alan Liss, New York.
Beigel, M. and Loyter, A. (1983). *Exp. Cell. Res.* **148**, 95–103.
Bennett, F., Busch, H., Lischwe, M. A. and Yeoman, L. C. (1983). *J. Cell Biol.* **97**, 1556–1572.
Bigelow, S., Hough, R. and Rechsteiner, M. (1981). *Cell* **25**, 83–93.
Boney, C., Finck, D., Schlichter, D., Carr, K. and Wicks, W. D. (1983). *J. Biol. Chem.* **258**, 4911–4918.
Boogard, C. and Dixon, G. (1983a). *Exp. Cell Res.* **143**, 175–190.
Boogard, C. and Dixon, G. (1983b). *Exp. Cell Res.* **143**, 191–205.
Bragman, K. S., Heath, T. D. and Papahadjopoulos, D. (1983). *Biochim. Biophys. Acta* **730**, 187–195.
Bravo, R. and Celis, J. E. (1980). *Exp. Cell Res.* **126**, 481–485.
Bravo, R., Fey, S. J., Small, J. V., Mose Larsen, P. and Celis, J. E. (1981). *Cell* **25**, 197–202.
Brown, D. B., Hank, S. K., Murphy, E. C. and Rao, P. N. (1985). *Exp. Cell Res.* **156**, 251–259.
Capecchi, M. (1980). *Cell* **22**, 479–488.
Capecchi, M. R., Vonder Haar, R. A., Capecchi, N. E. and Sveda, M. M. (1977). *Cell* **12**, 371–381.
Celis, J. E. (1977). *Brookhaven Symp. Biol.* **29**, 178–196.
Celis, J. E. (1984a). *Ciba Found. Symp.* **103**, 220–231.
Celis, J. E. (1984b). *Biochem. J.* **223**, 281–291.
Celis, J. E. and Bravo, R. (1981). *Trends Biochem. Sci.* **6**, 197–201.
Celis, J. E., Graessmann, M. and Loyter, A. eds (1980a). "Transfer of Cell Constituents into Eukaryotic Cells". Plenum Press, New York and London.
Celis, J. E., Kaltoft, K. and Bravo, R. (1980b). *In* "Introduction of Macromolecules into Viable Mammalian Cells" (R. Baserga, C. Croce and G. Rovera, eds), pp. 99–123. Alan Liss, New York.
Celis, J. E., Kaltoft, K., Celis, A., Fenwick, R. and Caskey, C. T. (1980c). *In* "Nonsense Mutations and tRNA Suppressors" (J. E. Celis and J. D. Smith, eds), pp. 254–276. Academic Press, London and New York.
Chejanovsky, N., Fridlender, B. and Loyter, A. (1985). *Biochim. Biophys. Acta*, in press.
Chin, D. T., Khuel, L. and Rechsteiner, M. (1982). *Proc. Natl. Acad. Sci. USA* **79**, 5857–5861.
Chu, G. and Sharpe, P. A. (1981). *Gene* **13**, 197–202.
Cooper, G. M. (1982). *Science* **218**, 801–806.
Diacumakos, E. G. (1973). *Methods Cell Biol.* **8**, 287–311.
Dimitriadis, G. T. (1978). *Nature* **274**, 923–924.
Einck, L., Soares, N. and Bustin, M. (1984). *Exp. Cell Res.* **152**, 287–301.
Evans, P. J. and Mayer, R. J. (1983). *Biochem. J.* **216**, 151–161.
Evans, P. J. and Mayer, R. J. (1984). *Biochem. J.* **219**, 61–72.
Eytan, G. and Eytan, E. (1980). *J. Biol. Chem.* **255**, 4992–4995.
Evered, D. and Whelan, J. eds (1984). "Cell Fusion"; *Ciba Found. Symp.* **103**.

Feramisco, J. R. (1979). *Proc. Natl. Acad. Sci. USA* **76**, 3967–3971.
Feramisco, J. R., Gross, M., Kamata, T., Rosenberg, M. and Sweet, R. W. (1984). *Cell* **38**, 109–117.
Finkelstein, M. and Weissmann, G. (1978). *J. Lipid Res.* **18**, 289–303.
Fraley, R. T., Fornari, C. S. and Kaplan, S. (1979). *Proc. Natl. Acad. Sci. USA* **76**, 3348–3353.
Fraley, R., Subramani, S., Berg, P. and Papahadjopoulos, D. (1980). *J. Biol. Chem.* **255**, 10431–10435.
Fraley, R., Straubinger, R. M., Rule, G., Springer, E. L. and Papahadjopoulos, D. (1981). *Biochemistry* **20**, 6978–6987.
Franke, W. E., Schmid, E., Mittnacht, S., Grund, C. and Jorcano, J. L. (1984). *Cell* **36**, 813–825.
Furusawa, M. (1980). *Int. Rev. Cytol.* **62**, 29–67.
Furusawa, M., Nishimura, T., Yamaizumi, M. and Okada, Y. (1974). *Nature* **249**, 449–450.
Furusawa, M., Yamaizumi, M., Nishimura, T., Uchida, T. and Okada, Y. (1976). *Methods Cell Biol.* **14**, 73–80.
Gad, A., Broza, R. and Eytan, G. (1979). *FEBS Lett.* **102**, 230–234.
Gersonde, K. and Nicolau, C. (1979). *Blut* **39**, 1–7.
Gitman, A. G., Kahane, I. and Loyter, A. (1985). *Biochemistry*, **24**, 2762–2768.
Glacy, S. D. (1983). *J. Cell Biol.* **97**, 1207–1213.
Godfrey, W., Dol, B. and Wofsy, L. (1983). *Proc. Natl. Acad. Sci. USA* **80**, 2267–2271.
Godfrey, W., Dol, B., Wallace, E. F., Breds, B. and Wofsy, L. (1981). *Exp. Cell Res.* **135**, 137–146.
Graessmann, A. (1968). Doctoral Dissertation, Free University of Berlin.
Graessmann, A. and Graessmann, M. (1971). *Hoppe-Seyler's Z. Physiol. Chem.* **352**, 527–532.
Graessmann, M. and Graessmann, A. (1976). *Proc. Natl. Acad. Sci. USA* **73**, 366–370.
Graessmann, M. and Graessmann, A. (1982). *EMBO J.* **1**, 1081–1088.
Graessmann, M. and Graessmann, A. (1983a). *Methods Enzymol.* **101**, 484–492.
Graessmann, A. and Graessmann, M. (1983b). *In* "Gene Expression in Normal and Transformed Cells" (J. E. Celis and R. Bravo, eds), pp. 247–261. Plenum Press, New York.
Graessmann, M. and Graessmann, A. (1984). *Miami Winter Symp.*, in press.
Graessmann, A., Graessmann, M., Hoffmann, E., Niebel, J., Brandner, G. and Mueller, N. (1974). *FEBS Lett.* **39**, 249–251.
Graessmann, A., Graessmann, M. and Mueller, C. (1976). *J. Virol.* **17**, 854–858.
Graessmann, A., Graessmann, M., Guhl, E. and Mueller, C. (1978). *J. Cell Biol.* **77**, 1–8.
Graessmann, M., Graessmann, A. and Mueller, C. (1979a). *Biochem. Biophys. Res. Commun.* **88**, 428–432.
Graessmann, A., Graessmann, M. and Mueller, C. (1979b). *Curr. Topics Microbiol. Immunol.* **81**, 1–21.
Graessmann, A., Graessmann, M. and Mueller, C. (1980a). *Methods Enzymol.* **65**, 816–825.
Graessmann, A., Graessmann, M., Tjian, R. and Topp, W. C. (1980b). *J. Virol.* **33**, 1182–1191.
Graessmann, A., Wolf, H. and Bornkamm, G. W. (1980c). *Proc. Natl. Acad. Sci. USA* **77**, 433–436.

Graessmann, A., Graessmann, M. and Mueller, C. (1981). *Adv. Cancer Res.* **35**, 111–146.
Graham, F. L. (1977). *Adv. Cancer Res.* **25**, 1–51.
Graham, F. L. and Bacchetti, S. (1983). *In* "Techniques in the Life Sciences", B5, Nucleic Acid Biochemistry, (R. A. Flavell, ed.), pp. 1–14. Elsevier, Ireland.
Graham, F. L. and van der Eb, A. J. (1973). *Virology* **52**, 456–467.
Graham, F. L., Bachetti, S. and McKinnon, R. (1980). *In* "Introduction of Macromolecules into Viable Mammalian Cells" (R. Baserga, C. Croce and G. Rovera, eds), pp. 3–25. Alan Liss, New York.
Gregoriadis, G. (1980). *In* "Transfer of Cell Constituents into Eukaryotic Cells" (J. E. Celis, A. Graessmann and A. Loyter, eds), pp. 173–199. Plenum Press, New York.
Gregoriadis, G. (1983). *Trends Pharmacol. Sci.* **4**, 304–307.
Gregoriadis, G., ed. (1984). "Liposome Technology". Vols I–III, CRC Press, Boca Raton.
Gregoriadis, G. and Allison, A. C., eds (1980). "Liposomes in Biological Systems". John Wiley, New York.
Gregoriadis, G. and Buckland, R. A. (1973). *Nature* **244**, 170–172.
Gregoriadis, G., Senior, J. and Trowet, A., eds (1982). "Targeting of Drugs". Plenum Press, New York.
Heath, D. T., Fraley, R. T. and Papahadjopoulos, D. (1981). *Science* **210**, 599–601.
Heath, D. T., Montgomery, J. A., Piper, J. A. and Papahadjopoulos, D. (1983). *Proc. Natl. Acad. Sci. USA* **80**, 1377–1381.
Huang, A., Kennel, S. J. and Huang, L. (1983). *J. Biol. Chem.* **258**, 14034–14040.
Hudziak, R. M., Laske, F. A., RajBhandary, U. L., Sharp, P. A. and Capecchi, M. (1982). *Cell* **31**, 137–146.
Huez, G., Bruck, C., Portetelle, D. and Cleuter, Y. (1980). *FEBS Lett.* **109**, 39–42.
Iino, T., Furusawa, M., Furusawa, I. and Obinata, M. (1983). *Exp. Cell. Res.* **148**, 475–480.
Izant, J. G. and Weintraub, H. (1984). *Cell* **36**, 1007–1015.
Jacobsen, K. and Wojciezyn, J. (1984). *Proc. Natl. Acad. Sci. USA* **81**, 6747–6751.
Kaltoft, K. and Celis, J. E. (1978). *Exp. Cell Res.* **115**, 423–428.
Kaltoft, K., Zeuthen, J., Engbaek, F., Piper, P. and Celis, J. E. (1976). *Proc. Natl. Acad. Sci. USA* **73**, 2793–2797.
Klimkowsky, M. W. (1981). *Nature* **291**, 249–251.
Kopchick, J. J. and Stacey, D. W. (1985). *Mol. Cell. Biol.*, in press.
Kopchick, J. J., Ju, G., Skalka, A. M. and Stacey, D. W. (1981). *Proc. Natl. Acad. Sci. USA* **78**, 4383–4387.
Kreis, T. E., Winterhalter, K. H. and Birchmeier (1979). *Proc. Natl. Acad. Sci. USA* **76**, 3814–3818.
Krieger, M. P., Griffin, J. D. and Livingston, D. M. (1978). *Cell* **14**, 983–994.
Kulka, R. G. and Loyter, A. (1979). *Curr. Topics Membr. Transport* **12**, 365–430.
Lewis, W. H., Srinivasan, P. R., Stokes, N. and Siminovitch, L. (1980). *Somatic Cell Genet.* **6**, 333–347.
Lin, J. J.-C. and Feramisco, J. R. (1981). *Cell* **24**, 185–193.
Liu, C. P., Slate, D. L., Gravel, R. and Ruddle, F. H. (1979). *Proc. Natl. Acad. Sci. USA* **766**, 4503–4506.
Loyter, A. and Volsky, D. J. (1979). *In* "Membrane Biogenesis" (S. P. Lee, G. Schatz and L. Ernster, eds), pp. 319–330. Addison-Wesley, London.
Loyter, A. and Volsky, D. J. (1982). *In* "Cell Surface Reviews" (G. Poste and G. L. Nicolson, eds), pp. 215–266. North-Holland, Amsterdam.

Loyter, A., Zakai, N. and Kulka, R. G. (1975). *J. Cell Biol.* **66**, 292–304.
Loyter, A., Volsky, D. J., Beigel, M., Ginsburg, H. and Cabantchik, Z. I. (1980). *In* "Transfer of Cell Constituents into Eukaryotic Cells" (J. E. Celis, A. Graessmann and A. Loyter, eds), pp. 143–154. Plenum Press, New York.
Loyter, A., Scangos, G., Juricek, D. and Keene, D. (1982). *Exp. Cell Res.* **139**, 223–234.
Loyter, A., Vainstein, A., Graessmann, M. and Graessmann, A. (1983). *Exp. Cell Res.* **143**, 415–425.
Loyter, A., Tomasi, M., Gitman, A. G., Etinger, L. and Nussbaum, O. (1984). *Ciba Found. Symp.* **103**, 163–175.
Machy, P. and Leserman, L. D. (1984). *EMBO J.* **3**, 1971–1977.
Martin, F. and McDonald, R. (1976). *J. Cell Biol.* **70**, 515–526.
Martin, F. J. and Papahadjopoulos, D. (1982). *J. Biol. Chem.* **257**, 286–288.
Martin, F. J., Hubbell, W. L. and Papahadjopoulos, D. (1981). *Biochemistry* **20**, 4229–4238.
Mayer, R. J., Evans, P., Russell, S. and Amenta, J. S. (1984). *Ciba Found. Symp.* **103**, 202–214.
McCutchan, J. H. and Pagano, J. S. (1968). *J. Natl. Cancer Inst.* **41**, 351–357.
McGarry, T., Hough, R., Rogers, S. and Rechsteiner, M. (1983). *J. Cell Biol.* **96**, 338–346.
Mercer, W. E., Avignolo, E. and Baserga, R. (1984). *Mol. Cell. Biol.* **4**, 267–281.
Mercer, E. W., Nelson, D., Hyland, J. K., Croce, C. and Baserga, R. (1983). *Virology* **127**, 149–158.
Mueller, C., Graessmann, A. and Graessmann, M. (1978). *Cell* **15**, 579–585.
Mukherjee, A. B., Orloff, S., Butler, J. D., Triche, T., Lalley, P. and Schulman, J. D. (1978). *Proc. Natl. Acad. Sci. USA* **75**, 1361–1365.
Mulcahy, L., Smith, M. R. and Stacey, D. W. (1985). *Nature* **313**, 241–243.
Nicolau, C. and Gersonde, K. (1979). *Naturwissenschaften* **66**, 561–564.
Nicolau, C. and Sene, C. (1982). *Biochim. Biophys. Acta* **721**, 185–190.
Nicolau, C., Le Pape, A., Soriano, P., Fargette, D., Juhel, M. F. and Muh, J. P. (1982). *In* "Proceedings of the FEBS Meeting on Cell Differentiation" (A. E. Evangelopoulos, ed.), pp. 321–331. Alan Liss, New York.
Nicolau, C., Soriano, P., Le Pape, A., Londos-Gagliardi, D., Legrand, A. and Grosse, E. (1983a). *Biol. Cell.* **47**, 121–130.
Nicolau, C., Le Pape, A., Soriano, P., Fargette, F. and Juhel, M. F. (1983b). *Proc. Natl. Acad. Sci. USA* **80**, 1068–1072.
Ohara, J., Sugi, M., Fugimoto, M. and Watanabe, T. (1982). *J. Immunol.* **129**, 1227–1232.
Okada, C. Y. and Rechsteiner, M. (1982). *Cell* **29**, 33–41.
Osawa, S., Betz, G. and Hall, P. F. (1984). *J. Cell Biol.* **99**, 1335–1342.
Ostro, M. C., Giacomini, D., Lavelle, D., Paxton, W. and Dray, S. (1978). *Nature* **274**, 921–923.
Ostro, M. C., Giacomini, D. and Dray, S. (1980). *In* "Introduction of Macromolecules into Viable Cells (R. Baserga, C. Croce and G. Rovera, eds), pp. 239–259. Alan Liss, New York.
Pagano, R. E. and Takeichi, M. (1977). *J. Cell. Biol.* **74**, 531–546.
Pagano, J. S. and Vaheri, A. (1965). *Arch. Gesamte Virusforch.* **17**, 456–464.
Pagano, R. E. and Weinstein, J. N. (1978). *Ann. Rev. Biophys. Bioeng.* **7**, 435–468.
Pagano, R., Huang, L. and Wey, C. (1974). *Nature* **252**, 166–167.
Papahadjopoulos, D. (1979). *Ann. Rep. Med. Chem.* **14**, 250–260.

Papahadjopoulos, D., Mayhew, R. and Poste, G. (1974a). *Nature* **252**, 163–166.
Papahadjopoulos, D., Poste, G. and Mayhew, E. (1974b). *Biochim. Biophys. Acta* **363**, 404–418.
Papahadjopoulos, D., Fraley, R. and Heath, T. (1980a). *In* "Liposomes and Immunobiology" (B. Tom and H. Six, eds), pp. 151–164. Elsevier/North Holland, New York.
Papahadjopoulos, D., Wilson, T. and Taber, R. (1980b). *In* "Transfer of Cell Constituents into Eukaryotic Cells" (J. E. Celis, A. Graessmann, and A. Loyter, eds), pp. 155–172. Plenum Press, New York.
Paraf, A. and Nicolau, C. eds (1981). "Liposomes in the Study of Drug Activity and Immunocompetent Cell Function". Academic Press, New York and London.
Perucho, M., Hanahan, D. and Wigler, M. (1980). *Cell* **22**, 309–317.
Poste, G. (1980). *In* "Liposomes in Biological Systems" (G. Gregoriadis and A. Allison, eds), pp. 101–151. John Wiley, New York.
Poste, G., Papahadjopoulos, D. and Vail, W. J. (1976). *Methods Cell Biol.* **14**, 33–71.
Pugatsch, T. and Stacey, D. W. (1982). *J. Virol.* **43**, 503–510.
Rassoulzadegan, M., Binetruy, B. and Cuzin, F. (1982). *Nature* **295**, 257–259.
Rechsteiner, M. C. (1982). *In* "Techniques in Somatic Cell Genetics" (J. W. Shay, ed), pp. 385–398. Plenum Press, New York.
Rechsteiner, M. and Kuehl, L. (1979). *Cell* **16**, 901–908.
Rechsteiner, M., Chin, D., Hough, R., McGarry, T., Rogers, S., Rote, K. and Wu, L. (1984). *Ciba Found. Symp.* **103**, 181–195.
Rubin, J. S., Joyner, A. L., Bernstein, A. and Whitmore, G. F. (1983). *Nature* **306**, 206–208.
Russell, S. and Mayer, R. J. (1983). *Biochem. J.* **216**, 163–175.
Scangos, G. and Ruddle, F. H. (1981). *Gene* **14**, 1–10.
Schäffer-Ridder, M., Wang, Y. and Hofschneider, P. H. (1982). *Science* **215**, 166–168.
Schlegel, R. A. (1984). *In* "Red Blood Cells as Carriers for Drugs" (J. R. DeLoach and U. Sprandel, eds). pp. 134–141. S. Karger, Basel.
Schlegel, R. A. and Mercer, W. E. (1980). *In* "Introduction of Macromolecules into Viable Mammalian Cells" (R. Baserga, C. Croce and G. Rovera, eds), pp. 145–155. Alan Liss, New York.
Schlegel, R. A. and Rechsteiner, M. (1975). *Cell* **5**, 371–379.
Schlegel, R. A. and Rechsteiner, M. C. (1978). *Methods Cell Biol.* **20**, 341–354.
Schlegel, R. A., Darrah, L. B. and Rechsteiner, M. C. (1976). *In* "Molecular Mechanisms in the Control of Gene Expression" (P. Nierlich, W. Rutter and C. F. Fox, eds), pp. 465–470. Academic Press, New York and London.
Schlegel, R. A., Iverson, P. and Rechsteiner, M. C. (1978). *Nucl. Acid. Res.* **5**, 3715–3729.
Shen, Y., Hirschhorn, R. R., Mercer, W. E., Surmacz, E., Tsutsui, Y., Soprano, K. J. and Baserga, R. (1982). *Mol. Cell. Biol.* **2**, 1145–1154.
Stacey, D. W. (1980a). *Cell* **21**, 811–820.
Stacey, D. W. (1980b). *In* "Transfer of Cell Constituents into Eukaryotic Cells" (J. E. Celis, A. Graessmann and A. Loyter, eds), pp. 29–60. Plenum Press, New York.
Stacey, D. W. (1981). *Methods Enzymol.* **79**, 76–78.
Stacey, D. W. and Allfrey, V. G. (1976). *Cell* **9**, 725–732.
Stacey, D. W. and Allfrey, V. G. (1977). *J. Cell Biol.* **75**, 807–817.
Stacey, D. W. and Allfrey, V. G. (1984). *Exp. Cell. Res.* **154**, 283–292.
Stacey, D. W. and Kung, H. F. (1984). *Nature* **310**, 508–511.

Stacey, D. W., Allfrey, V. G. and Hanafusa, H. (1977). *Proc. Natl. Acad. Sci. USA* **74**, 1614–1618.

Steinman, R. M., Silver, J. M. and Cohn, Z. A. (1974). *J. Cell Biol.* **63**, 949–969.

Straubinger, R. M. and Papahadjopoulos, D. (1983). *Methods Enzymol.* **101**, 512–527.

Straubinger, R. M., Hong, K., Friend, D. S. and Papahadjopoulos, D. (1983). *Cell* **32**, 1069–1079.

Straubinger, R. M., Düzgünes, N. and Papahadjopoulos, D. (1985). *FEBS Lett.* **1**, 148–154.

Struck, D. and Pagano, R. (1980). *J. Biol. Chem.* **255**, 5404–5410.

Szoka, F., Magnusson, K.-E., Wojcieszyn, J., Hou, Y., Derzko, Z. and Jacobsen, K. (1981). *Proc. Natl. Acad. Sci. USA* **78**, 1685–1689.

Timm, B., Kondor-Koch, C., Lehrach, H., Reidel, H., Edström, J. E. and Garoff, H. (1983). *Methods Enzymol.* **96**, 496–511.

Tjian, R., Fey, G. and Graessmann, A. (1978). *Proc. Natl. Acad. Sci. USA* **75**, 1279–1283.

Uchida, T., Yamaizumi, M. and Okada, Y. (1977). *Nature* **266**, 839–840.

Uchida, T., Yamaizumi, M., Mekada, E. and Okada, Y. (1980). *In* "Introduction of Macromolecules into Viable Mammalian Cells" (R. Baserga, C. Croce and G. Rovera, eds), pp. 169–185. Alan Liss, New York.

Uchida, T., Veda, S., Nakanishi, M., Miura, N. and Okada, Y. (1984). *Exp. Cell. Res.* **152**, 313–321.

Vainstain, A., Hershkovitz, M., Israel, S., Rabin, S. and Loyter, A. (1984). *Biochim. Biophys. Acta* **773**, 181–188.

Vainstain, A., Razin, A., Graessmann, A. and Loyter, A. (1983). *Methods Enzymol.* **101**, 492–512.

Vaheri, A. and Pagano, J. S. (1965). *Virology* **27**, 435–436.

Vogt, S. I., Snyder, J. A. and Mullins, J. M. (1983). *J. Cell. Biol.* **97**, 191a.

Volsky, D. J., Cabantchik, Z. I., Beigel, M. and Loyter, A. (1979). *Proc. Natl. Acad. Sci. USA* **76**, 5440–5444.

Volsky, D. J. and Loyter, A. (1978). *FEBS Lett.* **92**, 190–194.

Volsky, D. J., Shapiro, I. M. and Klein, G. (1980). *Proc. Natl. Acad. Sci. USA* **76**, 5453–5457.

Warden, D. and Thorne, H. V. (1968). *J. Gen. Virol.* **3**, 371–377.

Wasserman, M., Zakai, N., Loyter, A. and Kulka, R. G. (1976). *Cell* **7**, 551–556.

Wehland, J. and Weber, K. (1980). *Exp. Cell. Res.* **127**, 397–408.

Wiberg, F. C., Sunnerhagen, P., Kaltoft, K., Zeuthen, J. and Bjursell, G. (1983). *Nucl. Acid Res.* **11**, 7287–7302.

Wigler, M., Pellicer, A., Silverstein, S. and Axel, R. (1978). *Cell* **14**, 725–731.

Wille, W. and Willecke, K. (1980). *Exp. Cell. Res.* **130**, 95–99.

Willecke, K., Klomfass, M., Mierau, R. and Doehmer, J. (1979). *Mol. Gen. Genet.* **170**, 179–185.

Wilson, T., Papahadjopoulos, D. and Taber, R. (1979). *Cell* **17**, 77–84.

Wong, T. K., Nicolau, C. and Hofschneider, P. H. (1980). *Gene* **10**, 87–94.

Wu, R., Grossman, L. and Moldave, K., eds (1983). *Methods Enzymol.* **101C**.

Yamaizumi, M., Uchida, T., Mekada, E. and Okada, Y. (1979). *Cell* **18**, 1009–1014.

Yamamoto, F. and Furusawa, M. (1978). *Exp. Cell Res.* **117**, 441–445.

Yoshimori, T., Yamada, M., Sugawa, H., Mekada, E., Uchida, T. and Okada, Y. (1984). *Exp. Cell. Res.* **151**, 344–353.

Zavortink, M., Thacher, T. and Rechsteiner, M. C. (1979). *J. Cell Physiol.* **100**, 175–186.

13

Fusion of Cell Fragments: Studies on the Degradative Fate of Transplanted Mitochondrial and Karyoplastic Proteins

D. Fernig and R. J. Mayer

I. INTRODUCTION

It is intriguing that at a time when only some of the macromolecular components of the cellular genetic apparatus (nucleus) and energy transducing apparatus (mitochondria) had been identified by DNA and protein analytical techniques, biological scientists were already exploiting such knowledge in cellular and organellar-membrane reconstitution experiments. In the same year papers were published on the production of cell–cell hybrids (Barski *et al.*, 1960) and the reconstitution of energy-transducing mitochondrial inner membranes (Penefsky *et al.*, 1960).

At the cellular level it was envisioned that the fusion of cell fragments would permit a new approach to nucleocytoplasmic interactions, gene regulation and cell differentiation (Ringertz, 1978). Predictably, major genetic advances have stemmed from somatic cell fusion (Barski *et al.*, 1960; Ephrussi and Weiss, 1965), the fusion of karyoplasts (minicells), cytoplasts and microcells with cellular targets (Ringertz, 1978) and uptake of mitochondria into cells (Clark *et al.*, 1982).

Fragments of cell membranes have also been used to probe hormone–cell interactions. Initially, virally mediated fusion of one cell type, containing a specific receptor, with another cell type, containing only an intact adenyl cyclase system, demonstrated intercellular hormone receptor–adenyl cyclase coupling (Orly and Schramm, 1976). Subsequently, polyethylene glycol-mediated fusion of plasma membrane fragments containing specific receptors (Doyle *et al.*, 1979; Schramm, 1979; Neufeld *et al.*, 1980) and

Microinjection and Organelle Transplantation Techniques

ISBN: 0-12-164722-6
ISBN: 0-12-164723-4 Pbk

phospholipid vesicles containing purified receptors (Baumann *et al.*, 1980; Eimerl *et al.*, 1980) with receptorless target cells was achieved.

In short, these studies have provided insight into nuclear and mitochondrial genetics and hormone–cell membrane interactions which would have been otherwise difficult to achieve.

Cell fragments can be used in cellular reconstitutions (cell engineering) to study other poorly understood aspects of cell and molecular biology. One fundamental incompletely understood cell process which can be studied in this way is intracellular protein catabolism, particularly the cytoplasmic molecular events involved in the recognition and sequestration of cytosolic, membrane and organellar proteins into the cellular degradative systems. The principle is to bypass the complexities of labelling all cellular proteins with radiolabelled amino acids during protein biosynthesis (Evans *et al.*, 1983; Mayer *et al.*, 1984) so that their subsequent degradation can be studied. The bypass is effected by labelling proteins in the cell fragments of interest followed by introduction of the cell fragments into target cells. In this chapter the methods to introduce mitochondria, mitochondrial outer membrane and nuclei into target cells will be described. The methods and applications of organellar transplantation to study intracellular protein catabolism complement studies on erythrocyte-mediated transfer of proteins described earlier in Chapter 5.

II. TRANSPLANTATION OF MITOCHONDRIA AND MITOCHONDRIAL OUTER MEMBRANE

A. Mitochondria/mitochondrial outer membrane (MOM)–hepatocyte

(1) Methods

(a) Preparation of hepatocytes. Hepatocytes are prepared as previously described (Evans, 1981).

(b) Preparation and FITC (fluorescein isothiocyanate) labelling of mitochondria and mitochondrial outer membrane vesicles. Rat livers are perfused *in situ* (Evans, 1981) with 150 ml of Ca^{2+}-free Krebs and Henseleit (1932) bicarbonate buffer. Mitochondria are prepared from blood-free livers (Bustamante *et al.*, 1977). Mitochondrial outer membrane vesicles are prepared by the method of Martinez and McCauley (1977). Reductive methylation of both preparations is carried out as described by Evans and Mayer (1982).

A solution of FITC in Dulbecco's phosphate-buffered saline, pH 9.5 (Dulbecco and Vogt, 1954), is prepared by shaking FITC (1 mg/ml) for 1 h.

The suspension is centrifuged ($3000 \times g_{av.}$ for 30 min) and the clear supernatant used for fluorescent labelling of mitochondria. Each mitochondrial preparation (4 mg of protein) is resuspended in Dulbecco's phosphate-buffered saline, pH 7.4 and mixed with an equal volume of the FITC solution. The mixture is protected from light and intermittently shaken for 20 min at room temperature. The preparation is then dialysed against fresh changes (3×1 l) of Dulbecco's phosphate-buffered saline, pH 7.4, supplemented with newborn-calf serum (4%, v/v) for 15 h.

(c) Radiolabelling by reductive methylation [^{3}H]. Mitochondria and outer mitochondrial membranes (MOM) are prepared from the blood-free livers. Approximately 4 mg of the mitochondria or MOM are resuspended in 150 μl of 0.2 M sodium borate buffer, pH 9.9. The preparation is cooled on ice. Twenty microlitres of 20 mM formaldehyde are added and the contents mixed by means of a Pasteur pipette. After 30 s one crystal of [^{3}H]sodium borohydride is added and the preparation quickly mixed. One minute later 150 μl of 0.4 M sodium phosphate buffer, pH 5.8, containing 100 mM glycine is added. The methylated preparations are dialysed against fresh changes of phosphate-buffered saline for 15 h prior to use.

(d) Labelling of monoamine oxidase in mitochondrial outer membrane vesicles with [^{3}H]pargyline. Monoamine oxidase is labelled in mitochondrial outer membrane vesicles with [^{3}H]pargyline (Pintar *et al.*, 1979). Each preparation is dialysed against fresh changes (2×1 l) of Dulbecco's phosphate-buffered saline, pH 7.4, supplemented with pargyline (0.1 mM) and bovine serum albumin (1 mg/ml) and then against one change (1 l) of Dulbecco's phosphate-buffered saline, pH 7.4.

(e) Hepatocyte mitochondria/mitochondrial outer membrane vesicle fusions. Hepatocytes (3.5×10^7) are pelleted by low speed centrifugation ($100 \times g$ for 3 min). Mitochondrial outer membrane protein (1 mg) or mitochondrial protein (2 mg) is added in 200 μl of Dulbecco's phosphate-buffered saline, pH 7.4, and the tube (Sterilin Universal container, 30 ml) gently rotated to ensure thorough mixing. A 500 μl portion of polyethylene glycol (50%, v/v) in serum and antibiotic-free Leibovitz L-15 medium, supplemented with glucose (8.3 mM) and Hepes (25 mM), pH 7.4, is added and the tube gently rotated for 90 s. A 10 ml portion of polyethylene glycol-free supplemented medium is then slowly added. The cells are pelleted ($100 \times g$ for 3 min) and washed three times in culture medium, which consists of 10 ml of the L-15 medium, pH 7.4, supplemented with glucose (8.3 mM), Hepes (25 mM), heat-inactivated newborn-calf serum (10%) containing streptomycin and penicillin (100 units of each/ml). At each

wash the hepatocytes are redispersed by passage through a 10 ml pipette. Finally the cells are suspended in 10 ml of the culture medium. Preliminary experiments showed that, in the absence of polyethylene glycol, less than 10% of the radioactivity found in the presence of polyethylene glycol is associated with the cell pellet. Hepatocytes are cultured on an adsorbed collagen support (type III) in 60 mm diameter tissue culture dishes. Coated dishes are prepared by covering the bottom of each dish with sterile collagen (2 mg/ml) in 0.1% acetic acid. The dishes are left for 1 h, washed three times with sterile water and placed in a 37°C incubator for 48 h before use. Approximately 1.2×10^6 cells are added to 3 ml of culture medium, which contains insulin (0.8 mg/ml) and dexamethasone (1 μM). The medium is changed after 2.5 h and then at 24 h intervals, unless otherwise indicated.

(f) Cytochemical procedures

(i) Fluorescence microscopy. Glass coverslips (16 mm diameter) are cleaned aseptically by successive washes (5 min each) in ethanol (98%), HCl (1 M) and sterile water. Coverslips (three) are placed in 60 mm diameter tissue culture dishes. Finally the coverslips are rinsed with ethanol (98%) before being coated with collagen. Hepatocytes are cultured on these supports as described above. At the times indicated the culture medium is removed and the cells washed with phosphate-buffered saline, pH 7.4. The hepatocytes are fixed in 4% (v/v) formaldehyde in phosphate-buffered saline, pH 7.4, for 30 min. The coverslips are then mounted in a mixed glycerol/*p*-phenylenediamine solution, pH 8.0, to reduce photobleaching (Johnson and de C. Nogueira Aranjo, 1981).

(ii) Optical microscopy. Hepatocytes are cultured as above, fixed in glutaraldehyde (3%, v/v) in phosphate-buffered saline and stained with Toluidine Blue (2% in 50 mM sodium phosphate buffer, pH 7.4). Excess stain is removed from the cells with distilled water and finally with ethanol (98%).

(g) Cell homogenization and Percoll gradient centrifugation. Hepatocytes are harvested by treatment with trypsin, washed and resuspended in 0.25 M sucrose (1 ml). The cells are sonicated (one 10 s burst at amplitude 4 μm peak-to-peak with an MSE sonicator) and layered on 10 ml of Percoll (30%, v/v) in 0.25 M sucrose in 14 ml centrifuge tubes. Cell homogenates are centrifuged at 33000 rpm for 30 min in rotor 43114-121 (MSE Prepspin 75). Fractions (0.5 ml) are collected from the gradients.

(2) Cellular response to transplantation

The initial objective of these studies was to introduce mitochondria and MOM into target cells to study the degradation of incumbent proteins; the objective was not to transplant functional whole mitochondria or to surround endogenous mitochondrial inner membrane (mitoplast) with MOM, for example during mitochondrial biogenesis (which would be most unlikely from what is known of mitochondrial biogenesis). However, reductive methylation of whole mitochondria only impairs respiratory control by 50% and produces an upper limit of inhibition of the activity of mitochondrial enzymes tested of approximately 20% (monoamine oxidase, isocitrate dehydrogenase, cytochrome oxidase and malate dehydrogenase; Mayer *et al.*, 1984).

FITC-labelled mitochondria and MOM are internalized as demonstrated by fluorescence microscopy (Evans and Mayer, 1983, 1984) and Percoll gradient centrifugation of homogenized hepatocytes. Proteins in transplanted mitochondria and MOM retain their *in vitro* degradation characteristics. However, in all cases protein degradation at *in vivo* rates was only observed after a lag period of 24–30 h during which the transplanted material is internalized (average $t_{1/2}$ 1–6 h), and translocated to a perinuclear, frequently sided site similar to endogenous organelles. Initially internalized MOM is definitively not in lysosomes or around endogenous mitoplasts (Evans and Mayer, 1983), although subsequently lysosomes play at least a part in the degradation of mitochondrial and MOM proteins (Evans and Mayer, 1983, 1984). The effect of a spectrum of inhibitors of proteinolysis on the degradation of proteins in transplanted mitochondria is indistinguishable from their effects on the degradation of endogenous mitochondrial proteins, supporting the notion that the intracellular recognition and sequestration steps in the selection of mitochondrial proteins for destruction at *in vivo* rates are the same for proteins in endogenous and transplanted mitochondria (Mayer *et al.*, 1984).

B. Mitochondrial outer membrane (MOM)–hepatoma tissue culture (HTC) cell transplantation

(1) Methods

(a) Cell culture. HTC cells (derived from Morris hepatoma 7288c) purchased from Flow Laboratories (Irvine, Ayrshire, Scotland, UK) are cultured in EMEM-supplemented with MEM non-essential amino acids (Gibco, Paisley, Renfrewshire, Scotland, UK). Growth medium contains 10% (v/v) heat-inactivated newborn-calf serum and is replaced every 48–72 h. Cells are maintained as monolayer cultures on 90 mm diameter plastic culture dishes (Nunc, Roskilde, Denmark) at 37°C in an incubator under CO_2/air (1:19).

(b) Preparation of MOM fraction from rat liver. MOM vesicles are prepared from 180–200 g Wistar rats exactly as described by Martinez and McCauley (1977). The vesicles are washed after preparation in 1 M NaCl by sonication for 20 s at 70 W (Soniprobe; Dawe, London W3 UK) followed by centrifugation at 100000 × $g_{av.}$ for 30 min at 4°C. The membrane vesicles are labelled with [^{3}H]pargyline (15.3 Ci/mmol) by incubating resonicated MOM (10 mg of protein) in 20 mM potassium phosphate buffer, pH 7.4, with 30 μCi of [^{3}H]pargyline for 60 min at 30°C. After the incubation, the MOM vesicle suspension is exhaustively dialysed for 18 h at 4°C against HBSS without Ca^{2+} or Mg^{2+} supplemented with 5 μM pargyline. Reductively methylated MOM vesicles are prepared with NaB^3H_4 (5–20 Ci/mmol) by the method of Tack *et al.* (1980) modified by the use of 0.4 μmol of formaldehyde/mg of protein and 1 mCi of NaB^3H_4/mg of protein. After reductive methylation the MOM vesicles are washed by centrifugation in 40 ml of phosphate-buffered saline (Dulbecco and Vogt, 1954). Pelleting of the MOM vesicles is prevented by a 1 ml cushion of 2.2 M sucrose. The yellow layer of MOM vesicles is collected and exhaustively dialysed against HBSS without Ca^{2+} or Mg^{2+} for 18 h at 4°C. Fluorescein-labelled MOM vesicles are prepared by incubating vesicles (10 mg of protein) in 1 ml of 0.05 M Na_2CO_3 buffer, pH 8.5, with 0.1 mg of fluorescein isothiocyanate isomer I (Sigma) for 30 min at 0°C. The membranes are washed in 40 ml of phosphate-buffered saline and collected by centrifugation onto a cushion (1 ml) of 2.2 M sucrose. The fluorescein-labelled MOM was dialysed against HBSS without Ca^{2+} or Mg^{2+} at 4°C for 18 h.

(c) Fusion. MOM vesicles are fused to HTC cells by a modification of the method used by Baumann *et al.* (1980). In a typical fusion procedure, monolayer cultures of hepatoma cells (yielding approx. 10^8 cells) are treated with trypsin/EDTA solution (Gibco; 1 mg of trypsin/ml; 0.4 mg of EDTA/ml) for 2 min at 37°C. The suspended cells are washed once with growth medium and three times with phosphate-buffered saline (10 ml). To the packed cell pellet is added 0.2 ml of freshly prepared and dialysed MOM suspension (1–3 mg of MOM protein/10^8 cells per fusion). The components are mixed thoroughly by swirling and 0.6 ml of 50% (w/v) PEG-1000 (BDH Chemicals) in serum-free medium are added. The pH of the PEG-1000 solution is adjusted immediately before use to pH 7.2 with 0.1 M NaOH. The cell–MOM fusion mixture is incubated for 5 min at 37°C and then 15 ml of serum-free medium is added. After a further 2 min the cells are collected by centrifugation and washed twice with EMEM containing penicillin G (100 μg/ml) and streptomycin (60 μg/ml). The cells are then suspended in growth medium and plated out for monolayer culture. Viability of the cells after fusion (using the Trypan Blue exclusion test) is approximately 95%.

(d) Subfractionation of HTC cells after fusion. Subfractionation of the cells after fusion is achieved by (i) Percoll gradient centrifugation of sonicated cells and (ii) by differential centrifugation of homogenized cells.

(i) Percoll gradient centrifugation of sonicated cells. Cells are washed twice with serum-free medium and harvested by scraping into 0.25 M sucrose (0.5–1.0 ml). In preliminary experiments, several sonication conditions ranging from no sonication to 80 W for 30 s (Dawe Soniprobe) were tested to establish conditions giving optimum cell breakage with minimal damage to subcellular structures. Sonicated cells (70 W for 15 s) are layered on to 10 ml of Percoll in 0.25 M sucrose (mean density 1.075 g/ml) and centrifuged for $1.3 \times 10^6 g_{av.}$ min in rotor no. 43114-121 on the MSE 75 centrifuge (MSE Ltd., Crawley, Sussex, UK). The gradient is collected in 19–20 fractions and densities determined by fractionating an equivalent gradient containing density marker beads (Pharmacia, Uppsala, Sweden).

(ii) Differential centrifugation of homogenized cells. Cells are harvested as described above and washed by centrifugation in 0.25 M sucrose 3 mM imidazole buffer, pH 7.4. The cell pellet is resuspended in the same solution to a density of 2×10^7 cells/min. Experiments are performed with 10^7–10^9 cells. Cells are homogenized by 30–40 strokes of a 3 ml ground-glass homogenizer (Jencons, Hemel Hempstead, Herts, UK). Fractionation by differential centrifugation is performed as described by Lopez-Saura *et al.* (1978).

(e) Fluorescence microscopy. Cells for fluorescence microscopy were fixed by immersing them in glutaraldehyde (2%, v/v) for 5 min and then in glycerol (50%, v/v). Fluorescence microscopy was carried out with a Leitz SM-Lux microscope.

(2) Cellular response to transplantation

As indicated previously in Section A.2 recipient cells internalized transplanted MOM as observed by fluorescence microscopy, but with HTC cells, the transplanted MOM was first patched and capped (Russell and Mayer, 1983).

MOM–cell fusion was polyethylene glycol-dependent, occurred at 0°C and was not affected by pre-incubation of the cells with NaN_3 and 2-deoxyglucose. Percoll gradient and differential centrifugation showed that transplanted MOM is internalized into some intracellular membranous structures which are clearly distinct from endogenous mitochondria, lysosomes and plasma membrane (as in hepatocytes). However, in contrast to hepatocytes the transplanted MOM proteins are degraded approximately $2\frac{1}{2}$ times faster than *in vivo* i.e. $t_{1/2}$ av. 24 h. Interestingly, the transplantation of the same MOM into several genetically unrelated tissue culture cells showed the same alternative processing; with proteins in transplanted MOM degraded either with a $t_{1/2}$ of 24–28 h (MRC-5, human fibroblast, B82; mouse thymidine kinase deficient L cell; A549, human lung fibroblast) or $t_{1/2}$ of 55–70 h (CHO-K1, chinese hamster ovary, 3T3-L1; mouse preadipocyte) (Russell *et al.*, 1984). The latter slower rate is the same as for the proteins in endogenous and transplanted MOM in hepatocytes. Evidence for a similar alternative processing of a membrane protein (erythrocyte Band 3) in different cell types after transplantation in reconstituted Sendai virus envelopes has also been shown (Beigel and Loyter, 1983; see Chapter 10). Again (cf. hepatocytes, Section A.2) inhibitors of proteinolysis could not operationally distinguish the degradation of transplanted and endogenous MOM proteins in HTC cells, implying similar recognition and sequestration events in dealing with proteins in transplanted MOM (which is miscompartmentalized) and its endogenous counterpart (cf. hepatocytes). The same alternative processing, i.e. degradation at 24–28 h or 55–70 h of the same intracellular membrane (MOM) after transplantation into genetically distinct cell types, implies a selective sensitive intracellular recognition system which can deliver transplanted (and probably endogenous) membrane proteins into the endogenous protein destructive machinery at different alternative defined rates. The possibility exists that the recognition system distinguishes self from non-self during the course of a protein turn-over cycle (Mayer *et al.*, 1984). Such a recognition system alternatively, and not randomly, sequestering proteins for destruction would explain the small number (1–3) of populations of degradation rates for proteins in defined subcellular sites observed *in vivo* (Russell *et al.*, 1982). Clearly, these cytoplasmic events in membrane protein processing and destruction would not have been discovered without membrane transplantation.

C. Further applications

Membrane or cell fragments may be routinely introduced into tissue culture cells by the methods indicated above. The methods may be therefore used for the complete elucidation of the mechanism(s) of degradation of membrane proteins. The methods are easily extended to the transplantation of other intracellular membranes, e.g. smooth endoplasmic reticulum, Golgi vesicles or endosomes. In this way the cell can be used as a "natural" test tube in order to study the cell biological aspects of protein degradation, including the discovery of the nature of the macromolecules involved in protein recognition and sequestration for degradation, together with the role of cytoskeletal networks in the process.

III. TRANSPLANTATION OF KARYOPLASTS

(1) Methods

Cells may be enucleated in the presence of cytochalasin B by centrifugation either on coverslips (Poste, 1973; Prescott and Kirkpatrick, 1973; Lucas and Kates, 1977; Veomett, 1982) or through a discontinuous Ficoll gradient (Wigler and Weinstein, 1975). The latter method is preferred if large numbers of cytoplasts (anucleate cells) or karyoplasts (minicells) are to be prepared and will be described here for B82 cells (thymidine kinase deficient mouse L cells) together with techniques for purifying the cell fragments produced.

(a) Enucleation. Ficoll (50%, w/v) is dissolved in nanopure water by stirring overnight and sterilized by autoclaving. The 50% Ficoll is diluted with EMEM to the appropriate concentration and supplemented with cytochalasin B (10 μg/ml). Discontinuous Ficoll gradients are prepared the evening before use by carefully layering 25% (4 ml), 17.5% (5 ml), 15.5% (4 ml), 13% (3 ml) and 11% Ficoll (1 ml), all containing cytochalasin B (10 μg/ml) in 25 ml swing-out polypropylene centrifuge tubes (MSE, Crawley, Sussex, UK) previously sterilized by autoclaving. The gradients are placed in an incubator (37°C, 10% CO_2) overnight, along with 5 ml 11% Ficoll and 3 ml EMEM for each gradient.

Mouse B82 cells are collected by trypsinization and incubated for 1 h (37°C, 10% CO_2) in growth medium to allow the cells to recover from the effects of trypsinization. Cells are collected by centrifugation (800 × g, 1 min) and 1–3 × 10^7 cells are resuspended in 5 ml 11% Ficoll and layered on each gradient which is then overlayed with 3 ml EMEM. The gradients are loaded into a pre-warmed (24 h at 37°C) 3 × 25 ml MSE swing-out rotor and centrifuged for 60 min at 65 000 × $g_{av.}$ at 34°C. After centrifugation, bands are visible at the 13% (cell debris), 15.5% (cytoplasts, karyoplasts, cells) and 17.5% interfaces (karyoplasts, cytoplasts, some cells). Bands are collected with a Pasteur pipette, diluted with 20 ml DMEM and centrifuged at 800 × g for 10 min. Cytoplasts are concentrated in the 15.5% Ficoll band, karyoplasts in the 17.5% Ficoll band.

(b) Purification. A number of properties of cells and cell fragments may be exploited to purify cell fragments produced by enucleation. If the cell fragments differ from each other and from whole cells in size (e.g., lymphocytes) unit gravity sedimentation through linear gradients of bovine serum albumin may be exploited (Tulp *et al.*, 1980; Ohara *et al.*, 1981) as a separation technique.

However, B82 karyoplasts, collected from the 17.5% Ficoll band, must be purified by a combination of differential adhesion and Percoll density gradient centrifugation. The karyoplasts are plated out in 9 cm culture dishes in 5 ml growth medium supplemented with 0.001% (w/v) DNase (to prevent cell clumping, see below) and incubated for 90 min (37°C, 10% CO_2). Non-adherent material (karyoplasts) is collected with the plate washings (three times with 5 ml growth medium) and centrifuged at 800 × *g* for 1 min.

Percoll is sterilized by autoclaving and made iso-osmotic with 10 × concentrated Ca^{2+}/Mg^{2+} free Hanks Basic Salt Solution. The karyoplasts are resuspended in 10 ml 34% (w/v) Percoll [90% isoosmotic Percoll diluted with growth medium plus 5% (w/v) BSA] and centrifuged for 15 min at 23000 × $g_{av.}$ in an MSE 8 × 14 angle rotor at 25°C. Fractions are collected with a syringe and cannula from the bottom of the gradient, diluted with 20 ml DMEM and centrifuged at 800 × *g* for 10 min. Karyoplasts band at a density of 1.104 g/ml, while the cytoplasts and whole cells band at a density of 1.066 g/ml.

(c) Determination of karyoplast purity. (i) Whole cell contamination of the preparation is determined. Aliquots of karyoplasts are plated out and the number of whole cells present after 48 h (by which time all fragments have died) is counted. (ii) The macromolecular synthetic capabilities of the preparation are measured with suitable precursors (e.g. [^{3}H]leucine or [^{3}H]uridine) over 72 h. Incorporation of precursors after 48 h represents synthetic activity of contaminating whole cells. (iii) The contamination of karyoplasts by both cytoplasts and cells is measured after fixing the material for 3 h in 3% (v/v) glutaraldehyde, dehydration and embedding in epon. Thick sections are cut and stained with toluidine blue for examination under the light microscope. These methods show the B82 karyoplast preparation to be at least 95% pure.

(d) Karyoplast–cell fusion. Fusion of B82 karyoplasts to B82 cells is carried out with UV-inactivated Sendai virus in suspension.

Cells and karyoplasts are mixed in a ratio of 3:1, washed once (with DMEM by centrifugation; 800 × *g* for 1 min) and then washed once with fusion buffer (20 mM Tris-HCl, pH 7.4 containing 0.15 M NaCl, 1 mM $MnCl_2$ and 1 mM glucose). The final pellet is resuspended in 200 μl fusion buffer containing 100 HAU of UV-inactivated Sendai virus, placed on ice for 20 min, and then transferred to a shaking water bath at 37°C for 15 min. The fusion mixture is washed (by centrifugation) with 9 ml growth medium and the fusion products are plated into 6 cm culture dishes. In general two-thirds of the homokaryons produced have three or more nuclei.

(e) Comments on procedures. Enucleation appears to be cell specific: hepatoma tissue culture (HTC) cells and mouse adenocarcinoma (RAG) cells do not enucleate whilst mouse preadipocytes (3T3-L1) and B82 cells do. The enucleation process is very sensitive to the quality of the cells: freshly-trypsinized or over-trypsinized B82 cells enucleate very inefficiently. The composition of the Ficoll gradient does not appear to be important for enucleation in contrast to the overnight gassing in the incubator (to pH the Ficoll) and the temperature of the centrifugation (enucleation occurs only between 31°C and 37°C). Both the centrifugation time and *g* force as well as the cytochalasin B concentration are parameters which may be altered to improve the enucleation efficiency of a particular cell type (e.g., 3T3-L1 cells, 70 min centrifugation).

Cytoplasts cannot usually be purified by differential adhesion as they have similar adhesive properties to the parent cells, although both unit *g* sedimentation and Percoll density gradients are effective.

Clumping is often a serious problem on Percoll gradients. This can be reduced by the use of DNase to break up DNA strands (which are very adhesive) produced by cell lysis occurring on the Ficoll gradient. The presence of newborn-calf serum and BSA in the 34% Percoll prevents the clumping of material on the gradient itself.

Although polyethylene glycol is often quoted in the literature (Clark *et al.*, 1978) as the ideal fusogen, it has in our hands proved ineffectual in the transplantation of useful numbers (10–20%) of karyoplasts to cells. The fusogenicity of polyethylene glycol is also very variable between batches. From our experience, the best way to obtain an efficient cell-fragment transplantation system is to screen a number of cell lines for their fusogenicity, and then to take those cells having the highest fusion index (Shay and Clark, 1979) and test them for their susceptibility to enucleation.

(2) Cellular response to transplantation

Karyoplasts are made from B82 cells previously labelled with [^{3}H]leucine for 36 h (1 μCi/ml in growth medium containing only 10% of normal leucine). Karyoplasts are transplanted into unlabelled growing cells to study the degradation of nuclear proteins. The average rate of degradation of karyoplast proteins transplanted into growing B82 cells ($t_{1/2}$, 80 h) is similar to the average rate of degradation of endogenous B82 proteins in non-growing cells (Table I).

The data are explained by the fact that multinucleate heterokaryons (homokaryons in this case) do not grow. The rate of degradation of transplanted karyoplast proteins is therefore characteristic of average degradation rates of endogenous proteins in non-growing cells.

Table I. Degradation of endogenous proteins and transplanted karyoplast proteins in B82 cells.

	Averge $t_{1/2}$ (h)
Endogenous proteins in:	
growing B82 cells	160
confluent B82 cells	68
confluent B82 cells + NH_4Cl	130 (30% inhibition)
Transplanted karyoplast proteins in:	
B82 cells	80
B82 cells + NH_4Cl	150 (45% inhibition)

Autoradiographs of the multinucleate cells resulting from karyoplast transplantation show that the transplanted proteins remain in the karyoplast nucleus and do not migrate or exchange significantly with the nuclei of recipient cells. However, the NH_4Cl sensitivity of the degradation of karyoplast proteins suggests that karyoplast proteins are degraded in the lysosomal compartment, indicating that they must leave the nucleus to be degraded.

(3) Further applications

Transplantation of cell fragments in cell reconstruction (karyoplast–cytoplast fusion) or cybrid formation (cell–cytoplast fusion) has been used to study the interactions of nuclei and cytoplasm with respect to ageing (Muggleton-Harris, 1979; Nette *et al.*, 1982) and tumourogenicity (Shay and Clark, 1979). These types of experiments obviously have further applications in the study of other types of nucleo-cytoplasmic interactions. For example, the effects of the nucleus on the cytoskeleton and plasma membrane (and vice versa) could be examined.

ACKNOWLEDGEMENTS

We are indebted to the Medical Research Council and the Wellcome Trust for support of part of this work. We thank Jenny Paxton for typing the manuscript.

REFERENCES

Barski, G., Sorieul, S. and Cornefeit, F. (1960). *C. R. Acad. Sci.* **251**, 1825–1827.
Baumann, H., Hou, E. and Doyle, D. (1980). *J. Biol. Chem.* **255**, 10001–10012.
Beigel, M. and Loyter, A. (1983). *Exp. Cell Res.* **148**, 95–103.

Bustamente, E., Soper, J. W. and Pedersen, P. L. (1977). *Anal. Biochem.* **80**, 401–408.

Clark, M. A., Cremshaw, A. H. and Shay, J. W. (1978). *Tissue Culture Assoc. Manual* **4**, 801–804.

Clark, M. A., Reudelhuber, T. L. and Shay, J. W. (1982). *In* "Techniques in Somatic Cell Genetics" (J. W. Shay, ed.) pp. 203–209. Plenum Press, New York and London.

Doyle, D., Hou, E. and Warren, R. (1979). *J. Biol. Chem.* **254**, 6853–6867.

Dulbecco, R. and Vogt, M. (1954). *J. Exp. Med.* **99**, 167–182.

Eimerl, S., Neufeld, G., Korner, M. and Schramm, M. (1980). *Proc. Natl. Acad. Sci. USA* **77**, 760–764.

Ephrussi, B. and Weiss, M. (1965). *Proc. Natl. Acad. Sci. USA* **53**, 1040–1042.

Evans, P. J. (1981). *Biochim. Biophys. Acta* **677**, 433–444.

Evans, P. J. and Mayer, R. J. (1982). *Biochem. Biophys. Res. Commun.* **107**, 51–58.

Evans, P. J. and Mayer, R. J. (1983). *Biochem. J.* **216**, 151–161.

Evans, P. J. and Mayer, R. J. (1984). *Biochem. J.* **219**, 61–72.

Evans, P. J., Russell, S. M., Doherty, F. and Mayer, R. J. (1983). *In* "Proteinase Inhibitors" (N. Katunuma, H. Umezawa and H. Holzer, eds) pp. 283–292. Japan Scientific Societies Press, Tokyo; Springer Verlag, Berlin.

Johnston, G. D. and de C. Nogueira Aranjo, G. M. (1981). *J. Immunol. Methods* **43**, 349–350.

Krebs, W. A. and Henseleit, K. (1932). *Hoppe-Seyler's Z. Physiol. Chem.* **210**, 33–66.

Lopez-Saura, P., Trouet, A. and Tulkens, P. (1978). *Biochim. Biophys., Acta* **543**, 430–449.

Lucas, J. J. and Kates, J. R. (1977). *Methods Cell Biol.* **XV**, 359–370.

Martinez, P. and McCauley, R. (1977). *Biochim. Biophys., Acta* **497**, 437–446.

Mayer, R. J., Evans, P., Russell, S. and Amenta, J.L S. (1984). *In* "Cell Fusion", Ciba Foundation Symposium 103, pp. 202–219. Pitman, London.

Muggleton-Harris, A. L. (1979). *Int. Rev. Cytol. Suppl.* **9**, 279–301.

Nette, E. G., Sit, H. C. and King, D. W. (1982). *Mech. Ageing Devel.* **18**, 75–87.

Neufeld, G., Schramm, M. and Weinberg, N. (1980). *J. Biol. Chem.* **255**, 9268–9274.

Ohara, J., Sekigushi, T. and Watanabe, T. (1981). *J. Immunol. Methods* **45**, 239–248.

Orly, J. and Schramm, M. (1976). *Proc. Natl. Acad. Sci. USA* **73**, 4410–4414.

Penefsky, H. S., Pullman, M. E., Datta, A. and Racker, E. (1960). *J. Biol. Chem.* **235**, 3330–3336.

Pintar, J. E., Cawthon, R. M., Castro Costa, M. R. and Breakfield, X. O. (1979). *In* "Monoamine Oxidase: Structure, Functions and Altered Functions" (T. P. Singer, R. W. Van Korff and D. L. Murphy, eds) pp. 185–196. Academic Press, New York and London.

Poste, G. (1973). *Methods Cell Biol.* **VII**, 189–210.

Prescott, D. M. and Kirkpatrick, J. B. (1973). *Methods in Cell Biol.* **VII**, 189–202.

Ringertz, N. R. (1978). *Natl. Cancer Inst. Monograph* **48**, 31–36.

Russell, S. M. and Mayer, R. J. (1983). *Biochem. J.* **216**, 163–175.

Russell, S. M., Burgess, R. J. and Mayer, R. J. (1982). *Biochim. Biophys. Acta* **714**, 34–45.

Russell, S. M., Amenta, J. S. and Mayer, R. J. (1984). *Biochem. J.* **220**, 489–498.

Scramm, M. (1979). *Proc. Natl. Acad. Sci. USA* **76**, 1174–1178.

Shay, J. W. and Clark, M. A. (1979). *J. Supramol. Struct.* **11**, 33–49.

Tack, B. F., Dean, J., Eilot, D., Lorenz, P. E. and Schechter, A. N. (1980). *J. Biol. Chem.* **255**, 8842–8847.
Tulp, A., Collard, J. G., Hait, A. A. M. and Aten, J. A. (1980). *Anal. Biochem.* **105**, 246–256.
Veomett, G. E. (1982). *In* "Techniques in Somatic Cell Genetics" (J. W. Shay, ed.) pp. 67–79. Plenum Press, New York and London.
Wigler, M. H. and Weinstein, I. B. (1975). *Biochim. Biophys. Acta* **63**, 669–674.

14

Microdissection of Metaphase Chromosomes and Gene Transfer

D. Röhme

I. INTRODUCTION

Microtechniques for specific chromosome dissection and DNA extraction were first developed for the polytene chromosomes of *Drosophila* (Scalenghe *et al.*, 1981). By means of micromanipulation, a fragment comprising some 5 to 10 bands could be specifically dissected and the DNA (10–20 pg) extracted in a nanolitre volume. These investigators also demonstrated that the microextracted DNA could be cleaved with a restriction enzyme and used to construct recombinant molecules with phage lambda in this nanolitre volume. Thus, not only do these techniques allow microdissection of specific chromosome fragments, they could also be used to produce molecular clones derived from the DNA of this fragment.

In contrast to the polytene chromosomes where the DNA is present in 1000-fold copies, the amount of DNA and the size of metaphase chromosomes are correspondingly smaller. An average mammalian metaphase chromosome contains about 0.1 pg of DNA. However, using a minimum of about 100 pooled chromosomes dissected under high magnification, these techniques have been adapted for the handling of metaphase chromosomes (Röhme *et al.*, 1984).

The basis of the micromanipulation technique used here was described (de Fonbrune, 1949) using oil-filled chambers for both microdissection and microchemistry (Edström, 1964). The volumetry in the nanolitre range and micro-procedures for isolation and cloning of DNA have already been described in detail (Scalenghe *et al.*, 1981; Pirotta *et al.*, 1983). In this chapter, a detailed description is given of the microdissection and molecular cloning of specific metaphase chromosomes from mammalian cells and various applications are discussed.

Microinjection and Organelle Transplantation Techniques

ISBN: 0-12-164722-6
ISBN: 0-12-164723-4 Pbk

II. INSTRUMENTATION

A. Micromanipulator

Microdissection and microcloning are carried out with the aid of a micromanipulator adapted to a phase-contrast microscope. The principle of the micromanipulator is to reduce the amplitude of the movements of the hand to suit the dimensions of the microscope field. The smaller the object to be handled, the higher the movement reduction must be.

Microdissection of metaphase chromosomes must be carried out at the highest possible movement reduction and thus requires a pneumatically operated micromanipulator such as the de Fonbrune (Fig. 1). This micromanipulator is operated by the hand with a separate control stick, movements of which apply pressure to three orthogonal syringes. These in turn communicate with the tool holder or the receiver part by means of air-filled rubber tubing. The receiver part can also be adjusted by coarser screw controls, which is useful for proper positioning of the operating instruments (needles and micropipettes). To the receiver part, a second instrument can also be added. This can be a second needle which is in a fixed position and can be useful in microdissection in combination with the moveable needle operated pneumatically.

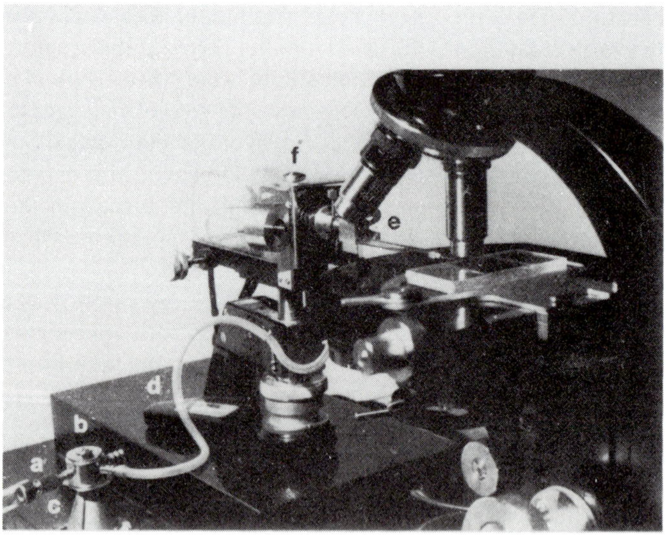

Fig. 1. The de Fonbrune micromanipulator. The set-up for handling of nanolitre volumes in the oil chamber. The syringe (a) is fastened to a three-way stopcock (b) and this in turn onto a wooden plate with a small metal stand (c). It connects with Teflon® tubing (d) to the holder of the micropipette (e) which is attached to the receptor part of the micromanipulator (f). From Timm *et al.* (1983).

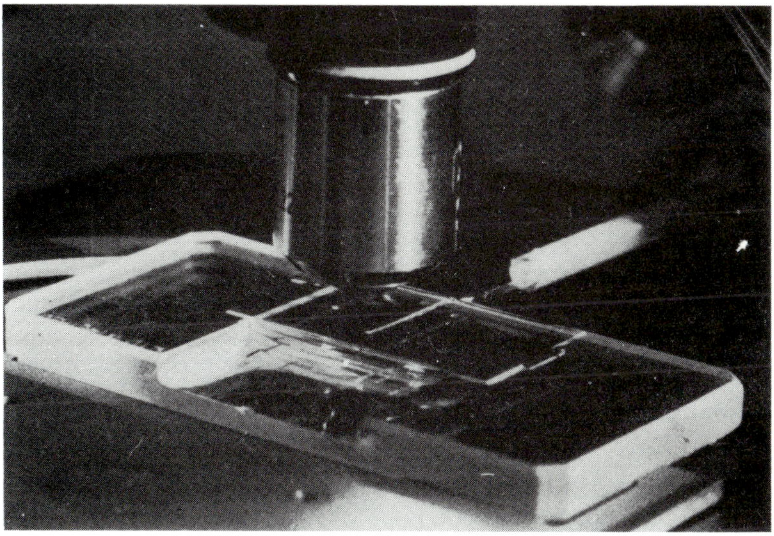

Fig. 2. An oil chamber seen on the microscope stage with an inserted micropipette. From Scalenghe *et al.* (1981).

B. Oil chamber and microscope

The oil chamber is a thick glass slide with a central slot over which are placed narrow glass coverslips (Fig. 2). The space between the slide and the coverslips can be filled with paraffin oil. The use of narrow coverslips (6 mm × 32 mm × 0.17 mm) is convenient, since it allows different liquids, chromosome material, etc. to be introduced into or removed from the chamber separately.

In the oil chamber, we distinguish between the front opening (away from the investigator) and the rear opening (towards the investigator). The instruments for the microhandling (needles and pipettes) enter the chamber through the front opening.

The underside of the coverslips, in contact with the oil, is the working surface for the micromanipulation. On this side of the coverslips the chromosomes are spread for microdissection, or small aqueous droplets hanging from the coverslip for use in biochemical manipulation.

The use of paraffin oil (Merck no. 7161, liquid paraffin, spectroscopic grade) allows the identification of the chromosomes at higher resolution in the phase-contrast microscope (Figs 6a and b). More importantly, it also prevents evaporation of the aqueous droplets without interfering with biochemical reactions required for the microcloning. The paraffin oil is kept over a layer of the so-called R buffer (50 mM KCl; 10 mM Tris, pH 7.5; 10 mM

$MgCl_2$; and 10 mM mercaptoethanol). The operations in the oil chamber are followed through a phase-contrast microscope with the following specifications: (1) focusing can be achieved by moving the objective lenses and not the microscope table; (2) it is equipped with a high focal length phase-contrast condenser allowing a focusing distance long enough for the oil chamber, 6 mm thick.

The glass material (oil chamber and coverslips) should be washed with hydrochloric acid before use. Coverslips used for extracting DNA from microdissected material and for further processing of the extract are siliconized before use. This is done by dipping the coverslips in a 1% solution of dimethyl diclorosilane in CCl_4 for 1 min followed by rinsing in 1 mM EDTA. That the correct siliconization has been obtained can be checked by applying a nanolitre drop to the surface in the oil chamber. If correct siliconization has been obtained, the wetting angle of the droplet should be about 90°.

II. PREPARATION OF TOOLS

The dissecting needles and micropipettes used for work in the oil chamber are prepared from glass rods and tubes using a de Fonbrune microforge (Fig. 3). This instrument permits controlled melting of glass by means of an electrically heated platinum filament. The operations in the microforge are followed under a low power microscope built into the instrument.

A. Dissecting needles

Needles are prepared from 2 mm rods of soft glass (soda glass). First the rod is heated and pulled to a length of 5 cm with a diameter of about 0.5 mm. The end of the thin part is then heated in the microforge by contact with the filament until the glass melts. The melted glass is pulled to make a cone, 1–2 mm long, at an angle of about 45° from the rod axis (Fig. 4). A sharp tip to the cone is obtained by using minimal heat when the tip is formed. As an alternative to this method, very sharp needles can be made by pulling glass rods (1 mm in diameter) in a standard electrode puller, adjusting the heat to give a tip which tapers sharply to a very fine point. The tip is bent in the microforge to an angle of about 45° from the axis. This is done by approaching the hot filament to the side of the needle, which then bends towards the heat. In our hands, however, the preparation of good needles is more difficult with the electrode puller than with the other method. This is due to difficulties in achieving independent control of the flexibility of the needle

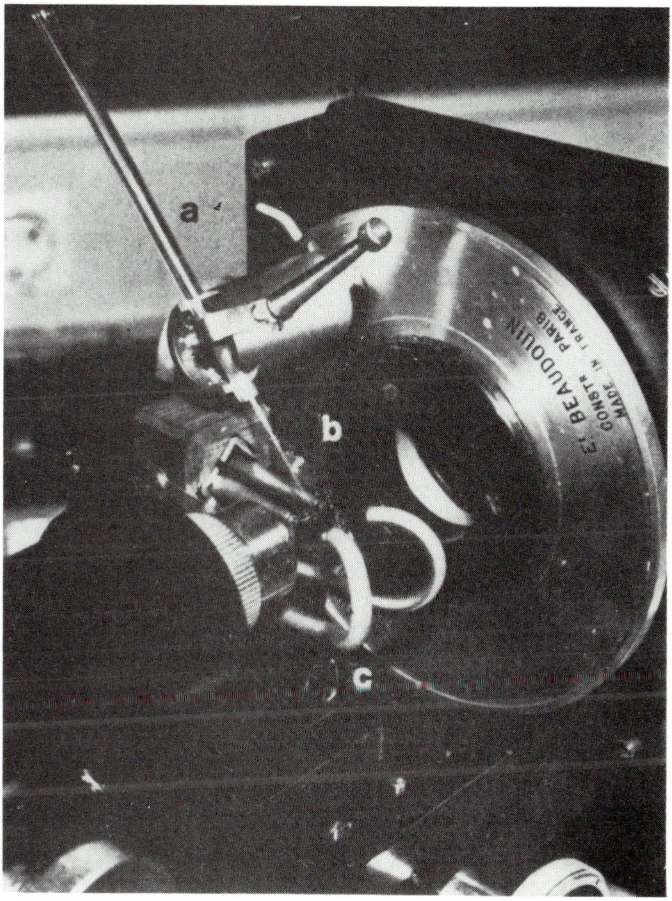

Fig. 3. The de Fonbrune microforge. The set-up demonstrates the preparation of a volumetric micropipette (cf. Fig. 5). (a) The pipette holder, (b) the capillary, and (c) a weight hooked on the tip of the capillary. From Pirotta *et al.* (1983).

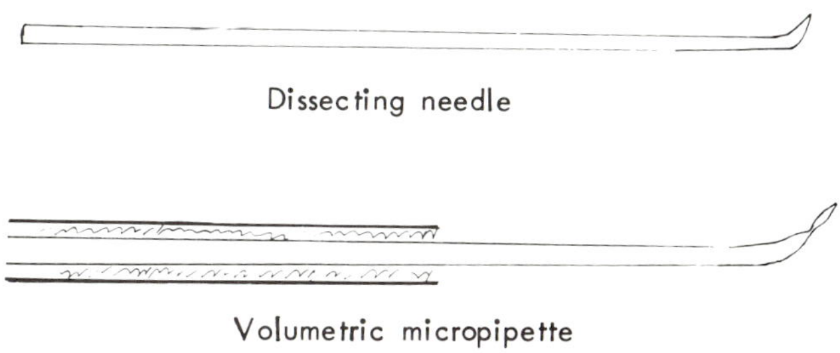

Fig. 4. Schematic representation of a dissecting needle. Note the ideal high cone angle of the tip.

and the sharpness and stability of the tip. Particularly when preparing very sharp needles with the electrode puller, less than 0.5 μm in tip diameter, the needles will be much too flexible to permit enough dissecting pressure on the tip of the needle. On the other hand, if the needle is too stiff, the tip has a high tendency to break when pressure is applied. Usually, a broken tip can be resharpened in the microforge, but the glass tends to become increasingly brittle when exposed to high temperature several times. It is difficult to give a general rule for preparing a good high resolution dissecting needle, well balanced between flexibility and sharpness. Usually the best needles are those which have a high cone angle but taper very sharply to a very thin tip.

B. Micropipettes

Volumetric micropipettes are used for transfer of liquids in the oil chamber. All pipettes are made from high melting point glass tubing (Pyrex and Duran). There are commercially available capillaries of about 1 mm diameter which may be used as a starting material for making volumetric pipettes. However, to obtain optimal pipettes, one has to start from a glass tube of 10 mm outer diameter and 1 mm wall thickness. First, these tubings are drawn out in a very hot flame to give capillaries of about 1 mm in diameter. The capillaries are cut in lengths of about 10 cm and are then heated over a small flame about 2 cm from the end to give a local thinning 0.2–0.3 mm in diameter (Fig. 5). The short end of the capillary is bent into a hook over the flame and is then inserted into a glass holder from the long end and fixed in place using melted paraffin, as shown in Fig. 5. The holder is mounted with the hook straight down on the microforge and a weight of about 1.5 g is added to the hook. The capillary is tilted 30° with the aid of the heating filament. The filament is shifted down to produce a local thinning and then

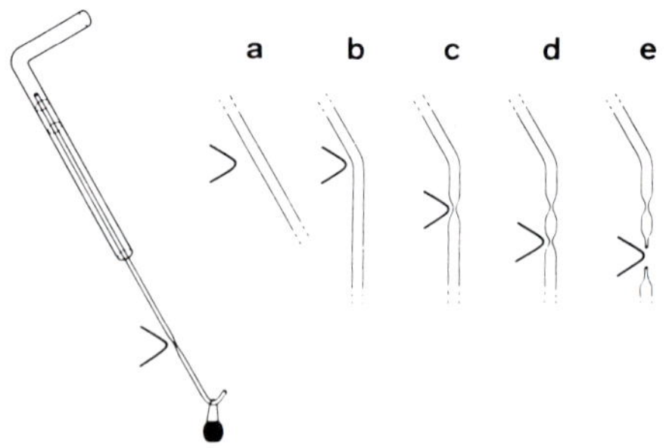

Fig. 5. Steps in preparing a volumetric nanolitre pipette, using an electrically heated platinum filament in the microforge. From Pirotta *et al.* (1983).

further down still to form the tip by heating the filament and letting the weight slowly extend the capillary until it breaks. Using a 1.5 g weight, the capillary will have an outside diameter of about 10 μm at the tip. Tips with smaller or larger openings can easily be made by using greater or lesser weights.

The micropipettes are connected with a rubber tubing to a 2 ml "Inaltera" glass syringe connected with a Luer-lock attachment to a three-way stopcock (both obtained from Henke-Sass Wolf GmbH, Kronenstrasse 16, Tuttlingen, FRG). The stopcock plug is fastened onto a cone-shaped brass stand fixed to a wooden platform on which both the microscope and the micromanipulator are placed. By sideways movements different outlets will be connected with the syringe, one for a rubber tube connected to the micropipette, another for intake or expulsion of air.

After being connected to the syringe and introduced into the oil chamber, the micropipette can be calibrated. This is done by filling the bulb with [^{3}H]uridine from a supply and depositing the contents on a separate coverslip. The coverslip is transferred to a scintillation vial and the radioactivity counted. The volume of the bulb is calculated by comparison with the radioactivity of a given volume of [^{3}H]uridine. After calibration the bulb should be siliconized using the same procedure as described for coverslips. As a rule each pipette should only be used for one purpose. Usually there is no need for special cleaning of the pipettes except filling and emptying them a couple of times with the solution to be pipetted.

IV. MICRODISSECTION OF METAPHASE CHROMOSOMES

A. Preparation of metaphase spreads

Metaphase chromosome spreads were prepared from mammalian cells (man, mouse, and Indian muntjac) grown as monolayer cultures as described (Röhme, 1981). Chromosome preparations were made by first treating the cells with colchemid (0.1 μg/ml for 1–1.5 h) and then detaching the cells from the culture flasks with a trypsin solution. After inactivation of trypsin with a 15% serum in nutrient medium, cells were pelleted by a brief spin (800 rpm for 5 min) and resuspended in 0.075 M KCl for 12–15 min. The cells were again pelleted and then resuspended in a fixation solution of methanol/acetic acid (in volumes 3:1). After three washes in this solution the cell suspension was dropped onto acid clean coverslips (marked to identify the cell side) and left to air-dry for 5 min. To avoid depurination of the DNA as much as possible the coverslips were washed several times in methanol to get rid of residual acid from the fixative. Until use, the coverslips were stored air-dried in dry dust-free boxes or left in methanol at −20°C.

In cases where mitotic enrichment was necessary, this was obtained by first transferring the cell culture to roller flasks (800 cm^2). After 1 day of growth, colchemid was added to a final concentration of 0.02–0.05 μg/ml, followed by further incubation for 4–12 h. Mitotic cells were harvested by rotating the roller flask at 300 rpm for 5 min in a specially constructed apparatus. After collection (10^7 cells/flask with more than 90% mitotic cells) chromosome spreads were made as above.

B. Microdissection of metaphase chromosomes

Coverslips containing the metaphase spreads were inverted over the oil chamber. Under the phase-contrast microscope the metaphase chromosomes appear inside the cell boundary surrounded by cytoplasm (Fig. 6a). After the addition of liquid paraffin, the cell boundary, as well as the cytoplasm, becomes almost invisible, whereas the resolution of the chromosomes is increased (Fig. 6b). The chromosomes shown in this figure are from the Indian muntjac which has a very low chromosome number ($2n = 6$ ♀; $2n = 7$ ♂). Individual chromosomes are dissected with two glass needles directed by the micromanipulator. For removing a chromosome from the cell (in this case the small Y chromosome), the tip is first moistened in a droplet of a few nanolitres of glycerol/phosphate (4 vol. 87% glycerol and 1 vol. 0.05 M sodium potassium phosphate buffer, pH 6.8). The needle is then put close to the chromosome and moved sideways towards the chromosome. The chromosome, together with some cytoplasm, is removed from the cell (Fig. 6d), adhering to the tip (Fig. 6e), and can be transferred through the liquid paraffin into the collection drop of glycerol/phosphate (Fig. 6f). The chromosomes usually leave the tip immediately when put into the drop, but when required, can be freed with a second needle (Fig. 6f).

To ensure the collection of pure uncontaminated chromosomes, dissections are made only in cells with well separated chromosomes and usually when the chromosomes of interest is located in the periphery of the metaphase spread. The peripheral location is particularly important when dissecting chromosome from complex karyotypes like those of man and mouse. In Fig. 7 is shown a dissection of a specific chromosome fragment comprising the proximal part of mouse chromosome 17. Although there has to be a selection of metaphase spreads suitable for dissection, having a high frequency of metaphases, this has only a very limited effect on the speed of

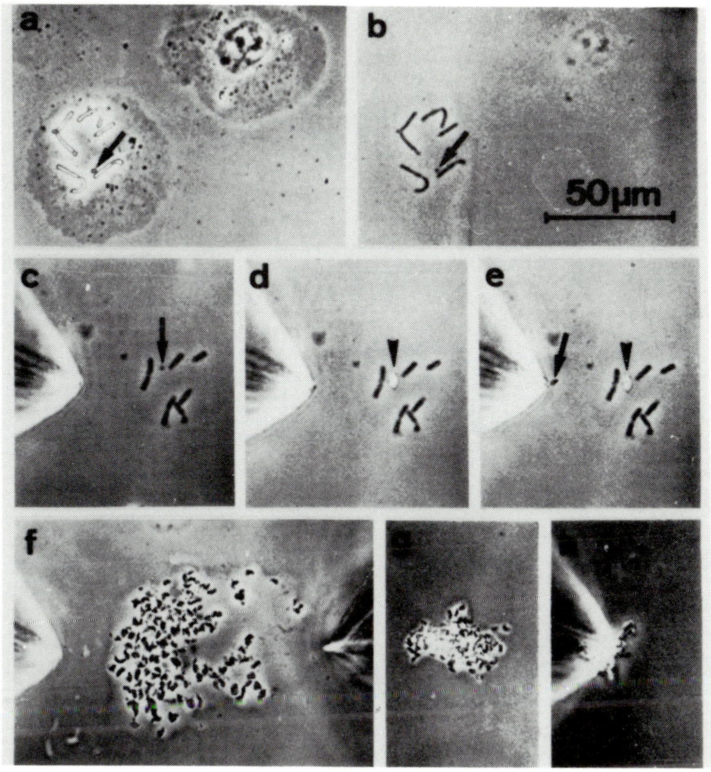

Fig. 6. Microdissection and collection of Y chromosomes from the Indian muntjac. Phase-contrast micrographs of mitotic chromosomes on slides inverted over the oil chamber before (a) and after (b) addition of liquid paraffin. Arrow shows the Y chromosome. A metaphase plate before (c) and after (d) the Y chromosome has been taken up on the tip of a glass needle. For demonstration it is placed back on the slide in front of the arrow (e). Note the empty position from which the chromosome was taken (arrowhead). For routine collection, single Y chromosomes were transferred on the tip of the needle through the oil and brought into a droplet of glycerol/phosphate (f). Excess glycerol/phosphate was micropipetted away (g) which allowed the pooled chromosomes to be put on the tip of the glass needle (h), and then be subjected to DNA extraction, restriction and cloning (Röhme, Jäckle and Edström; unpublished results).

dissection, usually 10 to 15 chromosomes or fragments can be dissected per hour.

The fact that each dissection leaves a clear zone in the surrounding cytoplasm allow an easy and reliable verification of the dissected chromosome. Chromosomes not clearly originating from the appropriate chromosome are immediately discarded. The specificity of the dissection has been verified with molecular hybridization using cloned DNA obtained from the dissected chromosome material as probes (Röhme *et al.*, 1984).

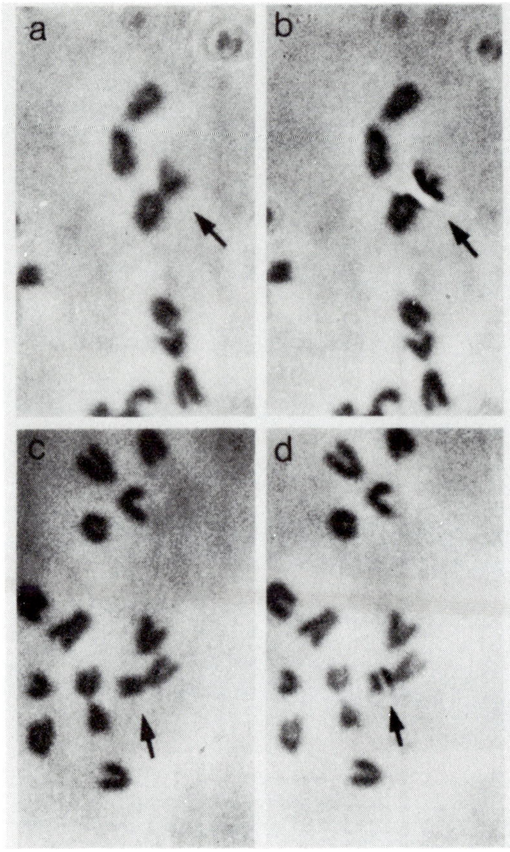

Fig. 7. Microdissection of a fragment from mouse chromosome 17. Parts of metaphase cells obtained from a mouse strain homozygous for the Robertsonian translocation Rb(8;17)65ic, as seen in the oil chamber before (a) and (c) and after (b) and (d) microdissection of the proximal fragment of chromosome 17 (arrows). From Röhme *et al.* (1984).

V. MICROEXTRACTION AND CLONING OF DNA

A. DNA extraction

DNA from the dissected chromosomes can be isolated in the oil chamber (Fig. 8). One or two hundred pooled chromosomes are sufficient for this procedure. After collection and pooling of chromosomes, excess glycerol/ phosphate solution is removed from the droplet with a micropipette (Fig. 6g). This allows the chromosomes to be collected in a cohering lump of

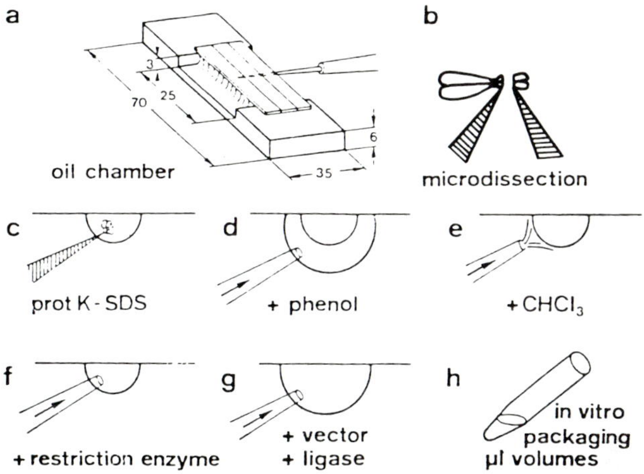

Fig. 8. Schematic illustration of the operations of microextraction and the molecular cloning in the oil chamber. Modified from Pirotta *et al.* (1983).

material which can be transferred in the oil chamber attached to the tip of the microneedle (Fig. 5h). The chromosome lump is then immersed into a one nanolitre drop of proteinase K-SDS solution (500 μl/ml proteinase K; 10 mM sodium chloride; 0.1% sodium dodecyl sulphate (SDS); and 10 mM Tris-HCl, pH 7.5). The oil chamber is placed in a moist chamber and incubated at 37°C. After 2 h incubation in the proteinase K-SDS solution, the oil chamber is put back into the microscope and the DNA is extracted three times by adding 4 volumes (i.e. 4 nl) of phenol to the aqueous drop. The phenol phase can easily be identified surrounding the aqueous drop (Fig. 8). The DNA is further extracted with chloroform to get rid of remaining traces of phenol (Fig. 8). Since phenol is somewhat soluble in the oil, the coverslip carrying the DNA drop is transferred to a new oil chamber.

B. Molecular cloning

The extracted DNA (of the order of 10 pg from 100–200 dissected chromosomes) could be digested with restriction enzymes in the nanolitre drop. The enzyme EcoRI is added to the DNA drop in large excess; to a 0.6 nl DNA drop is added 0.4 nl of 200 units/μl diluted with an equal volume of 2 × R buffer (1 × R buffer: 50 mM potassium chloride; 10 mM Tris-HCl, pH 7.5; 10 mM magnesium chloride; 10 mM mercaptoethanol). The oil chamber is placed in a moist chamber and incubated at 37°C for 90 min followed by 20 min incubation at 70°C to inactivate the enzyme.

The digested DNA is ligated to EcoRI cut lambda NM641 (Murray *et al.*,

1977), adding about a 10-fold excess vector DNA over the DNA fragments to be cloned in a reaction mixture of T4 ligase (1 unit/μl) in 1 × R buffer containing 0.4 mM ATP. The oil chamber is placed in a moist chamber and placed in 7°C for 12–18 h.

To obtain an efficient cloning, the ligated molecules are converted into infectious phage particles by the *in vitro* packaging technique (Hohn and Murray, 1977). The packaging is carried out in a microlitre volume. Thus, the nanolitre ligation drop has to be diluted to a microlitre volume. This is usually done by placing the oil chamber in a Petri dish filled with paraffin oil. The coverslip containing the ligation drop is inverted under the oil surface after which the Petri dish is placed under an ordinary dissecting microscope. Using a standard microlitre pipette, the ligation drop is diluted with 0.5–1 μl of TE buffer (10 mM Tris-HCl, pH 8.0; 1 mM EDTA) and the diluted ligation drop is then transferred to an Eppendorf tube. *In vitro* packaging extract, prepared as described (Scalenghe *et al.*, 1981), is added to the tube (2 μl of sonic extract and 10 μl of freeze–thaw lysate). After 60 min at room temperature, the extract is diluted with 100 μl phage buffer.

The recombinant phages were propagated in recK$^-$ met$^+$ bacterial strains such as Q358, derived from C600. Detection of the recombinant phages is based on the insertional inactivation of the cI gene of the vector, thus producing clear plaques as opposed to the turbid plaques produced by the intact vector. To eliminate the background of non-recombinant phages, we have as an alternative used the Hfl A host pop 101 (Lathe and Lecocq, 1977). This strain does not allow lytic growth of phage carrying an intact cI gene, but gives a normal plaque when infected with cI$^-$ phage. Thus, recombinant phages, but not the intact phage itself, will propagate on this host.

C. Yield of recombinants

The average size of the cloned fragments obtained was 3–4 kilobase pairs (kb), corresponding to the average EcoRI fragment size. The use of the vector NM641, which accepts inserts from 0–11 kb, thus optimizes the potential cloning of the vast majority of the DNA fragments obtained from the microdissected chromosomes.

Cloned DNA sequences from the microdissected metaphase chromosomes have now been obtained from three different chromosomes. The recoveries of cloned fragments were of the order of one cloned sequence per dissected chromosome in the more recent experiments. This corresponds to a cloning efficiency of 10–20 cloned sequences per picogram of DNA, which is the same efficiency as that obtained from cloning of microdissected chromosome fragments from dipteran polytene chromosomes (Pirotta *et al.*, 1983) and spermatocyte lampbrush loops (Hennig *et al.*, 1983).

Table I. Yields of recombinant phages from cloning of DNA from microdissected metaphase chromosomes or fragments.

Source of metaphase chromosomes	Amount of DNA per chromosome or fragment (pg)	Cloning efficiency plaques/pg of DNA
Indian muntjac		
Y-chromosome	0.035	4
Chromosome 1	0.8	8
Human		
Y-chromosome (euchromatic fragment)	0.015	13
Mouse		
Fragment of chromosome 17	0.03	13–25

VI. APPLICATIONS

Compared with other techniques for the isolation of specific chromosomes, such as chromosome sorting using flow cytofluormetry (Davies *et al.*, 1981; Sillar and Young, 1981), there are two major advantages at the microdissection technique discussed here. First, the microdissected chromosomes result in absolutely pure chromosome material without any contamination from other chromosomes. Not only can the desired chromosome be specifically dissected from the metaphase cells, but after each dissection the specificity of the dissected material is verified in the microscope and if doubtful discarded. Secondly, the technique can be used for dissection of specific subchromosomal regions. Applied to mouse chromosome 17, a fragment containing the proximal half of this small chromosome was specifically dissected and molecularly cloned (Röhme *et al.*, 1984). Further improvement in the microdissection of smaller chromosome fragments can be obtained by using high resolution banded chromosomes in prophase (Yunis, 1981) and even more in prematurely condensed chromosomes (Röhme and Heneen, 1982).

At present, the technique is particularly suitable for obtaining cloned sequences from defined regions of mammalian chromosomes. For this application, the requirement is not for a large yield of clones, but for precise localization of the dissected chromosome fragment. In particular, the combination of dissection from high resolution banded chromosomes with a genetic analysis using available defined deletions or translocations in the region of interest, would enable a localization of the cloned sequences with a very high precision. Such cloned sequences would be of interest as genetic markers, particularly if no other marker is available in the region. Applied to human genetics, these cloned sequences would be of particular interest for the localization and identification of disease genes using RFLP (restriction fragment length polymorphism) (Botstein *et al.*, 1980; Skolnick and White, 1982). Microdissection clones can also be used to screen a genomic library of large DNA fragments to initiate chromosome walking. These clones provide a selection of entry sites for simultaneous chromosomal walks into a limited chromosomal region. Due to the expected random distribution of the clones, the effort required to saturate the region with cloned sequences can thus be predicted. Using the microdissection clones isolated from the t region of the mouse chromosome 17 (Röhme *et al.*, 1984), such a procedure is currently being undertaken to cover this entire region.

Another principal type of application of this technique is the use of dissected chromosomes as a means for gene transfer. Microdissection-derived DNA could easily be injected into recipient cells using the same micromanipulation set-up as used for the dissection and cloning and which has been demonstrated for cloned DNA (Timm *et al.*, 1983). Due to the very limited amount of DNA that can be obtained with reasonable effort using microdissection, this is not practical at present. Potentially more interesting would be the ability to transfer intact dissected chromosomes directly into recipient cells by injection. This application is currently being considered, but it requires some modifications of the present technique for preservation of the chromosome structure and for permitting specific dissection of unfixed chromosomes.

REFERENCES

Botstein, D., White, R. L., Skolnick, M. and Davis, R. W. (1980). *Am. J. Hum. Genet.* **32**, 314–331.

Davies, K. E., Young, B. D., Elles, R. G., Hill, M. E. and Williamson, R. (1981). *Nature* **293**, 374–376.

Edström, J. E. (1964). *In* "Methods in Cell Physiology" (D. M. Prescott, ed.) pp. 417–447. Academic Press, New York and London.

de Fonbrune, P. (1949). "Technique de Micromanipulation", Monographes de l'Institut Pasteur. Masson, Paris.

Hennig, W., Huijser, P., Vogt, P., Jäckle, H. and Edström, J. E. (1983). *EMBO J* **2**, 1741–1746.

Hohn, B. and Murray, K. (1977). *Proc. Natl. Acad. Sci. USA* **74**, 3259–3263.

Lathe, R. and Lecocq, J. P. (1977). *Virology* **83**, 204–206.

Murray, N. E., Brammar, W. J. and Murray, K. (1977). *Mol. Gen. Genet.* **150**, 53–61.

Pirotta, V., Jäckle, H. and Edström, J. E. (1983). *In* "Genetic Engineering: Principles and Methods" (J. K. Setlow and A. Hollaender, eds) Vol. V, pp. 1–17. Plenum Press, New York.

Röhme, D. (1981). *Proc. Natl. Acad. Sci. USA* **78**, 5009–5013.

Röhme, D. and Heneen, K. (1982). *In* "Premature Chromosome Condensation" (P. N. Rao, R. T. Johnson and K. Sperling, eds) pp. 131–157. Academic Press, New York and London.

Röhme, D., Fox, H., Herrmann, B., Frischauf, A. M., Edström, J. E., Mains, P., Silver, L. M. and Lehrach, H. (1984). *Cell* **36**, 783–788.

Scalenghe, F., Turco, E., Edström, J. E., Pirrotta, V. and Melli, M. L. (1981). *Chromosoma (Berl.)* **82**, 205–216.

Sillar, R. and Young, B. D. (1981). *J. Histochem. Cytochem.* **29**, 74–78.

Skolnick, M. H. and White, R. (1982). *Cytogenet. Cell Genet.* **32**, 58–67.

Timm, B., Kondor-Koch, C., Lehrach, H., Riedel, H., Edström, J. E. and Garoff, H. (1983). *In* "Methods in Enzymology" (G. Blobel and D. Sabatini, eds) Vol. 96, pp. 496–511. Academic Press, New York and London.

Yunis, J. J. (1981). *Human Pathol.* **12**, 494–502.

Part II

Transfer of Macromolecules and Organelles into Eggs and Oocytes

15

Microinjection of Amphibian Oocytes and Eggs for the Analysis of Transcription

J. B. Gurdon and L. Wakefield

I. INTRODUCTION

The large size and easy availability of amphibian eggs and oocytes makes them particularly suitable for the microinjection of macromolecules (see also Chapters 16 and 17). By far the most commonly used Amphibian as a source of eggs and oocytes is *Xenopus*, and unless stated otherwise, all information in this contribution applies to *Xenopus laevis*. The technology of oocyte or egg injection is now in wide use, and relevant information is summarized here. A much more difficult problem is whether amphibian eggs or oocytes are likely to be useful for a particular purpose. We have therefore devoted the last few sections to the kinds of results and information which can be expected to come from their use.

II. PROPERTIES OF OOCYTES AND EGGS

A. Differences between oocytes and eggs

In Amphibia, an oocyte is a forming egg cell. It is located in the ovary, is closely surrounded by a few thousand follicle cells, and cannot be fertilized. It takes many months for a germ cell (about the same size as a somatic cell) to enlarge over 10^5 times to a 1 mm cell (Callen *et al.*, 1980). During this period its chromosomes are very active in RNA synthesis. Fully grown oocytes respond to pituitary hormone by undergoing "maturation". This involves the breakdown of the oocyte nucleus (the germinal vesicle), the

Microinjection and Organelle Transplantation Techniques

ISBN: 0-12-164722-6
ISBN: 0-12-164723-4 Pbk

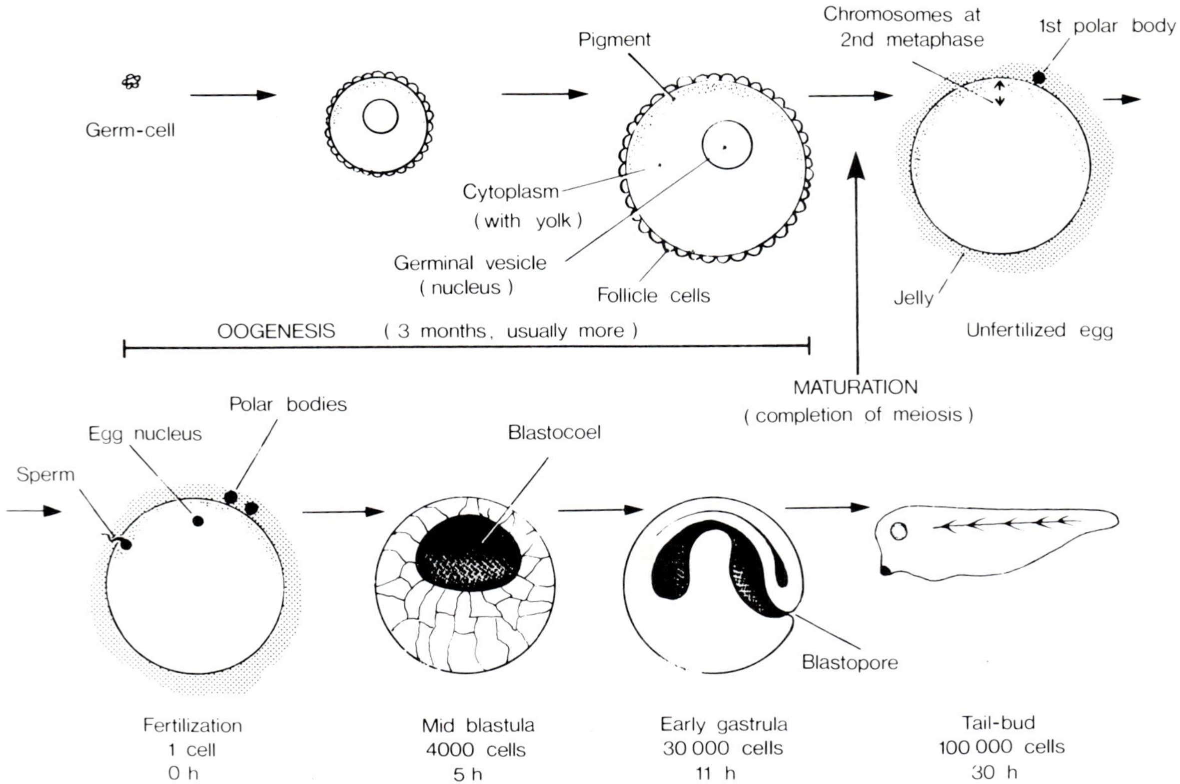

Fig. 1. Diagram of oogenesis and development in *Xenopus laevis*, at 23°C. Normal stages of oocyte growth and embryo development have been described by Dumont (1972) and Nieuwkoop and Faber (1956).

release of the oocyte from the ovary (ovulation), as well as the completion of the first meiotic division with arrest at the second meiotic metaphase. During the passage of the ovulated oocyte down the oviduct, it is covered with jelly. When released from the frog, the egg can be fertilized, and if so will develop very rapidly (3 days) into a free swimming larva. The great majority of amphibian injection experiments are carried out on fully grown oocytes, removed from the ovary of a female, or on recently fertilized eggs. The normal time scale of these developmental events is shown in Fig. 1.

B. Normal transcription of uninjected cells

The transcription of genes introduced into eggs or oocytes is influenced in several ways by the normal transcription of these cells. In particular, the background endogenous transcription must be taken into account when trying to assess the amount and kind of transcription from injected genes or nuclei. Figure 2 summarizes the main changes in RNA and DNA synthesis that take place in uninjected oocytes and eggs. It can be seen that each stage is characterized by a different pattern of RNA and DNA synthesis. The most important point is that an oocyte is a non-dividing cell with a nucleus which is immensely active in transcription. Conversely fertilized eggs and cleaving embryos up to the mid-blastula stage synthesize DNA and divide rapidly, but are inactive in transcription. Soon after the 12th division (4000 cells), cell division slows down due to the insertion of G1 and G2 phases into the lengthening cell cycle, and RNA synthesis starts. This stage is now referred to as the mid-blastula transition (Newport and Kirschner, 1982a), though it was Bachvarova and Davidson (1966) who first described the initiation of RNA synthesis at this stage. Although ribosomal DNA transcription appears to terminate correctly (Section VI.C), a common characteristic of oocyte gene expression seems to be for polymerase II transcription to read through from one gene to the next, without termination (Diaz *et al.*, 1981; working with a salamander), a result especially relevant to the transcription of injected genes (Section VI.C).

C. Major components of oocytes and eggs of *Xenopus*

The composition of an oocyte or egg indicates the amount of different substances present during biochemical extractions; these may be useful as carriers or inconvenient as contaminants. The content of nucleotides and amino acids can be used to calculate the specific activity of precursor pools in incorporation experiments.

The components of most general interest in an oocyte are listed in Table I. It is useful to regard one oocyte as having roughly the same volume and

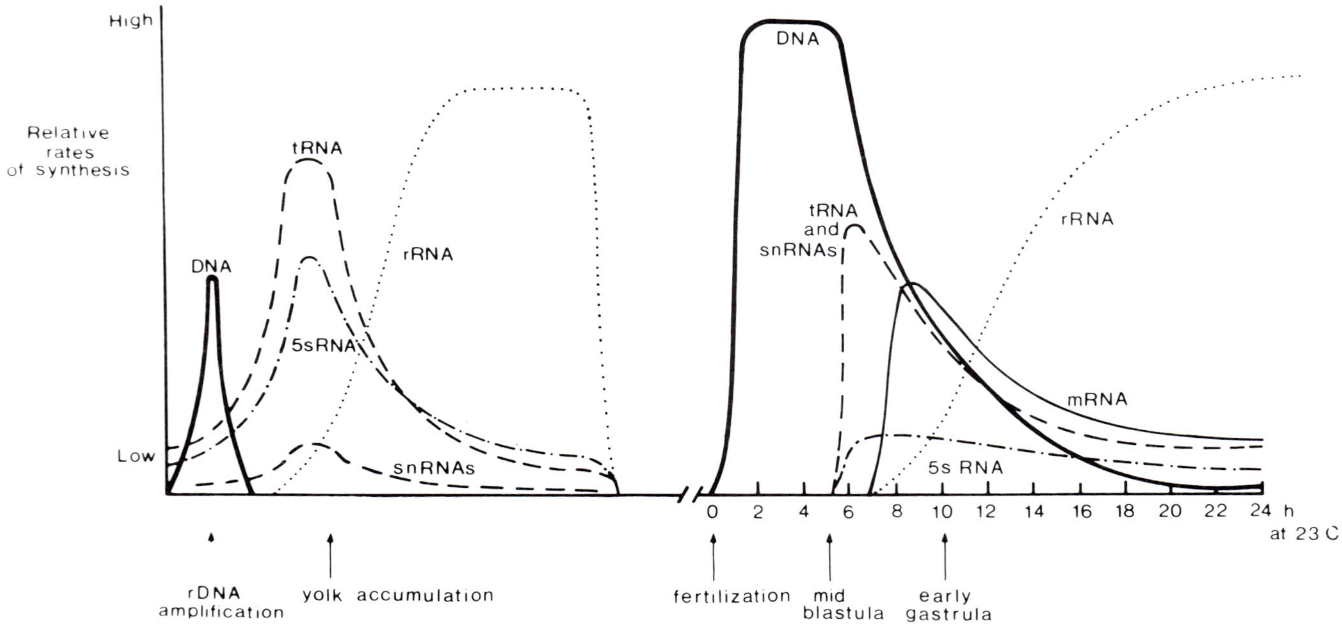

Fig. 2. Curves indicate relative rates of nucleic acid synthesis at different stages of oogenesis and development. Diagram based on Gurdon (1974), and modified in relation to results of Shiokawa *et al.* (1981), Forbes *et al.* (1983a,b) and Zeller *et al.* (1983).

Table I. Composition of a *Xenopus* oocyte, full grown and without follicle cells. Total volume, 1 μl; yolk-free volume 0.5 μl; GV volume 40 nl.

Component	Weight	Number of components	% of total in cytoplasm
DNA			
Oocyte chromosomal	12 pg	—	None
Nucleolar (rDNA)	25 pg	2×10^6 rDNA repeats	None
Mitochondrial	4000 pg	$\sim 10^8$ genomes	100%
RNA			
Ribosomal	5 μg	10^{12} ribosomes	99%
5S	60 ng	10^{12}	99%
tRNA	60 ng	1.5×10^{12}	99%
snRNA U1	0.07 ng	8×10^8	99%
polyA + RNA	80 ng	5×10^{10} (if 2500 bases long)	90%
Ribosomal protein mRNA	10 ng	2×10^{10}	—
Actin mRNA	~1 ng	5×10^8	—
Heat-shock 70 mRNA	0.004 ng	10^6	—
Protein			
Yolk	250 μg	—	100%
Non-yolk	25 μg	5×10^{14} (30 K protein)	90%
Histones	140 ng	5×10^{12}	50%
Nucleoplasmin	250 ng	5×10^{12}	98%
RNA polymerase I and II		$\sim 10^5 \times$ somatic cell	—
RNA polymerase III		$5 \times 10^5 \times$ somatic cell	—
Precursors			
dTTP	10 pmol	—	—
rGTP	250 pmol	—	—
Methionine	40 pmol	—	—

The content of an uncleaved egg is likely to be the same as above. This table is based on Gurdon and Wickens (1983), with additional information from Forbes *et al.* (1983a), Pierandrei-Amaldi *et al.* (1982), Bienz (1984a) and Zeller *et al.* (1983).

overall composition as 200 000 somatic cells. It is also useful to know that about half the volume of an oocyte is solid yolk (dispersed as platelets) and is unavailable space for injected substances. It is not generally appreciated that an oocyte has a huge amount of DNA in its cytoplasm (as mitochondria), and in the surrounding 5000 follicle cells. An egg has much the same composition as an oocyte except that it is entirely devoid of follicle cells (which are left in the ovary during ovulation), and has a large amount of surrounding jelly which can be removed (see below).

D. Rates of synthesis and precursor pool sizes

The most commonly used precursors for RNA and protein synthesis are ^{32}P-GTP and ^{35}S-methionine respectively, each with pool sizes in the oocyte as listed in Table I. If 1 μCi of ^{32}P-GTP is injected into an oocyte, this will usually yield, within 24 h, about 10^5 cpm of ^{32}P-RNA from endogenous transcription and up to a similar amount from injected genes, as discussed in detail by Gurdon and Wickens (1983). Another useful guide to synthetic activity is that an uninjected oocyte normally synthesizes 20 ng total RNA and 400 ng total protein per day (Gurdon and Wickens, 1983; Table II).

The rates at which various steps in gene expression take place in oocytes are listed in Table II. It can be seen that, in oocytes as in most other cell types, the limiting (or regulated) step in RNA and protein synthesis is initiation. Other steps all take place relatively rapidly in relation to the time-scale over which injection experiments are usually carried out (one day or more).

Table II. Rates of gene activity in *Xenopus* oocytes (19°C).

Process	Rate	Regulated
RNA synthesis		
Initiation	1 RNA polymerase every 100–200 nucleotides	Yes
Elongation	15 nucleotides/s	No
Termination	Generally little; subsequent trimming	No
Overall synthesis	20 ng stable RNA accumulated per day. Max rate = 10 000 transcripts/gene/day	—
Nucleus to cytoplasm transport		
rRNA		
tRNA	Fast (few min)	—
polyA + RNA		
Protein synthesis		
Initiation	1 ribosome every 100 nucleotides	Yes
Elongation	3 nucleotides (1 codon)/s	No
Termination	Run off	No
Overall synthesis	400 ng accumulated per day. Max rate = 2500 proteins/mRNA/day	—
DNA synthesis (for comparison)		
Elongation	~10 nucleotides/s	No

The values above are documented in Gurdon and Wickens (1983) and in Davidson (1976). Additional information from Callan (1973); Richter *et al.* (1982); Woodland and Old (1984).

III. SOURCES OF MATERIALS, MEDIA AND EQUIPMENT

A. How to obtain oocytes and eggs

Adult *Xenopus* are obtainable commercially from many sources, such as Xenopus Ltd., Holmesdale Nursery, Mid Street, South Nutfield, Redhill RH1 4JY, UK (Europe), Nasco Inc., 901 Jamesville Avenue, Fort Atkinson, Wisconsin 53538 (USA), or African Xenopus Facility, PO Box 2263, Clareinch, Republic of South Africa 7740.

To obtain oocytes, an adult female (no previous hormone treatment is necessary) is anaesthetized in tap water containing 0.1% ethyl *m*-aminobenzoate for 20–30 min. When it no longer moves having been turned upside down, it is placed on its back on damp paper. The ventral surface is wiped with Hibitane (10% in 75% ethanol) and an incision about 4 mm long is made in the region shown in Fig. 3 by cutting through the layers of skin and muscle. Part of the ovary is pulled out, cut off, and placed in MBS (see below). One gram of ovary will contain about 500 fully grown oocytes. The incision should be sewn together through both layers with one or two stitches of non-self-digesting surgical thread. After 10 days the stitches should be removed. The frog will recover within about 2 h if placed in tap water. The same female can be used at frequent intervals to obtain oocytes, as long as each incision is not too close to previous ones. Pieces of ovary divided into fragments, each containing not more than about 20 oocytes washed free of organic material, can be kept for several days in MBS, if the MBS is changed daily. They are best maintained at 19°C.

Eggs can be obtained from females in good condition by injecting 500 International Units of chorionic gonadotropin (LH) under the skin. Egg-lay-

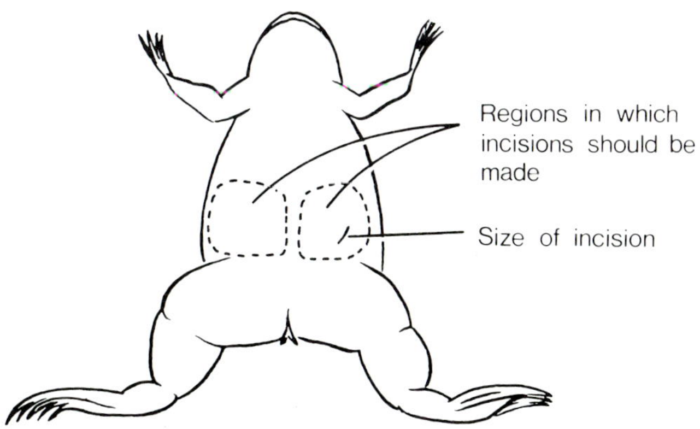

Fig. 3. Ventral view of female *Xenopus*, showing, outlined in dots, where an incision should be made to remove parts of ovary for oocytes.

ing will commence about 12 h later. If this procedure does not result in egg-laying, it will be helpful to give a female an initial injection of 200 units of gonadotropin, and then a further 400–500 units 6–8 h later. Egg-laying should commence about 6 h after the second injection. If this does not succeed, 100 units of a follicle-stimulating hormone such as Folligon should be given 4–7 days before commencing the gonadotropin injections specified above. It is important to remember that egg-laying is strongly inhibited by cool temperatures; 23°C is thought to be optimal. To obtain fertilized eggs, a male is placed in the same tank as a female at the time of the last hormone injection. A male should have black nuptial pads on its fore-arms and upper arms if it is to fertilize eggs successfully; if its black pads are not this well developed, it should be given 100–200 units of chorionic gonadotropin about one week earlier, thereby causing black pads to appear. *In vitro* fertilization can be used to obtain large numbers of accurately and similarly staged embryos using methods described by Wolf and Hedrick (1971). A female induced to lay eggs by hormone treatment is best rested for at least 3 months before being induced by hormone to lay again.

Sometimes it is necessary to make injected oocytes undergo maturation into eggs *in vitro*. There is great variability among females in the proportion of their oocytes which will undergo maturation. Only fully grown oocytes are capable of undergoing maturation. Pieces of ovary containing such oocytes are placed overnight in MBS containing 1 μg/ml progesterone (for further information, see Cicirelli *et al.*, 1983). The next day oocytes which underwent maturation will have been released from the pieces of ovary, and will have a pale area in the middle of the animal hemisphere pigment (as have unfertilized eggs), due to material released by the germinal vesicle.

Table III. Modified Barth Solution (from Gurdon, 1977) for oocyte and embryo culture (MBS).

Component	Concentration (mM)
NaCl	88
KCl	1
$NaHCO_3$	2.4
$Ca(NO_3)_2$	0.33
$CaCl_2$	0.41
$MgSO_4$	0.82
Hepes buffer	10
Benzyl penicillin	10 (mg/l)
Streptomycin sulphate	10 (mg/l)

Can be made up as 10 × stock and stored for long periods at 4°C, if sterilized and antibiotics added when diluted for use. Overall pH with NaOH, 7.5.

Table IV. High salt MBS for accumulation of unactivated eggs.

Component	Concentration (mM)
NaCl	88
KCl	1
$NaHCO_3$	2.4
$MgSO_4$	0.8
Na_2HPO_4	0.5
Tris buffer	15

Antibiotics may be added if required. Overall pH with acetic acid, 7.6. Can be made up as 8 × stock and stored at 4°C.

B. Culture media

A commonly used medium is Modified Barth Solution (MBS) — see Table III. In full strength, this is suitable for culturing oocytes and eggs or embryos. However if embryos are required to gastrulate normally, they must be transferred before gastrulation to 1/10 MBS. Oocytes will continue to synthesize RNA and protein for over two weeks if maintained in MBS which is changed daily. Survival is best when oocytes or embryos are kept well dispersed; a 5 cm Petri dish with 15 ml medium is suitable for 50 oocytes.

Wallace and colleagues (Table V) have designed a medium called OR2 in which oocytes will *grow* by uptake of vitellogenin. In comparison, MBS is a simpler medium for maintenance but not growth.

It is often desirable to accumulate unfertilized eggs in large numbers for bulk extraction. Frogs placed in a high salt calcium-free medium (Table IV)

Table V. OR2 medium for protein uptake and oocyte growth *in vitro*. From Wallace *et al.* (1973) and Wallace and Misulovin (1978).

Component	Concentration (mM)
NaCl	82.5
KCl	2.5
$CaCl_2$	1
$MgCl_2$	1
NaH_2PO_4	1
Hepes buffer	5

Overall pH with NaOH, 7.8. For long term growth, use above solution in 50% Leibovitz L-15 medium, with 5 mg/ml vitellogenin, 1 mM glutamine, 100 μg/ml gentamycin, and 50 units/ml nystatin.

will continue to lay eggs which remain in an unactivated but fertilizable state for several hours.

C. Microinjection equipment

Two types of injection procedure are in general use for amphibian oocytes and eggs. In one the injection pipette is calibrated, such that the meniscus of the fluid being injected is seen under the microscope to move from one calibration mark to the next. This has the advantage of making it certain that the desired volume is in fact injected. In the second procedure, mechanical or air pressure is used for a carefully controlled amount of time to expel the required volume. The advantage of the second procedure is that pipettes need not be calibrated (and ones made with conventional pipette pullers are satisfactory); on the other hand, pipettes can become partially blocked and a given duration of pressure application does not deliver a required volume as reliably as direct observation of fluid moving in a calibrated pipette.

Suitable components for the first type of outfit include a syringe (such as the Agla type, Wellcome Reagents, Beckenham, Kent, UK) filled with light paraffin oil. The syringe is connected by plastic tubing (1 mm diameter) to the injection pipette, which is in turn held in an appropriate manipulator. The most convenient manipulator is one which moves in three dimensions, directly reducing hand movements by about five times [e.g. Microdissector, of Singer Instruments, Treborough Lodge, Roadwater, Watchet, Somerset, UK, or Micro Techniques (Oxford) Ltd., 7 Little Clarendon Street, Oxford OX1 2HP, UK]. A cheaper alternative is to use a two-dimensional "mechanical stage" manipulator [such as Narushige, Optical Instrument Services (Croydon) Ltd., 166 Anerly Road, London SE20 8BD, UK, or Prior, Prior Scientific Instruments Ltd., London Road, Bishops Stortford, Herts CM23 5NB, UK]; this should be mounted at 45° to give diagonal movement. Apparatus of the second type has been described by Stephens *et al.* (1981). The latter paper gives full details of equipment in which a continuous air stream is deflected either down a micropipette (for injection) or away from it (whenever the pipette is not in an egg or oocyte). This design of equipment has the advantage of avoiding any suck-back of cytoplasm or yolk into the pipette and consequent blockage.

The injection pipettes required for the second type of equipment mentioned above can be made on any electrophysiological pipette puller. These pipettes, which usually taper sharply to a point, are unsuitable for the first type of injection equipment. For the latter, a pipette with a shaft of about 0.3 mm is needed, so that this can be calibrated (see Fig. 4). For these pipettes a sharpened tip on a fairly wide bore can be made by use of a suitable microforge (de Fonbrune, Metallurgical Service Laboratories Ltd., Reliant

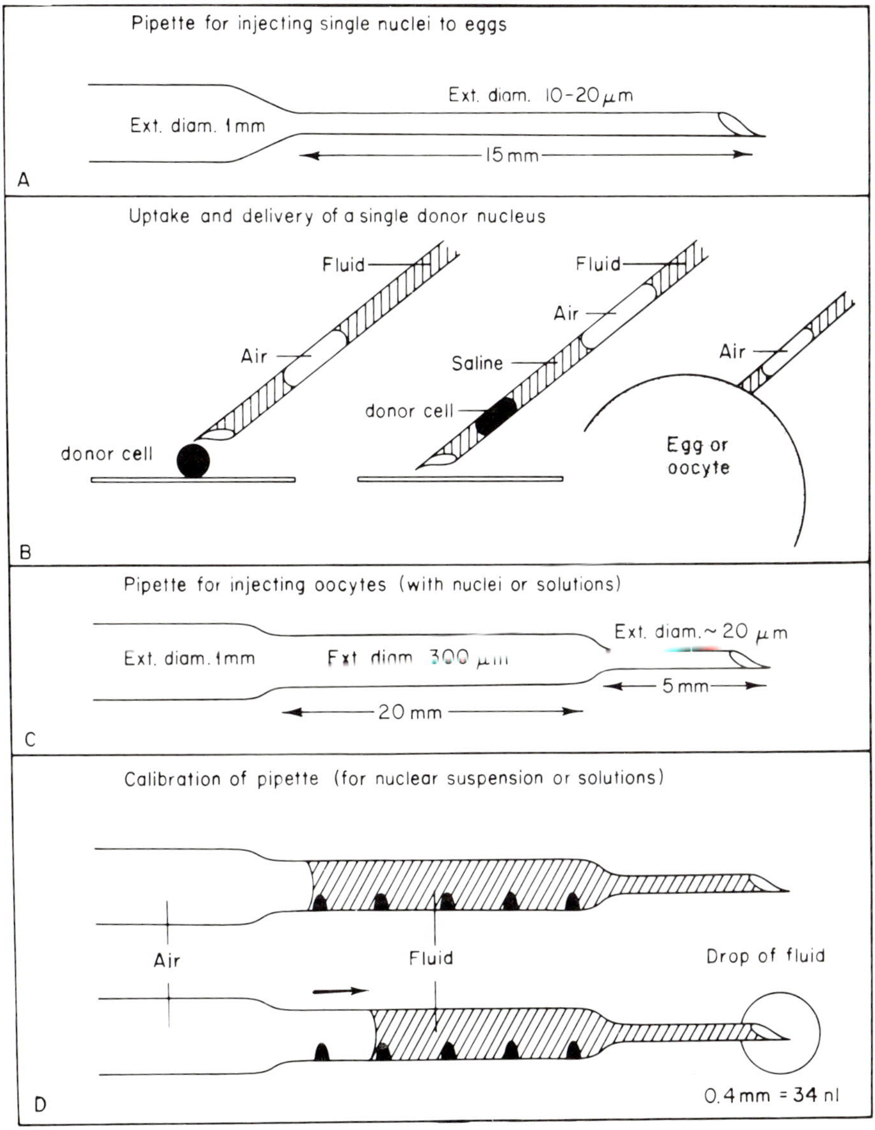

Fig. 4. Construction of micropipettes for injection of amphibian oocytes and eggs. (A) A pipette for transplanting single nuclei to unfertilized eggs. (B) Operation of the single-nucleus transfer pipette and its air bubble marker. (C) A pipette for injecting oocytes with solutions or suspensions of nuclei. (D) Calibration of the oocyte pipette shown in (C). Diagram taken from Gurdon (1977).

Works, Brockham, Betchworth, Surrey RH3 7HW, UK or Research Instruments Ltd., Kernick Road, Penryn, Cornwall TR10 9DQ, UK).

D. Injection procedure

(1) Oocytes

Single oocytes or small groups of up to 5 in the same ovarian fragment may be injected in MBS or in air on damp filter paper. Each oocyte needs to be held with forceps in one hand, while the injection pipette is inserted into the oocyte, using the manipulator with the other hand. The hand which holds the forceps (now not needed) is used to operate the syringe or other injection mechanism. Difficulty in making the injection needle enter the oocyte through the follicle cells is usually caused by the last part of the pipette being too long and flexible. This part should not exceed 5 mm (see Fig. 4C).

The injection of material (e.g. DNA) into an oocyte's nucleus (germinal vesicle, GV) is not as simple as injecting into the cytoplasm because pigment and yolk obscure the GV. One procedure (Gurdon, 1976) is to aim the micropipette tip to a position slightly nearer to the animal pole (centre of pigmented region) than to the centre of the oocyte. With experience the GV can be injected by this means in 80% of all attempts. In most experiments, the uninjected 20% does not matter, since DNA is not transcribed in the cytoplasm. This is the quickest and simplest procedure. If, however, it is important that over 95% of oocytes have material deposited in the GV, they may be lightly centrifuged (500 $\times$ *g*, 10 min) to bring the GV near the surface (Kressmann *et al.*, 1978). To do this single oocytes are placed on a nylon mesh with holes about 1 mm across. If they have been placed on the grid with the pigmented hemisphere uppermost, a circular discoloration appears where the GV has displaced pigment. This procedure takes longer but can achieve a higher success rate of GV injection.

The medium in which a sample is dissolved for injection is not critical, and distilled water is entirely satisfactory. High salt, such as traces of CsCl, are very toxic. The volume of injected fluid which can be tolerated is not more than 100 nl for the cytoplasm and 50 nl for the GV. It is generally best, however, to inject no more than 50 nl into the cytoplasm and 25 nl into the GV.

(2) Eggs

The jelly which surrounds eggs impedes injection and tends to block pipettes, but helps by sealing the injection wound. The jelly can be partly removed by a few seconds' exposure to a low wavelength UV, or completely removed by leaving eggs in MBS containing 2% cysteine hydrochloride, pH 8.0 with NaOH, for 5 min. De-jellied eggs will develop normally if well washed with MBS. If jelly is completely removed, leakage tends to occur after injection. This problem can be alleviated by placing eggs or embryos for a few minutes before, during, and after injection in MBS containing 2% Ficoll (Pharmacia, rel. mol. mass 400 000).

Additional technical information on manipulative and embryological procedures applicable to amphibian oocytes and eggs may be found in Gurdon (1974; 1977), Gurdon and Wickens (1983).

IV. NUCLEAR TRANSFER TO EGGS

The nucleus of a single somatic cell can be injected into an enucleated egg, and will promote development of the egg into an embryo and sometimes into a larva or adult frog. In *Xenopus*, the nucleus of an embryonic cell (up to the neurula stage) will generally yield swimming tadpoles in about 30%, and fertile adults in about 25% of all nuclear transfers (Gurdon, 1974). The more differentiated the cell from which a nucleus is taken, the less is the probability that normal development will be obtained. It has not yet been possible to obtain a normal adult animal by the transplantation of the nucleus of an adult animal's cell into an egg; the nuclei of adult cells have, however, yielded swimming tadpoles with functional differentiated cells of most kinds (Gurdon *et al.*, 1975; Wabl *et al.*, 1975; Di Berardino and Hoffner, 1983).

The main technical demands of these experiments are to enucleate the recipient eggs and to handle the donor nucleus correctly. Enucleation of *Xenopus* eggs can be reliably achieved by ultraviolet light, emitted at 1.6×10^4 J/s/cm^2 (Gurdon, 1977). There are two genetic markers which can be used in these experiments to provide direct proof that the egg nucleus has been eliminated. These are the periodic albino mutant (Hoperskaya, 1975) and the *1-nu* nucleolar mutation (Elsdale *et al.*, 1958). Since unfertilized eggs are used, there is no need to remove a sperm nucleus. The handling of the donor nucleus requires skill. It is necessary to construct pipettes with a smooth opening but also a sharp point (Figs 4A and B). A dissociated donor cell is then gently sucked into a pipette tip sufficiently small to break the cell, but not the nucleus. The donor nucleus is transplanted with its surrounding cytoplasm; there is no documented success of an animal cell nucleus, devoid of cytoplasm, being able to promote normal development of an egg.

It is technically straightforward to inject a suspension of nuclei into an unfertilized egg. This is useful for experiments in which an immediate response of nuclei to egg cytoplasm is required; for example, nuclei are induced to commence DNA synthesis within 1–2 h of injection into eggs, even if the nuclei are taken from non-dividing cells such as brain cells or erythrocytes. Eggs injected with multiple nuclei do not cleave, but remain viable and synthetically active for about 12 h. It has not yet been shown that gene expression, i.e mRNA and protein synthesis, is promoted by multiple nuclei injected into eggs, though this is certainly the case for single nuclei in enucleated eggs.

V. NUCLEAR TRANSFER TO OOCYTES

A. Gene expression

When somatic nuclei are injected into oocytes, whether into the oocyte nucleus (GV) or cytoplasm, they do not replicate; instead they enlarge and become increasingly active in RNA synthesis (Gurdon, 1976). The injected nuclei, as well as the host oocyte's own GV, continue to synthesize RNA for as long as the oocytes remain healthy. This experimental situation is of potential value since it involves the transfer of genes in their normal chromosomal environment into another cell, where they are more likely to be correctly regulated than when transferred as cloned DNA.

Some genes in oocyte-injected nuclei are expressed. At the level of RNA synthesis, genes transcribed by RNA polymerase III are very active (Korn and Gurdon, 1981). The injection of somatic nuclei, usually about 500, causes a 2- to 3-fold increase in the total amount of RNA synthesized by an oocyte, and much of this increase is due to the activity of RNA polymerase III (Wakefield *et al.*, 1983). The new polymerase III activity results from the activation of genes such as oocyte-type 5S and OAX which are not expressed in somatic cells, and from an increased transcription of tRNA genes. These genes are very active in an oocyte's own chromosomes. It is known that oocytes have a very large amount of RNA polymerase III, in fact the amount contained in 5×10^5 cultured cells (Roeder, 1974), most of which cannot be engaged in transcription in an uninjected oocyte, with only a tetraploid chromosome set. Oocytes evidently have considerable spare capacity in respect of RNA polymerase III, and must also have an excess supply of other factors required for activation as well as maintenance of polymerase III transcription, such as the TFIIIA needed for 5S gene transcription (Engelke *et al.*, 1980). The absolute amount of such factors is subject to considerable variation between individual animals (see Section VIII.B).

Some genes in injected nuclei are known to be expressed at the levels of protein synthesis and enzyme activity. Two-dimensional gels have been used to recognize human HeLa cell and adenovirus proteins in *Xenopus* oocytes injected with HeLa cell and adenovirus-infected nuclei. Similarly *Xenopus* proteins have been seen in the oocytes of another amphibian, *Pleurodeles*, injected with *Xenopus* nuclei (De Robertis and Gurdon, 1977). In some cases, as in the case of LDH enzyme (Etkin, 1976), the injected nuclei continue to synthesize in oocytes the same proteins which they were making in the donor cells. In other cases, genes not expressed in the donor cells are activated in injected oocytes, or genes expressed in the donor cells become inactive after nuclear injection.

The general rule which emerges from all reported nuclear-transfer-to-oocyte experiments is that the injected nuclei change their pattern of gene expression to some extent so as to conform to that characteristic of an oocyte. Thus the genes activated appear to be those typically expressed in oocytes. These experiments have established that gene expression of mammalian (and presumably of other vertebrate) nuclei can be maintained or activated in amphibian oocytes. Gene expression appears to continue for several days, and translatable mRNA seems to accumulate, since proteins coded for by somatic nuclei appear several days after injection. The efficiency of gene expression is not known, since the number of copies of the expressed genes has not been determined. It is not yet clear whether the expression of a single copy gene in somatic nuclei can be detected after injection into oocytes. The maximum rate of gene transcription in amphibian cells is believed to be about 10 transcripts/gene/min (Table II). An oocyte injected with 300 diploid nuclei might therefore accumulate 10^7 transcripts, if totally stable, in two days; this would be detectable by sensitive transcript assays.

B. Techniques

The following technical aspects of these nuclear injection experiments may be useful. Best results have been obtained with nuclei prepared by a very mild procedure. This involves the incubation of intact cells with a low concentration of lysolecithin, just sufficient to permeabilize the cells. The lysolecithin treatment is controlled by serum albumin. For details see Gurdon (1976).

The type of pipette required for transfer of multiple nuclei is important since the dense suspension of nuclei (500 per 50 nl or 10^7/ml) can easily block a pipette with a very fine or constricted opening. An orifice of 25 μm diameter is desirable, and the microforging of the tip (see Fig. 4C) is essential. The tendency of a dense suspension of nuclei to form aggregates and to block a pipette is greatly reduced by including 3% bovine serum albumin in the nuclear resuspension medium (Gurdon, 1976).

VI. GENE INJECTION TO OOCYTES

A. Uses and special techniques

Almost all kinds of DNA when injected into the nucleus of an oocyte are transcribed to a greater or lesser extent into complementary RNA (Mertz and Gurdon, 1977). DNA starts to be transcribed within one to three hours of injection (Gurdon and Brown, 1978; Miller and Mertz, 1982) and does not integrate into the host oocyte's chromosomes. It is usual to inject about 2 ng of DNA (equivalent to 5×10^8 copies of 5 kb DNA) into a single oocyte nucleus. Injected DNA provides a transient assay system for any cloned DNA sequence. In particular, injected oocytes can be used to identify *cis*-acting DNA sequences as well as *trans*-acting proteins or other molecules. Each application requires a knowledge of the accuracy and efficiency with which injected genes are transcribed and expressed.

It is essential to inject DNA into the oocyte nucleus if it is to be transcribed (see Section III.D). DNA-injected oocytes can be labelled either by mixing label with DNA before injection, or by a second injection at any desired time. ^{32}P-GTP, the most commonly used label, spreads rapidly through the oocyte and enters the nucleus. It may therefore by injected into the cytoplasm, unless mixed with DNA.

B. α-Amanitin sensitivity and types of RNA polymerase activity

Oocytes show about the same sensitivity to α-amanitin as do cell-free systems, and this gives a clear indication of the type of RNA polymerase involved in any particular transcriptional activity. Fig. 5 summarizes this information. It has always turned out so far that the type of polymerase used to transcribe an injected gene in an oocyte is the same as that used to transcribe this gene in cells where it is normally expressed, irrespective of species (see Fig. 5 for summary).

C. Initiation and termination

It is most convenient to inject cloned eukaryote genes into oocytes in the vector in which they have been grown. It has been found that much of the RNA complementary to an injected gene may be a result of read-through from the vector, certain regions of which happen to serve as transcription initiation sites in an oocyte (e.g. Wickens *et al.*, 1980). If this happens, an oocyte clearly would not provide a satisfactory assay for the effect on transcription of sequences in and around an injected gene. The success with which injected genes are transcribed in oocytes differs, and is discussed below, according to the type of RNA polymerase used.

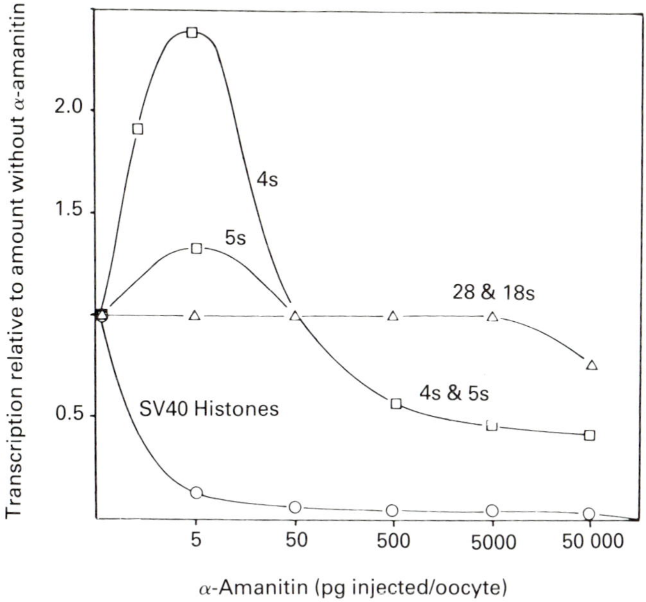

Fig. 5. α-Amanitin sensitivity of transcription in DNA-injected oocytes. Diagram from Gurdon and Wickens (1983).

Genes transcribed by polymerase III work particularly well in oocytes. 5S, tRNA, and OAX genes all yield abundant transcripts of the correct length and composition (e.g. Brown and Gurdon, 1977; Cortese *et al.*, 1978; Kressmann *et al.*, 1978; Melton and Cortese, 1979; Andrews *et al.*, 1984). Some tRNA gene transcripts are known to undergo progressive trimming at the 5′ and 3′ ends and splicing of a precursor (Melton *et al.*, 1980) and all of these steps proceed satisfactorily in an oocyte. 5S and OAX genes are thought to be transcribed directly into the final RNA product, in injected oocytes and in other cells. In either case, injected oocytes give a high yield of correct transcripts from this class of genes and have been widely used to define important DNA sequences such as promoters (review by Ciliberto *et al.*, 1983).

The transcription of injected ribosomal genes (rDNA) by polymerase I is hard to investigate because of the great activity of the amplified endogenous ribosomal genes (2×10^6 per oocyte). Nevertheless the combination of suitable probes with the injection of *Xenopus laevis* genes into *X. borealis* oocytes has shown that accurately initiated transcripts are obtained from the injected genes in sufficient abundance to carry out promoter mapping experiments (e.g. Moss, 1982; Sollner-Webb *et al.*, 1983). The large size of ribosomal genes has made them especially suitable for the EM analysis of nuclear spreads (e.g. Trendelenburg and Gurdon, 1978; Bakken *et al.*, 1982). The injected ribosomal DNA genes and vector DNA are seen as small circles, and are therefore immediately distinguishable from the host oocyte's genes (including the amplified ones) which are present as tandem arrays of several hundred genes.

The transcription of injected genes by polymerase II is more complicated; almost all possible results seem to have been observed. The so-called housekeeping genes, expressed in most cell types, seem usually to initiate and terminate correctly. For example, transcripts with the correct 5′ and 3′ ends, or overall size, have been described for some sea urchin histone genes (Probst *et al.*, 1979; Etkin and Maxson, 1980), for *Xenopus* histones H1 and H4 (Clerc *et al.*, 1983; Turner *et al.*, 1983), and for human and *Xenopus* sn RNAs U1 and U2 (Murphy *et al.*, 1982; Mattaj and Zeller, 1983; Zeller *et al.*, 1984). Other sea urchin histone genes fail to initiate and/or terminate correctly (Hentschel *et al.*, 1980). The correct 3′ end of some sea urchin histone transcripts may arise by the processing back of a long primary transcript; such an activity exists in the nucleus but not cytoplasm of oocytes (Birchmeier *et al.*, 1984). Inducible heat shock genes of *Drosophila* and *Xenopus* give RNA with correct 5′ and 3′ ends (see Section VI.F). Animal virus genes such as Herpes virus thymidine kinase, SV40 T antigen and virion proteins, and mouse Moloney leukaemia virus DNA, usually yield some stable transcripts with correct 5′ ends (Laskey *et al.*, 1978; Rungger and Türler, 1978; McKnight *et al.*, 1981; Breindl *et al.*, 1983; Wickens and Gurdon, 1983; Fradin *et al.*, 1984). Cellular genes whose expression is normally cell-type specific, on the other hand (such as chick ovalbumin, Wickens *et al.*, 1980; human β- and γ-globin genes, Partington *et al.*, 1984), do not usually produce RNA with correct 5′ and 3′ ends. The one exception, so far, is a human ζ- (embryonic α-) globin gene which gives predominantly correct cap-site initiation in injected oocytes (Proudfoot *et al.*, 1984). In this last case, the same gene and vector failed to give RNA with a correct 5′ end in HeLa cells or Cos cells. It will be interesting to see whether cell-type specific genes which are normally expressed in embryos are more correctly expressed in injected oocytes than genes normally active only in adult cells and if cell-type specific genes can be made to initiate correctly by complementation with cell-type specific factors.

D. Post-transcriptional events

Most post-transcriptional events in gene expression take place, at least to some extent, in injected oocytes. At the 5′ end, snRNAs are modified by the addition of the special snRNA cap (Murphy *et al.*, 1982). mRNAs from injected genes have not been examined at their 5′ ends, but are assumed to be correctly capped, because uncapped globin mRNA is very unstable (Green *et al.*, 1983). Accurate splicing is inferred in those cases where correct proteins are detected (see below) and has been shown to occur for SV40 transcripts (Wickens and Gurdon, 1983). Oocytes differ from SV40- and adeno-infected somatic cells in their preferential use of different, legitimate splice sites (Jones *et al.*, 1983). 3′ polyadenylation has been documented for transcripts of *Drosophila* hsp 70 (Voellmy and Rungger, 1982) and of SV40 (Wickens and Gurdon, 1983; Fradin *et al.*, 1984), though over half the SV40 RNAs are not polyadenylated compared to infected cells (Miller *et al.*, 1982). Evidently the mechanism for polyA addition exists but is not always fully efficient for some kinds of RNA. 3′ polyA addition is not required for splicing (Green *et al.*, 1983). For several tRNAs, base modifications have been analysed; most bases are correctly modified in *Xenopus* oocytes, even if the tRNA genes are from nematodes or sea urchins (reviewed by Gurdon and Melton, 1981). Yeast and prokaryote tRNAs are modified in a vertebrate manner, modifications specific to yeast and prokaryotes being absent (Nishikura and De Robertis, 1981; Bossi and Ciampi, 1983).

Nuclear to cytoplasmic transport of RNA transcribed from injected genes has been found whenever looked for, though the majority of the RNA complementary to an injected gene remains in the oocyte nucleus and is turned-over rapidly ($\frac{1}{4}$ h half life); polyA + RNA which reaches the cytoplasm is transported from the nucleus within 1 h (Miller *et al.*, 1982). The high rate of nuclear RNA turnover may well represent the normal fate of an oocyte's endogenous nuclear RNA (Anderson and Smith, 1977). For injected genes, it has been found that only those transcripts with correct 3′ ends are transported to the cytoplasm (Probst *et al.*, 1979; Wickens and Gurdon, 1983); those with incorrect 3′ ends, if injected to the cytoplasm, do not migrate back to the nucleus nor are they subsequently trimmed to a correct 3′ end (Krieg and Melton, 1984). Several authors (Green *et al.*, 1983; Wickens and Gurdon, 1983) have observed the transport of unspliced transcripts to the cytoplasm, a situation which may well apply to an oocyte's endogenous transcripts (Anderson *et al.*, 1982). It is important to know that abnormal transcripts (as from mutated genes) may be very unstable, disappearing within a few hours (Traboni *et al.*, 1984). This possibility must be kept in mind if genes are modified in order to distinguish their products from endogenous RNAs.

The synthesis of proteins coded for by injected DNA has been seen for a variety of genes including histones of several species, SV40 and other viral proteins (refs. in Gurdon and Melton, 1981; also Old *et al.*, 1982). In most of these cases the yield of protein is very small compared to the amount of complementary RNA synthesized (e.g. 2% for chick ovalbumin; Wickens *et al.*, 1980), even when much of this RNA has been correctly initiated (Breindl *et al.*, 1983). It has been suggested that the low yield of protein may result from the low efficiency of splicing or of RNA transport from nucleus to cytoplasm. As we have seen, almost every step in the expression of injected genes which has been carefully investigated takes place at a 50% or lower efficiency compared to cells in which these genes are normally expressed. It should be remembered that gene expression in an oocyte takes place over at least 100 days, and there is no reason to believe that any of these steps are as fast in oocytes as in somatic cells. It has not been possible to examine the rate of each step in the synthesis of proteins coded for by an oocyte's own genes, because of the low copy number of these genes. It could be that the expression of injected genes reflects that of an oocyte's own genes, or that the large number of genes that has to be injected to permit gene products to be detected overloads the oocyte, causing each step to take place less efficiently than normal.

E. Are injected genes efficiently transcribed?

Table VI summarizes rates of transcription from injected genes. The values given refer to transcripts accumulated over 24 h, after the injection of large numbers of genes. As judged from experience with 5S and ribosomal RNA genes, a lower number of genes injected would have resulted in a higher average efficiency for genes transcribed by polymerase II, had such a test been possible. Nevertheless, by comparison with an oocyte's endogenous transcription rate (Table II), most injected genes are transcribed by polymerase II at a very low rate. It is not known whether this low rate represents a small loading of polymerases on many injected genes, or a maximum loading on very few, as seems more probable from electron microscope studies (Trendelenburg *et al.*, 1980). In either case, this situation is potentially favourable for assaying *trans*-acting factors (as explained below, Section VIII). Some injected genes are transcribed with an efficiency approaching that of the same endogenous genes (see Table VI).

F. Are injected genes correctly regulated?

5S, tRNA, ribosomal, and histone genes are all correctly transcribed (though at very different rates) when injected into oocytes, and in this respect they conform to the activity of the same genes of the host cell. This could either mean that the injected genes are correctly regulated in an oocyte, or that all kinds of injected DNA are assembled into an active state even if the equivalent host genes are not expressed. If we assume that

Table VI. Typical rates of transcription of genes injected into a *Xenopus* oocyte nucleus.

Type of gene	Type of RNA polymerase	Injected genes: average accumulated transcripts/ gene/day*	Reference (injected genes)
tRNA	III	500–1000	Gurdon and Melton (1981)
5S	III	"	" " "
rDNA	I	100–200	Moss (1982)
Sea urchin histones	II	1–2	Probst *et al.* (1979) Etkin and Maxson (1980)
Thymidine kinase	II	3	McKnight *et al.* (1981)
SV40	II	2	Miller *et al.* (1982) Gurdon and Wickens (1983)
snRNA U1	II	20–100	Murphy *et al.* (1982) and authors' unpub. res.
Ovalbumin chick			
(plasmid initiation)	II	<2	Wickens *et al.* (1980)
(correct 5′ initiation)	II	None	Gurdon and Wickens (1981)
Xenopus adult globin	II	0.005–0.1	Bendig and Williams (1984)
Murine Moloney Virus DNA	II	0.5	Breindl *et al.* (1983)

* Only transcripts with correct 5′ ends have been scored, except where indicated. All analyses result from oocytes with about 5 ng DNA per oocyte and incubated for 24 h. Estimates of the rates of endogenous gene transcription for rDNA, 5S, tRNA, and snRNA U1 genes range from 1000–10000 transcripts/gene/day.

adult globin genes and the amphibian equivalent of ovalbumin genes are not normally transcribed in oocytes, the lack of cap-site initiation on injected globin and ovalbumin genes could be regarded as conforming to the host cell's pattern of gene regulation. This may mean that oocytes lack cell-type specific factors needed for transcription or for assembly of genes into a transcribable form of chromatin. It is also possible that an oocyte has the required components, but not in sufficient abundance for the accurate transcription of the large numbers of genes injected.

In contrast to the lack of evidence for regulation of cell-type specific genes introduced into oocytes, some inducible genes appear to be correctly regulated. This is the case for the *Xenopus* hsp 70 heat-shock genes which are normally expressed at cool temperatures in *Xenopus* oocytes (Bienz and Gurdon, 1982; Bienz, 1984a). When a cloned *Xenopus* hsp 70 gene is injected into oocytes, it is also transcribed at cool temperatures (Bienz, 1984b). In contrast, a *Drosophila* hsp 70 gene, which is transcribed in

Drosophila only after a heat-shock, is not transcribed at a cold temperature in *Xenopus* oocytes but is induced after a heat-shock (Bienz and Pelham, 1982; Voellmy and Rungger, 1982). Therefore the *Xenopus* gene comes under the correct regulation of a *Xenopus* oocyte, and the *Drosophila* gene is inducible.

G. Configuration and composition of DNA for injection

Any form of circular DNA is suitable for injection, since all are converted in an oocyte nucleus to supercoiled closed circles. Single stranded DNA, as in M13, is made double-stranded (Cortese *et al.*, 1980) and nicks in circular DNA are repaired. Linear DNA, whether single- or double-stranded, is gradually degraded in oocyte nuclei, apparently by an exonuclease activity. These and other matters concerning DNA conformation are reviewed by Gurdon and Melton (1981). For transcription to occur it seems to be necessary for DNA to be assembled into chromatin in a supercoiled form. Linear DNA (unless of very great length) does not become supercoiled or assembled into chromatin, and is transcribed about 100 times less well, if at all, compared to circular DNA (Mertz, 1982; Harland *et al.*, 1983; Pruitt and Reeder, 1984).

An important question is whether the kind or amount of vector DNA surrounding a cloned segment of eukaryotic DNA interferes with transcription. In microinjected oocytes, as in other assay systems, vector sequences may affect the efficiency with which cloned control sequences function (Kressmann and Birnstiel, 1979; Bienz and Pelham, 1982; Breindl *et al.*, 1983). Most commonly used vectors, such as pBR322, λ, and the replicative form of M13 contain sequences which act as weak promoters for polymerase II, which may read through into a promoterless segment of cloned DNA. In other cases (e.g. Clerc *et al.*, 1983) transcription is unaffected by vector sequences. When injected genes are to be transcribed by polymerases I or III, the amount of transcription is improved by including sufficient α-amanitin to suppress polymerase II activity (Fig. 5).

Eukaryotic DNA which has been cloned in bacteria is methylated at sites which differ from those methylated in its own species. Whether the state of methylation affects transcription in an oocyte seems to depend on the type of DNA and the sites methylated. Vardimon *et al.* (1982a) have convincingly shown that methylation of HpaII sites (CCGG) in the E2a region of adenovirus DNA inhibits its transcription in injected oocytes. This region is well transcribed if unmethylated, or if methylated at Bsu R1 sites (GGCC) (Vardimon *et al.*, 1982b). HpaII methylation of pBR322 has no effect on its transcription in oocytes. Another instance in which HpaII methylation does not affect transcription is that of ribosomal DNA (Pennock and Reeder,

1984). In the adenovirus E2a work referred to above, the state of methylation, assayed by HpaII/MspI, was unchanged over a 24 hour period in DNA injected into oocytes.

VII. GENE INJECTION TO EGGS

A. Uses and special techniques

DNA injected into fertilized eggs is replicated, but most of it remains unintegrated into the host cell chromosomes for the first day or two of development (review Gurdon and Melton, 1981). Since 10^7 genes can be injected into a single *Xenopus* egg, this is an especially favourable opportunity to study the expression of introduced genes independently of any adjacent host genes. In a "transient" expression system of this kind, the role of *cis*-acting DNA sequences should become clear. Though a small proportion of the injected and replicated DNA eventually integrates into chromosomes, this also happens in mice and *Drosophila*, which have the advantage over frogs of a much shorter life cycle, and are therefore more commonly used to study injected genes in an integrated state.

If more than 1 ng of DNA is injected into fertilized eggs, this causes abnormal cleavage. The DNA is best deposited in the animal (pigmented) hemisphere. The egg and sperm pronuclei cannot be seen among the yolk platelets and cannot therefore be injected directly.

B. Fate of injected DNA

In complete contrast to what happens in oocytes, DNA injected into fertilized eggs is extensively replicated. The amount of amplification varies greatly from one sample of eggs to another, ranging from a very little to over 50 times. All of this increase takes place during cleavage. The highest value is reached at the late blastula stage, and this is maintained until the end of gastrulation when copies of the injected DNA progressively disappear over the next few days (Rusconi and Schaffner, 1981). Almost all of this amplified DNA of the injected kind is not integrated; some exists as single molecules of the same length and composition as the DNA injected (Gurdon and Smith, 1984), though some concatemers are formed (e.g. Bendig, 1981). The injected DNA is seen in host cell nuclei as well as in nucleus-like structures formed around the DNA (Forbes *et al.*, 1983b). Analyses of growing tadpoles and frogs have shown that a small fraction of the injected and amplified DNA is stably integrated into host chromosomal DNA, averaging 1–10 copies per somatic cell genome (Rusconi and Schaffner,

1981), as has been also found for other organisms in which DNA has been injected into fertilized eggs.

Changes in DNA configuration that follow injection are similar to those observed in oocytes (Section VI.G). It has been found by several authors that the methylated state of injected DNA is propagated without changes during its amplification (Busby and Reeder, 1982; Harland, 1982; Bendig and Williams, 1983).

C. Transcription of injected DNA

Almost all kinds of DNA injected into eggs, whether fertilized or unfertilized, are transcribed into RNA. 5S and tRNA genes are transcribed sufficiently strongly for direct measurement of labelled RNA synthesized in a few hours (Gurdon and Brown, 1977). On the other hand, more sensitive assays are needed to detect the products of genes transcribed by polymerase II. Estimates of the rate of transcription of injected genes must take into account the substantial amplification of injected DNA (see above). When this is allowed for, the rate of transcription ranges from 0.01 to 0.1 transcript per gene per day for *Xenopus* globin (Bendig and Williams, 1984b) to about 1 for rabbit globin (Rusconi and Schaffner, 1981). It appears that 5S and tRNA are transcribed much more efficiently than cell-type specific genes, such as globin (see Table VI).

The accuracy of transcription of genes in eggs or embryos is generally good for housekeeping genes. Most 5S and tRNA transcripts are correctly initiated and terminated (whether by processing or not). At least some transcripts of genes read by polymerase II are correctly initiated, as with *Xenopus* α- and β-globins (Bendig and Williams, 1983, 1984b), and spliced, as with rabbit β-globin (Rusconi and Schaffner, 1981). The latter authors saw an improvement in the fidelity of transcription, when the β-globin gene was removed from its vector and religated. Some correct initiation has been reported for *Drosophila* ADH and certain sea urchin histone genes (Etkin *et al.*, 1984).

The regulation of injected genes has only been assessed so far in respect of temporal control. Gene transcription normally starts in *Xenopus* development at the mid-blastula stage (Section II). Newport and Kirschner (1982b) found that injected yeast tRNA genes start transcription at this stage, even though the genes were transcribed incorrectly for the first 2 h after injection. It is suggested that it may require about 2 h for injected genes to be assembled into chromatin and only then to be shut down, thus conforming to the host cells' transcriptional controls. Busby and Reeder (1983) have found that injected rDNA first gives detectable transcripts at the late blastula stage, just as in normal development (Shiokawa *et al.*, 1981). One other possible indication of gene regulation rests on the observation that, when adult and tadpole globin genes of *Xenopus* are coinjected, the tadpole genes are first transcribed at about the normal time in development (tail-bud; Bendig and Williams, 1984a). In the same embryos, the injected adult globin genes are clearly not correctly regulated, since they are transcribed throughout embryonic life, though endogenous adult globin genes are not transcribed until metamorphosis.

VIII. OOCYTE ASSAYS FOR *TRANS*-ACTING FACTORS

A. Nuclear migration of proteins and RNAs

Xenopus oocytes have the characteristic that nuclear proteins and RNAs of oocytes and somatic cells, if injected into the cytoplasm, will migrate into, and concentrate in, the oocyte nucleus. The migratory behaviour of nuclear molecules in oocytes was first shown for histones (Gurdon, 1970), but has now been established for many other proteins, as well as for RNAs and nucleoprotein complexes (reviewed by De Robertis, 1983). Furthermore, when a mixture of normally nuclear and cytoplasmic molecules are injected into oocyte cytoplasm, they soon take up their normal intracellular distribution, whether nuclear, cytoplasmic, or equally concentrated in both parts (De Robertis *et al.*, 1978). The tendency of molecules to be correctly localized is probably true of all cell types, but is particularly useful in the case of oocytes. This is because a large volume of an impure cell fraction can be injected; after a day, the oocyte will have concentrated nuclear molecules into its nucleus, leaving in the cytoplasm all other components which do not have a nuclear function. Proteins with a high nuclear affinity, such as histones and nucleoplasmin, will become at least 10 times more concentrated in the nucleus than in the cytoplasm. It is then possible to inject genes into the nucleus of a previously injected oocyte, so that these genes are assembled into chromatin with the migrated nuclear proteins.

The potential value of this procedure has been demonstrated (Weisbrod *et al.*, 1982). ^{3}H-labelled non-histone nuclear proteins known as HMG proteins 14 and 17, characteristically associated with transcriptionally active chromatin, were injected into oocyte cytoplasm. Two days later, ^{32}P-SV40 DNA was injected into the oocyte nucleus. One day later, minichromosomes were extracted and shown to contain ^{3}H-proteins associated with ^{32}P-DNA. This procedure therefore offers the prospect of an assay for the transcriptional effect of *trans*-acting factors present in crude cell extracts.

B. An oocyte complementation test

The experimental design described has been used very successfully to identify a type of RNA required for the correct termination of gene transcription (Galli *et al.*, 1983). Sea urchin histone H3 genes do not terminate their transcription correctly in injected *Xenopus* oocytes. Oocytes were therefore injected, into their cytoplasm with a fraction of sea urchin chromatin, and in their nuclei with histone H3 genes. This assay was used to purify a 60-nucleotide RNA required to make a correct 3′ terminus.

Oocytes can be used to identify genes whose products influence the expression of other genes. This has been demonstrated in an experiment where the adenovirus promoter E3 is influenced by the product of another adenovirus gene E1a. Jones *et al.* (1983) coinjected DNA containing the E3 promoter attached to a CAT gene with DNA of another plasmid containing the E1a gene. This led to increased CAT activity, not observed when a mutant E1a gene was used. This effect appears to be due to the E1a gene product affecting the E3 promoter, since the transcription of this promoter was affected in other experiments involving the direct injection of E1a protein (Ferguson *et al.*, 1984).

In principle, this oocyte complementation test can be used to purify not only components which oocytes do not possess, such as a sea urchin histone termination factor, but also components of which they have a limited supply. For example, a few hundred somatic nuclei each containing 40000 inactive oocyte-type 5S genes can be injected into an oocyte. It has been found that the oocytes of certain females possess enough "activating" factor to cause extensive transcription of these genes, while the oocytes of other females do not (Korn and Gurdon, 1981). By injecting somatic nuclei together with extracts of activating oocytes into non-activating oocytes, it was possible to show that a protein exists which can activate developmentally repressed 5S genes. In conclusion, it seems likely that oocytes will prove to be a valuable assay for a wide range of *trans*-acting factors.

C. DNA competition experiments

If a factor is required for the transcription of different genes, this will become obvious in a competition experiment. If a constant amount of gene A is coinjected into an oocyte nucleus with increasing amounts of gene B, the transcription of gene A will be decreased if they share the need for a factor in limited supply. This design of experiment was used to demonstrate that SV40 and 5S are not in competition with each other, since they are transcribed in oocytes by different polymerases (Gurdon and Brown, 1978). The same design of experiment has been used to compare the transcriptional requirements of 5S and OAX genes (Andrews *et al.*, 1984). By the use of suitably deleted genes, it should be possible to determine the exact region of two genes which compete, and hence to deduce a sequence of DNA for which a *trans*-acting factor must exist. DNA competition experiments have also been used to determine the relative strengths of natural or modified promoters (McKnight and Kingsbury, 1982; Reeder *et al.*, 1983).

When planning competition experiments, the following considerations should be kept in mind. If less than 5 ng of DNA is injected, this may adversely affect assembly of DNA into chromatin (Gargiulo and Worcel, 1983); however amounts substantially less than 1 ng are nevertheless efficiently transcribed (e.g. Sollner-Webb and McKnight, 1982). In coinjection experiments, a 2:1 competitive advantage of one gene over another at low doses (1 ng) may become a 20:1 advantage at high doses (10 ng). In sequential injection experiments, the first DNA to be injected has a strong competitive advantage, even if it has none in a coinjection experiment (Reeder *et al.*, 1983; Gargiulo *et al.*, 1984), a situation very reminiscent of one already described for an *in vitro* transcription system based on oocyte nuclei (Brown, 1984).

IX. USE OF OOCYTES FOR GENE CLONING

From limited experience so far, it appears that cDNA is not expressed as RNA or protein when injected into oocytes; it is not surprising that this applies to cDNAs of genes with intervening sequences, such as ovalbumin (Wickens *et al.*, 1980), since introns have been found to have a function for transport from nucleus to cytoplasm. However, in another respect, oocytes are particularly valuable for identifying fractions of mRNA from which it is useful to prepare cDNA.

Unlike most cell-free mRNA translation systems, oocytes will assemble the appropriate products of different mRNAs into a normal structure. This has been demonstrated most impressively by Barnard and colleagues, who injected total polyA + RNA from various sources, such as *Torpedo* electric organ (Barnard *et al.*, 1982) or rat brain (Gundersen *et al.*, 1983), and observed within 2 days the formation of functional nicotinic acetylcholine receptors and serotonin receptors. Since a functional membrane receptor requires the correct assembly of different proteins, several mRNAs must have been translated, and their products transported and sufficiently well assembled to respond to an electrophysiological assay. The conclusion of general significance which emerges from these experiments is that injected oocytes can be used to recognize unknown mRNAs, where the only assay for them depends on the assembly of products from several different messages.

The same advantage applies when the only assay for an mRNA is an antibody against an antigen formed by the assembly of the product of this mRNA with one or more different cell components.

Once an RNA fraction has been shown to contain a desired kind or kinds of mRNA, oocyte translation can be used to identify the species concerned. A suitable procedure would be to make a cDNA library from the RNA fraction, and use random subdivisions of this to isolate mRNAs for injection and assay. If two or more mRNAs are needed to produce the structure which is assayed, this could require numerous tests. However, there is a significant chance that a complex structure for which an assay exists may be formed by the product of one kind of injected mRNA in combination with other components already present in an oocyte, a situation which is much less likely to exist in cell-free systems.

REFERENCES

Anderson, D. M. and Smith, L. D. (1977). *Cell* **11**, 663–671.
Anderson, D. M., Richter, J. D., Chamberlin, M. E., Price, D. H., Britten, R. J., Smith, L. D. and Davidson, E. H. (1982). *J. Mol. Biol.* **155**, 281–309.
Andrews, D. L., Millstein, L., Hamkalo, B. A. and Gottesfeld, J. M. (1984). *Nucl. Acids Res.* **12**, 7753–7769.
Bachvarova, R. and Davidson, E. H. (1966). *J. Exp. Zool.* **163**, 285–296.
Bakken, A., Morgan, G., Sollner-Webb, B., Roan, J., Busby, S. and Reeder, R. H. (1982). *Proc. Natl. Acad. Sci. USA* **79**, 56–60.
Barnard, E. A., Miledi, R. and Sumikawa, K. (1982). *Proc. Roy. Soc. B* **215**, 241–246.
Bendig, M. M. (1981). *Nature* **292**, 65–67.
Bendig, M. M. and Williams, J. G. (1983). *Proc. Natl. Acad. Sci. USA* **80**, 6197–6201.
Bendig, M. M. and Williams, J. G. (1984a). *Mol. Cell Biol.* **4**, 567–570.
Bendig, M. M. and Williams, J. G. (1984b). *Mol. Cell Biol.* **4**, 2109–2119.
Bienz, M. (1984a). *Proc. Natl. Acad. Sci. USA* **81**, 3138–3142.
Bienz, M. (1984b). *EMBO J.* **3**, 2477–2483.
Bienz, M. and Gurdon, J. B. (1982). *Cell* **29**, 811–819.
Bienz, M. and Pelham, H. R. B. (1982). *EMBO J.* **1**, 1583–1588.
Birchmeier, C., Schumperli, D., Sconzo, G. and Birnstiel, M. L. (1984). *Proc. Natl. Acad. Sci. USA* **81**, 1057–1061.
Bossi, L. and Ciampi, M. S. (1983). *Nucl. Acids Res.* **11**, 3207–3226.
Breindl, M., Kalthoff, H. and Jaenisch, R. (1983). *Nucl. Acids Res.* **11**, 3989–4006.
Brown, D. D. (1984). *Cell* **37**, 359–365.
Brown, D. D. and Gurdon, J. B. (1977). *Proc. Natl. Acad. Sci. USA* **74**, 2064–2068.
Busby, S. J. and Reeder, R. H. (1982). *Devel. Biol.* **91**, 458–467.
Busby, S. J. and Reeder, R. H. (1983). *Cell* **34**, 989–996.
Callan, H. G. (1973). *Cold Spring Harbor Symp. Quant. Biol.* **38**, 195–203.
Callen, J. C., Dennebouy, N. and Mounolou, J. C. (1980). *Devel. Growth Diff.* **22**, 831–840.
Cicirelli, M. F., Robinson, K. R. and Smith, L. D. (1983). *Devel. Biol.* **100**, 133–146.

Ciliberto, G., Castagnoli, L. and Cortese, R. (1983). *Curr. Topics Dev. Biol.* **18**, 59–87.

Clerc, R. G., Bucher, P., Strub, K. and Birnstiel, M. L. (1983). *Nucl. Acids Res.* **11**, 8641–8657.

Cortese, R., Melton, D., Tranquilla, T. and Smith, J. D. (1978). *Nucleic Acids Res.* **5**, 4593–4611.

Cortese, R., Harland, R. and Melton, D. (1980). *Proc. Natl. Acad. Sci. USA* **77**, 4147–4151.

Davidson, E. H. (1976). "Gene Activity in Early Development". Academic Press, New York and London.

De Robertis, E. M. (1983). *Cell* **32**, 1021–1025.

De Robertis, E. M. and Gurdon, J. B. (1977). *Proc. Natl. Acad. Sci. USA* **74**, 2470–2474.

De Robertis, E. M., Longthorne, R. F. and Gurdon, J. B. (1978). *Nature* **272**, 254–256.

Diaz, M. O., Barsacchi-Pilone, G., Mahon, K. A. and Gall, J. G. (1981). *Cell* **24**, 649–659.

Di Berardino, M. A. and Hoffner, N. J. (1983). *Science* **219**, 862–864.

Dumont, J. N. (1972). *J. Morphol.* **136**, 153–180.

Elsdale, T. R., Fischberg, M. and Smith, S. (1958). *Exp. Cell Res.* **14**, 642–643.

Engelke, D. R., Ng, S.-Y., Shastry, B. S. and Roeder, R. G. (1980). *Cell* **19**, 717–728.

Etkin, L. D. (1976). *Devel. Biol.* **52**, 201–209.

Etkin, L. D. and Maxson, R. E. (1980). *Devel. Biol.* **75**, 13–25.

Etkin, L. D., Pearman, B., Roberts, M. and Bektesh, S. L. (1984). *Differentiation* **26**, 194–202.

Ferguson, B., Jones, N., Richter, J. and Rosenberg, M. (1984). *Science* **224**, 1343–1345.

Forbes, D. J., Kornberg, T. B. and Kirschner, M. W. (1983a). *J. Cell Biol.* **97**, 62–72.

Forbes, D. J., Kirschner, M. W. and Newport, J. W. (1983b). *Cell* **34**, 13–23.

Fradin, A., Jove, R., Hemenway, C., Keiser, H. D., Manley, J. L. and Prives, C. (1984). *Cell* **37**, 927–936.

Galli, G., Hofstetter, H., Stunnenberg, H. G. and Birnstiel, M. L. (1983). *Cell* **34**, 823–828.

Gargiulo, G. and Worcel, A. (1983). *J. Mol. Biol.* **170**, 699–722.

Gargiulo, G., Razvi, F. and Worcel, A. (1984). *Cell* **38**, 511–521.

Green, M. R., Maniatis, T. and Melton, D. A. (1983). *Cell* **32**, 681–694.

Gundersen, C. B., Miledi, R. and Parker, I. (1983). *Proc. Roy. Soc. B* **219**, 103–109.

Gurdon, J. B. (1970). *Proc. Roy. Soc. B* **176**, 303–314.

Gurdon, J. B. (1974). "The Control of Gene Expression in Animal Development". Oxford and Harvard University Presses, Oxford, UK and Cambridge, MA.

Gurdon, J. B. (1976). *J. Embryol. Exp. Morph.* **36**, 523–540.

Gurdon, J. B. (1977). *Methods in Cell Biol.* **16**, 125–139.

Gurdon, J. B. and Brown, D. D. (1977). *In* "The Molecular Biology of the Mammalian Genetic Apparatus" (P. T'so, ed.) Vol. 2, pp. 111–123. North-Holland, Amsterdam.

Gurdon, J. B. and Brown, D. D. (1978). *Devel. Biol.* **67**, 346–356.

Gurdon, J. B. and Melton, D. A. (1981). *Ann. Rev. Genet.* **15**, 189–218.

Gurdon, J. B. and Smith, D. (1984). *In* "Transfer and Expression of Eukaryotic Genes", P. and S. Symposium, New York, June 1984 (H. S. Ginsberg and H. J. Vogel, eds) pp. 143–151.

Gurdon, J. B. and Wickens, M. P. (1983). *Methods Enzymol.* **101**, 370–386.
Gurdon, J. B., Laskey, R. A. and Reeves, O. R. (1975). *J. Embryol. Exp. Morph.* **34**, 93–112.
Harland, R. M. (1982). *Proc. Natl. Acad. Sci. USA* **79**, 2323–2327.
Harland, R. M., Weintraub, H. and McKnight, S. L. (1983). *Nature* **302**, 38–43.
Hentschel, Ch., Probst, E. and Birnstiel, M. L. (1980). *Nature* **288**, 100–102.
Hoperskaya, O. A. (1975). *J. Embryol. Exp. Morph.* **34**, 253–264.
Jones, N. C., Richter, J. D., Weeks, D. L. and Smith, L. D. (1983). *Mol. Cell. Biol.* **3**, 2131–2142.
Korn, L. J. and Gurdon, J. B. (1981). *Nature* **289**, 461–465.
Kressmann, A. and Birnstiel, M. L. (1979). *In* "Transfer of Cell Constituents into Eukaryotic Cells" (J. E. Celis, A. Graessmann and A. Loyter, eds) pp. 383–407. Plenum Press, New York.
Kressmann, A., Clarkson, S. G., Pirrotta, V. and Birnstiel, M. L. (1978). *Proc. Natl. Acad. Sci. USA* **75**, 1176–1180.
Krieg, P. A. and Melton, D. A. (1984). *Nature* **308**, 203–206.
Laskey, R. A., Honda, B. M., Mills, A. D., Morris, N. R., Wyllie, A. H., Mertz, J. E., De Robertis, E. M. and Gurdon, J. B. (1978). *Cold Spring Harbor Symp. Quant. Biol.* **42**, 171–178.
Mattaj, I. W. and Zeller, R. (1983). *EMBO J.* **2**, 1883–1891.
McKnight, S. L. and Kingsbury, R. (1982). *Science* **217**, 316–324.
McKnight, S. L., Gavis, E. R. and Kingsbury, R. (1981). *Cell* **25**, 385–398.
Melton, D. A. and Cortese, R. (1979). *Cell* **18**, 1165–1172.
Melton, D. A., De Robertis, E. M. and Cortese, R. (1980). *Nature* **284**, 143–148.
Mertz, J. E. (1982). *Mol. Cell. Biol.* **2**, 1608–1618.
Mertz, J. E. and Gurdon, J. B. (1977). *Proc. Natl. Acad. Sci. USA* **74**, 1502–1506.
Miller, T. J. and Mertz, J. E. (1982). *Mol. Cell. Biol.* **2**, 1595–1607.
Miller, T. J., Stephens, D. L. and Mertz, J. E. (1982). *Mol. Cell. Biol.* **2**, 1581–1594.
Moss, T. (1982). *Cell* **30**, 835–842.
Murphy, J. T., Burgess, R. R., Dahlberg, J. E. and Lund, E. (1982). *Cell* **29**, 265–274.
Newport, J. and Kirschner, M. (1982a). *Cell* **30**, 675–686.
Newport, J. and Kirschner, M. (1982b). *Cell* **30**, 687–696.
Nieuwkoop, P. D. and Faber, J. (1956). "Normal Table of *Xenopus laevis*" (Daudin). North-Holland, Amsterdam.
Nishikura, K. and De Robertis, E. M. (1981). *J. Mol. Biol.* **145**, 405–420.
Old, R. W., Woodland, H. R., Ballantine, J. E. M., Aldridge, T. C., Newton, C. A., Bains, W. A. and Turner, P. C. (1982). *Nucl. Acids Res.* **10**, 7561–7580.
Partington, G. A., Yarwood, N. J. and Rutherford, T. R. (1984). *EMBO J.* **3**, 2787–2792.
Pennock, D. G. and Reeder, R. H. (1984). *Nucl. Acids Res.* **12**, 2225–2232.
Pierandrei-Amaldi, P., Campioni, N., Beccari, E., Bozzoni, D. and Amaldi, F. (1982). *Cell* **30**, 163–171.
Probst, E., Kressmann, A. and Birnstiel, M. L. (1979). *J. Mol. Biol.* **135**, 709–732.
Proudfoot, N. J., Rutherford, T. R. and Partington, G. A. (1984). *EMBO J.* **3**, 1533–1540.
Pruitt, S. C. and Reeder, R. H. (1984). *J. Mol. Biol.* **174**, 121–139.
Reeder, R. H., Roan, J. G. and Dunaway, M. (1983). *Cell* **35**, 449–456.
Richter, J. D., Wasserman, W. J. and Smith, L. D. (1982). *Devel. Biol.* **89**, 159–167.
Roeder, R. G. (1974). *J. Biol. Chem.* **249**, 249–256.

Rungger, D. and Türler, H. (1978). *Proc. Natl. Acad. Sci. USA* **75**, 6073–6077.
Rusconi, S. and Schaffner, W. (1981). *Proc. Natl. Acad. Sci. USA* **78**, 5051–5055.
Shiokawa, K., Tashiro, K., Misumi, Y. and Yamana, K. (1981). *Devel. Growth Diff.* **23**, 589–597.
Sollner-Webb, B. and McKnight, S. (1982). *Nucl. Acids Res.* **10**, 3391–3405.
Sollner-Webb, B., Wilkinson, J. A. K., Roan, J. and Reeder, R. H. (1983). *Cell* **35**, 199–206.
Stephens, D. L., Miller, T. J., Silver, L., Zipser, D. and Mertz, J. E. (1981). *Anal. Biochem.* **114**, 299–309.
Traboni, C., Ciliberto, G. and Cortese, R. (1984). *Cell* **36**, 179–187.
Trendelenburg, M. F. and Gurdon, J. B. (1978). *Nature* **276**, 292–294.
Trendelenburg, M. F., Mathis, D. and Oudet, P. (1980). *Proc. Natl. Acad. Sci. USA* **77**, 5984–5988.
Turner, P. C., Aldridge, T. C., Woodland, H. R. and Old, R. W. (1983). *Nucl. Acids. Res.* **11**, 4093–4107.
Vardimon, L., Kressmann, A., Cedar, H., Maechler, M. and Doerfler, W. (1982a). *Proc. Natl. Acad. Sci. USA* **79**, 1073–1077.
Vardimon, L., Gunthert, U. and Doerfler, W. (1982b). *Mol. Cell. Biol.* **2**, 1574–1580.
Voellmy, R. and Rungger, D. (1982). *Proc. Natl. Acad. Sci. USA* **79**, 1776–1780.
Wabl, M. R., Brun, R. B. and Du Pasquier, L. (1975). *Science* **190**, 1310–1312.
Wakefield, L., Ackerman, E. and Gurdon, J. B. (1983). *Devel. Biol.* **95**, 468–475.
Wallace, R. A. and Misulovin, Z. (1978). *Proc. Natl. Acad. Sci. USA* **75**, 5534–5538.
Wallace, R. A., Jared, D. W., Dumont, J. N. and Sega, M. W. (1973). *J. Exp. Zool.* **184**, 321–333.
Weisbrod, S., Wickens, M. P., Whytock, S. and Gurdon, J. B. (1982). *Devel. Biol.* **94**, 216–229.
Wickens, M. P. and Gurdon, J. B. (1983). *J. Mol. Biol.* **163**, 1–26.
Wickens, M. P., Woo, S., O'Malley, B. W. and Gurdon, J. B. (1980). *Nature* **285**, 628–634.
Wolf, D. P. and Hedrick, J. L. (1971). *Devel. Biol.* **25**, 348–359.
Woodland, H. R. and Old, R. W. (1984). *In* "Developmental Control in Animals and Plants" (C. F. Graham and P. F. Wareing, eds) 2nd Ed., pp. 422–504. Blackwell Scientific, Oxford.
Zeller, R., Nyffenegger, T. and De Robertis, E. M. (1983). *Cell* **32**, 425–434.
Zeller, R., Carri, M.-T., Mattaj, I. W. and De Robertis, E. M. (1984). *EMBO J.* **3**, 1075–1081.

16

Functional Aspects of tRNAs Microinjected into Xenopus laevis *Oocytes: Results and Perspectives*

H. Grosjean and E. Kubli

I. INTRODUCTION

The oocytes of the South-African clawed toad, *Xenopus laevis*, are giant cells that allow, through direct microinjection, the introduction of various natural or synthetic macromolecules into either the cytoplasm or the nucleus. This unique system has been widely used to study translation, stability and subcellular compartmentation of injected heterologous messenger RNA, as well as transcription, processing and maturation of various foreign genes and their RNA transcripts (see also Chapters 15 and 17). Curiously, much less has been published on the microinjection of other macromolecules of high biological interest, such as proteins with particular structural or specific catalytic functions, or transfer RNAs (tRNA). It is the purpose of this chapter to review the literature on microinjection of foreign tRNAs into *Xenopus laevis* oocytes with special emphasis on protein synthesis and related problems. Furthermore, we would like not only to demonstrate the potential of this approach in the study of structure and function relationships, or of the role of this important class of nucleic acids in a variety of cellular processes, but also draw attention to certain pecularities of the complex organization of the oocyte itself.

A. The multifunctional character of the tRNA molecule, biosynthesis and genetic engineering

The most obvious and best documented role of the mature tRNA molecule in the cytoplasm of a living cell is the transport of the amino acids to the site

Microinjection and Organelle Transplantation Techniques

ISBN: 0-12-164722-6
ISBN: 0-12-164723-4 Pbk

of protein synthesis, the ribosome. This central role already implies that the tRNA molecule interacts specifically with various components of the protein synthesis machinery, i.e. the aminoacyl-tRNA ligases, the initiation or elongation factors, proteins and nucleic acids in the acceptor and peptidyl sites of the mRNA–ribosome complex, and the termination factors. In higher eukaryotes it is now becoming evident that the large majority of aminoacyl-tRNA ligases, as well as other components of the protein synthesis apparatus (e.g. certain modifying enzymes), can be part of very high relative molecular mass complexes, which themselves may be part of a supramolecular organization of the whole *in vivo* protein synthesizing machinery. The transfer of amino acids along such multi-enzyme complexes has not been elucidated so far (Agris *et al.*, 1983; Deutscher, 1984).

In addition to their direct role in protein synthesis, tRNAs have been implicated in a variety of cellular processes which are not known yet in detail at the molecular level. In prokaryotes, the regulatory role of the tRNA molecule on the efficiency of protein synthesis has become clear; similar roles are postulated in eukaryotes. In addition, a role in the regulation of activity of certain enzymes (involved in amino acid and DNA synthesis), in packaging of some viral RNAs into virions, in amino acid transport as well as participation as phosphoseryl donors in reactions not involving ribosomes, and serving as primers for reverse transcriptase, have been demonstrated (for details see La Rossa and Söll, 1978; Cortese, 1979).

The biosynthesis of tRNA is also an extraordinarily complex process. It involves transcription of the corresponding tRNA gene by polymerase III with the participation of additional protein components. But many subsequent enzymatic steps are needed before the matured, highly modified tRNA appears in the cytoplasm. About 60–80 enzymes are involved in the maturation processes for all tRNAs, some present in the nucleus, others in the cytoplasm. Here again, the detailed molecular mechanisms, as well as the regulation of these multi-enzymatic processes, are largely unknown (Clarkson, 1983; Sharp *et al.*, 1985).

The development of recombinant DNA technology, and more recently of recombinant RNA technology, permits now the alteration almost at will of the nucleotide sequence of a tRNA gene or the mature tRNA. The combination of these new techniques with the subsequent microinjection of the recombinant nucleic acids into a living cell, offers the opportunity to change quantitatively the population of a specific tRNA in a single cell. Furthermore, the effect of various mutations on the synthesis of this important class of macromolecules and its various functions can now be studied.

B. Transfer RNA synthesis, storage and content

Xenopus oocytes provide a real *in vivo* assay system; they make it possible to perform experiments under conditions existing within living cells. It should not be forgotten, however, that the oocytes are programmed to fulfil a function of their own, which is not to serve as test tubes for eager biochemists, but to prepare for fertilization and embryogenesis. It is the aim of this section to provide the biological background necessary to enable the experimenter to take into account the physiological and biochemical particularities of the growing and full grown oocyte with respect to tRNA metabolism (see also Chapter 15).

The logistics of tRNA in the oocyte can best be understood by considering two important aspects of oocyte growth. First, as already mentioned above, the aim of this process is to provide the egg with all the necessary compounds for early embryogenesis. Due to the enormous size of the *Xenopus* egg, the time needed to synthesize these components is considerable (see below). Second, the synthesis of the stable RNAs of the egg occurs in two steps (see Fig. 2 of Chapter 15). In short, the small RNAs (4S and 5S) are synthesized during the pre-vitellogenic stage, while the ribosomal RNAs 18S + 28S, and mRNAs are accumulated during the vitellogenic phase.

The *Xenopus laevis* egg contains 4–6 μg of total RNA, of which about 1–2% is tRNA (Mairy and Denis, 1971, Clarkson *et al.*, 1973). This represents an enormous amount of tRNA for a single cell. The genes coding for tRNA are not amplified in the oocytes, although they are highly redundant. Assuming a reiteration of 4×10^4 tRNA genes in the tetraploid oocyte nucleus, it can be calculated that to reach the amount of 40 ng of tRNA per full grown oocyte, transcription would require just over one year (Clarkson *et al.*, 1973). The imbalance in the synthesis of small and large stable RNAs during oocyte growth is exemplified by the fact that 40% of the RNA content of pre-vitellogenic (150 μm diameter) oocytes is tRNA (Mairy and Denis, 1971), whereas in the full grown oocyte the tRNA represents only 1–2% of the total RNA as mentioned above. Small RNAs are synthesized throughout oogenesis, whereas the genes for 18S + 28S RNA are fully active only after the beginning of vitellogenesis. Thus, at the end of oogenesis the oocyte has accumulated approximately equal amounts of tRNA, 5S, 18S + 28S molecules with vastly different numbers of genes coding for tRNA, 5S, and 18S + 28S RNA.

A large proportion of tRNA synthesized in the pre-vitellogenic stage is associated with a cytoplasmic 42S nucleoprotein particle (Ford, 1971; Denis and Mairy, 1972), i.e. does not exist as free molecules in the cytoplasm. These particles, named thesaurisomes by Denis and Lemaire (1983), probably have a tetrameric structure, the fundamental unit being a seven-component, 15S particle. The monomer contains one molecule of 5S RNA associated with a protein *b* (rel. mol. mass 40000), and three tRNA molecules less tightly bound to two identical proteins *a* (rel. mol. mass 50000; Picard *et al.*, 1980). Additional proteins are associated in non-stoichiometric amounts, among them the aminoacyl-tRNA ligases. The composition in tRNA isoacceptors and in aminoacyl-tRNA ligases in the 42S particles seems to be random (Denis and Mairy, 1972). An interesting peculiarity is that each bound tRNA is constantly maintained fully charged, probably by the aminoacyl-tRNA ligases present in the thesaurisomes; this enzymatic process costs a lot of energy (ATP) to the oocyte (Wegnez and Denis, 1979; Denis and Lemaire, 1985). With the onset of vitellogenesis the 42S particles disappear and the aminoacyl-tRNAs are released into the cytoplasm (Denis and Mairy, 1972; Dixon and Ford, 1982; Barrett *et al.*, 1983). It is not clear whether all the aminoacyl-tRNA present in the full grown oocyte is available for protein synthesis. Compartmentation has been demonstrated for phenylalanyl-tRNA ligase in the *Xenopus* oocyte by Gatica *et al.* (1980). These authors suggested that a large proportion of the phenylalanyl-tRNA ligase present in the oocytes is not available to injected tRNAs.

A comparison between tRNAs isolated from somatic cells and oocytes has been made by Denis *et al.* (1975). Reversed-phase chromatography profiles for phenylalanyl-, methionyl-, and leucyl-tRNAs isolated from small and large oocytes, eggs, and liver- and kidney-cells have been compared. Striking differences were observed between isoacceptor profiles of tRNAs extracted from small oocytes and somatic cells. Isoacceptor patterns from large oocytes differ much less when compared with somatic patterns, and the egg profiles were almost identical. The molecular basis for these findings is not yet established, although it seems reasonable to assume that most are due to differences in degree of modification. These data are especially interesting considering the activity of modification enzymes during oogenesis. It seems that some enzymes are only active during the pre-vitellogenic phase, while others might persist until the fully grown oocyte is formed.

The concentration of single isoacceptors has only been determined for the $tRNA^{Met}_{init.}$ (Wegnez *et al.*, 1975). A single fully grown *Xenopus* oocyte contains at least 2.5 ng of initiator tRNA. Methods as those developed by Kleiman *et al.* (1983) might be adequate to determine the amount of single isoacceptors. Some tRNAs isolated from oocytes and *Xenopus* tRNA genes have been sequenced. A compilation is found in the article by Sprinzl *et al.* (1985).

Finally an important biological aspect of oogenesis shall be mentioned. Oogenesis is a continuous process. From this it follows that immature females contain a large number of small oocytes, whereas mature females contain oocytes at all stages. It has been observed that in a growing female more than half of the oocytes belong to a relatively homogeneous size class (Mairy and Denis, 1971). Thus, there exists a positive correlation between the size of a growing female and the abundance of oocytes of a given size. Under laboratory conditions females often do not lay eggs (oocytes are removed by surgery), or egg-laying is interrupted by long intervals. Mairy and Denis (1971) have shown that the rate and pattern of RNA synthesis is strikingly affected by the timing of egg-laying. Similar effects might result from irregular removal of oocytes by surgery. Thus the frequency of egg-laying or surgery may influence the metabolism of the ovary, an important aspect that has to be taken into account in the interpretation of oocyte microinjection experiments.

II. MICROINJECTION OF FOREIGN tRNAs INTO FULLY GROWN OOCYTES

Known amounts of individual tRNA species can easily be microinjected, into either the cytoplasm or the nucleus of fully grown oocytes, as defined above. Depending on how the experiment is conducted (see Fig. 1 and Table I), the microinjected tRNA can serve as a probe for several molecular processes in which the injected nucleic acid might be involved.

A. Microinjected tRNAs are stable

Microinjection is an obvious means of studying nucleic acid degradation within a natural environment, whether it be the cytoplasm or the nucleus of the oocyte. So far, most efforts have been devoted to studies of the stability of microinjected messenger RNA and viral RNA (see Chapter 17). Allende *et al.* (1974) have reported on the stability of microinjected transfer RNA into *X. laevis* oocytes. By microinjecting ^{32}P-labelled yeast bulk tRNA and purified *Escherichia coli* UAG suppressor $tRNA^{Tyr}_{sup\text{-}3}$ into the cytoplasm of fully grown oocytes, they estimated the half-life of these nucleic acids to be approximately 2–3 days. This remarkable stability was intrinsic to the tRNA molecules since other microinjected ribonucleic acids, such as ribosomal RNAs and most synthetic ribopolynucleotides, were rapidly degraded by ribonucleases. However, it should be emphasized that in growing oocytes the half-life of tRNAs in the thesaurisomes can be several months (Denis and Lemaire, 1983).

The possibility of labelling tRNA with [^{32}P]orthophosphate now permits a more systematic investigation into the stability of various *individual*

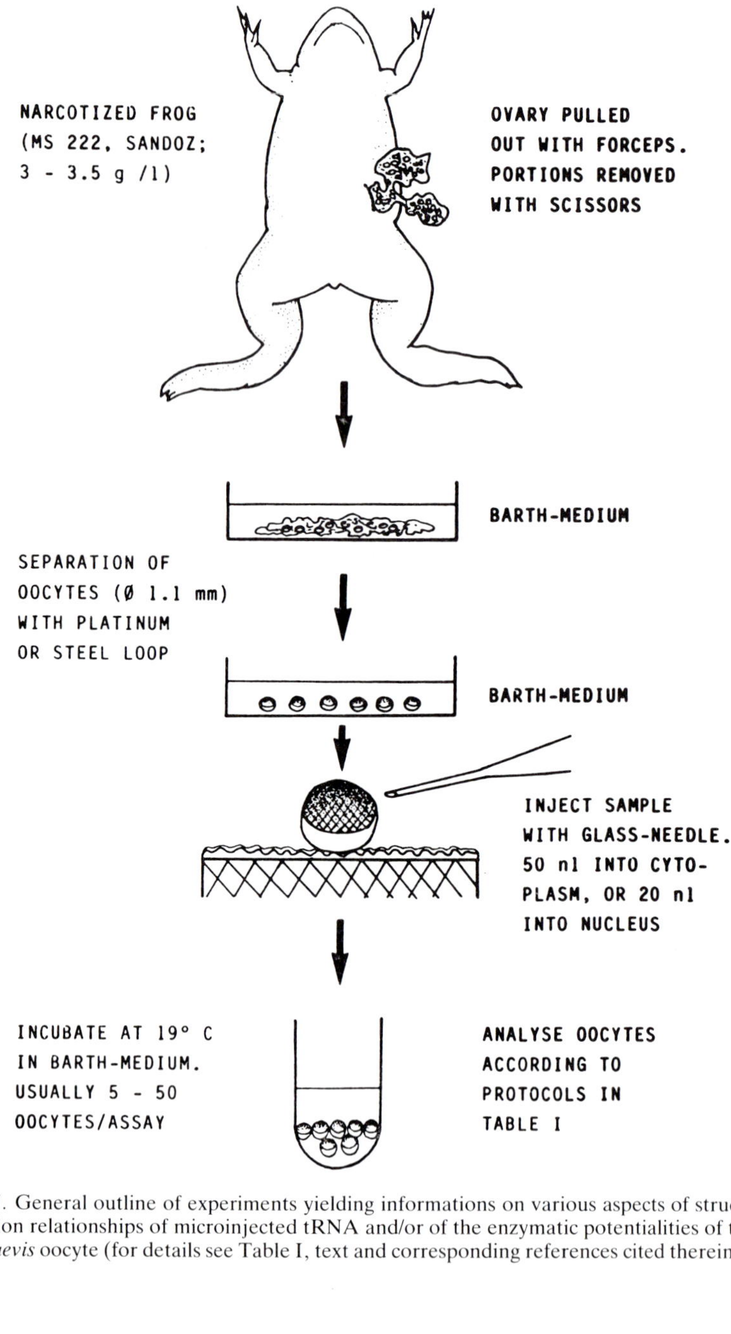

Fig. 1. General outline of experiments yielding informations on various aspects of structure–function relationships of microinjected tRNA and/or of the enzymatic potentialities of the *X. laevis* oocyte (for details see Table I, text and corresponding references cited therein).

Table I. General outline of experimental protocols for structure–function studies of tRNA using *Xenopus* oocytes as *in vivo* assay system.

Injection	Incubation	Analysis
A. tRNA stability, minoacylation, nucleotide modification		
Inject [^{32}P]tRNA into the cytoplasm or nucleus	15 min–80 h	Phenol extract total RNA at pH 4.5 Precipitate RNA with ethanol Separate by electrophoresis on PAA-gels Elute labelled tRNA and count cpm (Fig. 2) Hydrolyse tRNA completely with nuclease T-2 or P-1 Chromatograph nucleotides on 2-D TLC Form Tu-GTP complex or let react phenoxyacetyl-*N*-hydroxysuccinimide and gel-chromatograph
B. tRNA aminoacylation		
Inject pure isoacceptor tRNA into cytoplasm, if necessary with cognate synthetase	15 min–6 h with labelled amino acid	Phenol extract RNA at pH 4.5 Precipitate tRNA with cold TCA and count cpm in the precipitate (Fig. 3)
C. Nonsense suppression		
Inject suppressor tRNA into cytoplasm (if necessary with cognate synthetase) together with mRNA	1–24 h with labelled amino acid	Extract soluble, labelled proteins Separate by PAA electrophoresis Autoradiograph (Fig. 5) Elute protein bands and count radioactivity Calculate % read-through
D. Codon recognition		
Inject [^{3}H] or [^{14}C]-labelled aminoacyl tRNA into cytoplasm together with mRNA	4 h	Extract soluble, labelled proteins Separate by PAA electrophoresis Elute protein, cleave protein Separate peptides on PAA-gels Elute peptides and count cpm Normalize data
E. tRNA gene transcription and tRNA maturation		
Inject tRNA gene together with α[^{32}P]-labelled nucleoside tri-phosphate	15 min–6 h	Phenol extract total RNA Precipitate with ethanol Separate by PAA gel-electrophoresis autoradiograph Autoradiograph Elute radioactive bands Determine base composition or nucleotide sequence

purified tRNAs from various origins, including those of *X. laevis*. Such information is already available for the following tRNAs: $tRNA^{Tyr}_{sup\text{-}3}$ (as stated above); *E. coli* $tRNA^{Met}_{f}$; purified wild-type tRNAs from yeast specific for aspartic acid, arginine, cysteine, leucine, phenylalanine and tryptophan; and tRNA recombinants constructed from those purified tRNAs (with one or two oligonucleotides in the anticodon altered; Carbon *et al.*, 1982; Fournier, Vacher, Doi, Haumont, Droogmans, and Grosjean, unpub. res.). These results clearly point out two important aspects of tRNA stability. First, all wild-type tRNAs are rather stable but not equally stable in the cytoplasm of the *Xenopus* oocyte, the least stable in the above series being *E. coli* $tRNA^{Met}_{f}$ with a half-life of approximately one day, the most stable being yeast $tRNA^{Asp}$ with a half-life of more than seven days. Second, certain minor changes in the anticodon of some of those tRNAs (split anticodon or nucleotide replaced leading to a mutated tRNA) result in a considerable decrease in stability (half-line of a few hours instead of days, Fig. 2), an important aspect to be considered in genetic engineering experiments. These views are supported by experiments of Schlegel *et al.* (1978) studying tRNA turn-over using the technique of red cell-mediated microinjection (see Chapter 5).

A similar situation might exist inside the nucleus of the oocyte during the complex process of maturation of the tRNA precursor after transcription of the tRNA gene. Indeed, one base substitution at a specific location in the microinjected $tRNA^{Pro}$ gene of *Caenor habditis elegans* destabilizes the primary transcriptional product leading to a half-life considerably shorter than that of the wild-type molecule (Traboni *et al.*, 1984).

How can such a spectacular differential stability of two tRNA molecules differing only by one base be explained? One interesting possible interpretation is that only *functional* tRNA molecules are stable, due to continuous transient association with many components of the translation machinery and other proteins interacting with tRNAs, thus protecting the tRNAs from nucleases. The interplay of biosynthetic and degradative enzymes (specific or not) may be important in limiting the production and/or the accumulation of "aberrant", possibly functionally defective, macromolecules in a cell or even in a specific compartment of a cell (Gurevitz and Apirion, 1983). Specialized nucleases may also recognize structurally altered tRNA molecules (Ghosh and Deutscher, 1978); thus, inside the living cell, there might exist several mechanisms that selectively degrade "aberrant" tRNAs. Supporting this general idea are the observations that the turn-over of most tRNAs is not the same in resting or growing cells (Abelson *et al.*, 1974), during cellular differentiation (Kleiman *et al.*, 1980), or during tumorization (Borek *et al.*, 1977, 1981). It is generally believed that the increased degradation of a given endogenous tRNA inside a mammalian cell under-

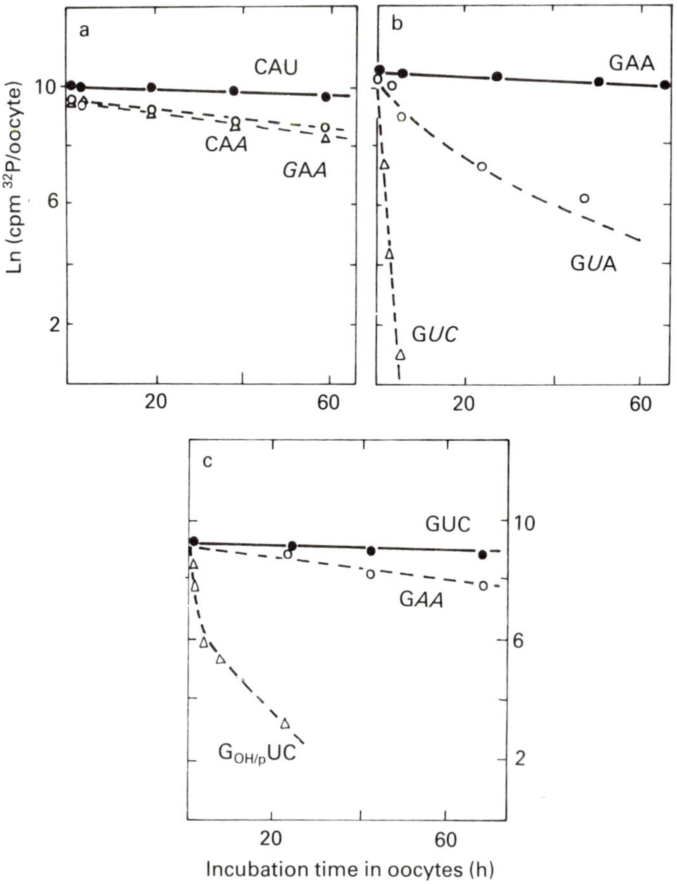

Fig. 2. Stability of microinjected tRNAs (natural or chimeric) in the *X. laevis* oocytes. A given amount (fmol level) of purified ^{32}P-labelled tRNA was microinjected into the cytoplasm of the oocyte. At the indicated time after microinjection, the residual amount of isotope found in the tRNA fraction of the oocyte was determined after electrophoresis on polyacrylamide gels under denaturing conditions (see protocol A, Table I, and more details in Carbon *et al.*, 1982). Solid circles give results for natural tRNA, open symbols for chimeric tRNAs mutated or altered in their anticodons. (a) Shows results obtained by injecting *E. coli* $tRNA^{Met}_{init.}$ with its original anticodon CAU or a mutated anticodon CA*A* or *GAA* (Doi and de Henau, unpubl. res.). (b) Shows results for yeast $tRNA^{Phe}$ with its original anticodon G_mAA (except for a G_{37} instead of a Y_{37}) or a mutated anticodon G*U*A or G*UC* (Droogmans, unpubl. res.). (c) Shows results for yeast $tRNA^{Asp}$ with its normal anticodon GUC or a mutated G*AA* (Haumont, unpubl. res.). The results for $G_{OH/p}UC$ were obtained by microinjecting yeast $tRNA^{Asp}$ in which the anticodon was split between nucleosides 34 and 35 (see Carbon *et al.*, 1982). The results are expressed as Ln of [^{32}P] cpm recovered in tRNA after the indicated period of time inside the oocyte. Clearly, each of the natural tRNAs from *E. coli* or yeast are stable in oocytes while certain mutants derived from these tRNAs with one or two base changes in the anticodon are particularly unstable. Up to now we have no clear rationale for these experimental observations. Reproduced with permission of the authors.

going different physiological states is largely dependent on the degree of certain specific natural nucleoside modifications, the undermodified tRNA being less stable than the fully matured one. An interesting speculation concerning the possible relationships between undermodified "aberrant" tRNAs induced by a variety of factors, increases in tRNA turn-over and levels of tRNA modifying enzymes can be found in Randerath *et al.* (1983, Fig. 12).

Fully grown *Xenopus laevis* oocytes may not be the best suited system to study the *regulation* of tRNA turn-over, because of the "storage function" of the oocyte. But it may be that a systematic study of the stability of various tRNAs (wild-type and mutants) could at least help to elucidate which features of the molecule makes them stable or unstable. The results of such studies might give a clue to our understanding of why certain nucleic acids with specific characteristics have been highly conserved during evolution. Also, they can help guide experiments with the aim of modifying the genetic potentialities of a given cell using a genetic engineering approach.

B. Microinjected tRNA is aminoacylated

Microinjection of tRNA into fully grown oocytes permits the study of aminoacylation catalysed by the oocyte aminoacyl-tRNA ligases under *in vivo* conditions. In their pioneer work, Gatica *et al.* (1975) microinjected *bulk* non-acylated yeast [^{3}H]tRNA (100 ng, i.e. 2.4 pmol/oocyte, which is about 2.5 times the amount of endogenous tRNA). After 5 h of incubation, about 80% of the injected yeast [^{3}H]tRNA was aminoacylated, thus demonstrating that the great majority of the yeast tRNA can be aminoacylated by the living oocyte. This result was obtained in an indirect way, by measuring *in vitro* the capacity of the recovered [^{3}H]tRNA to form a ternary complex with GTP and purified elongation factor 1 (isolated from wheat germ embryos). The separation of the aminoacylated from the non-acylated tRNA was done by Sephadex G-200 column chromatography. A more direct quantification of *in vivo* aminoacylation was possible by injection of *purified* yeast tRNA^{Phe}, incubating the oocytes for 3 h with [^{14}C]phenylalanine (high specific activity: 300–450 μCi/mM) in the medium, followed by phenol extraction and cold TCA precipitation (Gatica *et al.*, 1979, 1980; see also protocol C in Table I). Due to the low amount of endogenous tRNA^{Phe} and to low levels of protein synthesis, uninjected oocytes (or cells injected with tRNA lacking accepting capacity for phenylalanine) synthesized only negligible amounts of ^{14}C-labelled cold TCA products. This is in contrast to oocytes injected with large amounts of purified tRNA^{Phe}. After 3 h of incubation they show a considerable amount of incorporation into the tRNA fraction. The incorporation was proportional to the amount of injected yeast

$tRNA^{Phe}$ up to 4 pmol/oocyte (which corresponds to about 50 times the normal concentration of the endogenous $tRNA^{Phe}$, assuming that 1/20 of the tRNA is specific for phenylalanine).

Gatica *et al.* (1979, 1980) have carried out a comparative study between the *in vivo* and *in vitro* assay systems. A very interesting observation was that, despite the high efficiency of $tRNA^{Phe}$ aminoacylation, the specific activity of the oocyte phenylalanine-tRNA ligase, as assayed under *in vivo* conditions, was less than 10% of the same enzyme activity when tested *in vitro*. The cellular conditions were not inhibiting the activity of the endogenous enzyme as assayed by microinjection of additional exogenous phenylalanyl-tRNA ligase purified from *X. laevis* ovaries. Clearly a large fraction of the phenylalanyl-tRNA ligase present in oocytes is in a physical state which is normally not available to the injected tRNA. Together with other proteins it could be sequestered in large macromolecular structures or in specific subcellular compartments (Allende *et al.*, 1981; Deutscher, 1984). Therefore, it is possible that in fully grown oocytes most enzymes needed for protein synthesis or tRNA processing exist in a storage form until required by the demands of protein synthesis at a later stage of oocyte development or early embryogenesis. Nevertheless, it is clear from the above experiments that "active" (free?) phenylalanyl-tRNA ligase is able to aminoacylate about 4 pmol (10^{10} molecules) or foreign microinjected $tRNA^{Phe}$ per oocyte per hour. This is at least 10 times more than the ligase activity needed to provide the necessary amount of aminoacyl-tRNA for the nascent endogenous peptide chains (about 0.3–0.4 pmol of [^{14}C]phenylalanine/h, Allende *et al.*, 1981).

From our experience in microinjecting several pure tRNA species from different origins (mainly eukaryotes), we can say that the methodology initially developed by Allende's group for assaying microinjected yeast $tRNA^{Phe}$ was always successful, provided that high specific activity amino acids were used. This does not hold for the incorporation of aspartic acid and glutamic acid into tRNA (or proteins), mainly because both amino acids are very poorly taken up by the oocyte from the external medium, and also because their internal pools are exceptionally large (Bravo and Allende, 1976). Another limitation is that certain injected heterologous tRNAs are not efficiently charged by the aminoacyl-tRNA ligases of the oocytes; this is often observed with tRNAs from procaryotes (see Fig. 3) or from mitochondria. An easy way of overcoming this situation consists of coinjecting cognate aminoacyl-tRNA ligases known to charge the relevant tRNAs *in vitro*. Using this stratagem we succeeded in aminoacylating yeast mitochondrial $tRNA^{Trp}$ by coinjecting partially purified *E. coli* tryptophanyl-tRNA ligase (Grosjean *et al.*, 1981; Martin *et al.*, 1981).

The capacity of the oocyte to aminoacylate microinjected tRNA can be

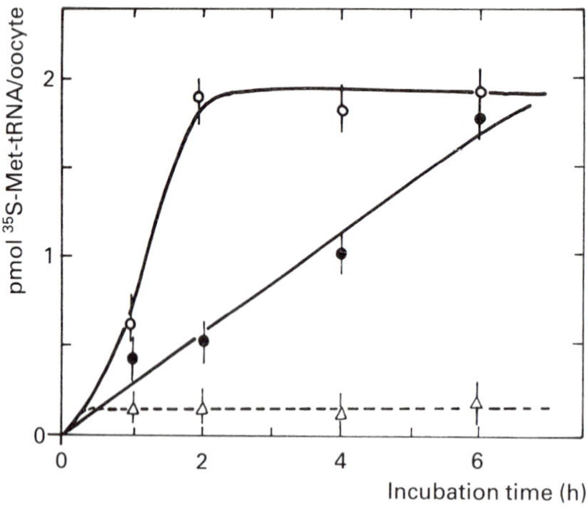

Fig. 3. In vivo aminoacylation of $tRNA^{Met}_{init.}$ microinjected into *X. laevis* oocytes. Aminoacylations were determined according to protocol B in Table I, i.e. after extraction of total RNA from the oocyte by phenol (at pH 4.5), acid precipitation and counting the radioactivity in the precipitated [^{35}S]Met-tRNA. The amount of tRNA microinjected per oocyte was about 3 pmoles, the specific radioactivity of [^{35}S]Met, about 26 Ci/mmol. Symbols are: (○) for microinjected rabbit liver $tRNA_{Met}$, (●) for microinjected *E. coli* $tRNA^{Met}_{init.}$ and (△) for non-injected oocytes. Clearly, *E. coli* $tRNA^{Met}_{init.}$ is more slowly aminoacylated than the rabbit liver $tRNA^{Met}_{init.}$ by the oocyte acylating enzyme. Notice that the level of aminoacylation of microinjected $tRNA^{Met}$ is much higher than the level of the endogenous $tRNA^{Met}$ determined under identical experimental conditions, but without microinjection of heterologous tRNA. Unpublished results of Doi, de Henau and Grosjean, reproduced with permission.

taken as a means of measuring the functional integrity of different individual tRNAs. Ginzburg *et al.* (1979) demonstrated that the aminoacylation of tRNA from ethionine (an ethyl analogue of methionine) treated rats was impaired when assayed in oocytes. By contrast, using oocyte extracts (an *in vitro* system) as the source of aminoacyl-tRNA ligases, they could not observe significant differences between the tRNA preparations from normal and ethionine-treated animals. Thus, the *in vivo* system is far more sensitive to minor modifications of the tRNA and could be used to study more systematically, for example, the role of modified nucleosides in tRNA.

The microinjection of a large amount (about 10^8–10^9 copies) of an appropriate tRNA gene together with [^{32}P]α-nucleotide triphosphates of very high specific activity (3000 Ci/mM) into the oocyte nucleus followed by an overnight incubation eventually leads to the appearance of very small amounts (fmol levels) of the corresponding gene products: the precursor or/and the fully mature tRNA. These are generally detected *in vivo* only because of their high radioactivity and also because they are almost the only gene transcript in the fully grown oocyte. Exploiting the radiochemical purity of the exogenous gene transcripts, Corbo *et al.* (1982) evaluated the consequence of several single point mutations in *C. elegans* $tDNA^{Pro}$ for its ability to become aminoacylated in the cytoplasm of the *Xenopus* oocyte. The assay was based on the specific binding of aminoacyl-tRNA (but not uncharged tRNA) to purified *E. coli* elongation factors, i.e. a procedure similar to that previously used by Gatica *et al.* (1975). Corbo *et al.* showed, for example, that a mutant carrying an insertion of a single base in the anticodon loop (having 8 instead of 7 nucleotides) was not aminoacylated *in vivo*. This demonstrates the importance of the anticodon loop structure for the interaction of the heterologous $tRNA^{Pro}$ with the prolyl-tRNA ligase of *Xenopus* oocytes. In a similar way, but using recombinant RNA technology, we have constructed many variants of several yeast tRNAs (Carbon *et al.*, 1982; Fournier *et al.*, 1983; Vacher *et al.*, 1984). Usually the amounts of such chimeric tRNAs obtained are very low. However, this drawback is partially overcome by the possibility of labelling the nucleic acid with ^{32}P of very high specific activity (3000 Ci/mM) during the *in vitro* construction procedure. The aminoacylation of very small amounts of such ^{32}P-labelled tRNAs inside the cytoplasm of the oocyte can be assayed as described by Gatica *et al.* (1975) or Corbo *et al.* (1982), but we preferred the following less tedious procedure (Beauchemin, Cedergren, and Grosjean, submitted). After phenol extraction and ethanol precipitation of the injected ^{32}P-labelled tRNA, the nucleic acid is treated with phenoxyacetyl-carbodiimide (Gillam and Tener, 1971). The resulting phenoxy-acetylated aminoacyl-tRNA is then quantified by a two-step elution using BD-cellulose chromatography column in an Eppendorf-tip. For the three aromatic amino acids the quantification procedure is even simpler, since the phenoxyacetylation step is not needed. While this method leads to a very rapid estimation of the aminoacylation level of the chimeric tRNA in the oocyte, it does not give any information on the kind of amino acid attached to the tRNA. Thus, a potential misacylation of the chimeric tRNA cannot be determined by this procedure.

It is interesting to note that a fragment of Turnip yellow mosaic virus-RNA (TYMV-RNA), the so-called 3′ terminal "tRNA-like" structure that appears in the cytoplasm of the oocyte after microinjection of the whole genome of TYMV, is aminoacylated with valine, probably by the oocyte valyl-tRNA ligase. However, the extent of this "misacylation" reaction is extremely low (Joshi *et al.*, 1978).

Misacylations of certain tRNAs under *in vitro* conditions have been characterized some time ago. They occur especially between tRNAs and certain aminoacyl-tRNA ligases originating from different sources (yeast, *E. coli*, *Bacillus stearothermophilus*; Giégé *et al.*, 1974; Grosjean *et al.*, 1976). It would therefore be of interest to test whether similar misacylations of microinjected heterologous tRNAs also occur at significant rates *in vivo*, and if so, how the oocyte eliminates the faulty aminoacyl-tRNA.

Last but not least, it is possible to inhibit almost completely one particular aminoacylation reaction *in vivo* by incubating and/or microinjecting the oocytes with an appropriate amino acid analogue or other specific inhibitors of a given aminoacyl-tRNA ligase. The endogenous aminoacylation of the $tRNA^{His}$ can be inhibited for at least 4 h by injecting histidinol (Meier *et al.*, 1985). Similarly, the oocyte tyrosyl-tRNA ligase was almost completely inhibited by the injection of tyrosinyl-adenylate (Grosjean, unpub. res.). The latter approach could in principle be used for any amino acid.

C. Microinjected tRNAs are involved in protein synthesis

Aminoacylated tRNA microinjected into oocytes is used very efficiently for endogenous protein synthesis. Aminoacyl transfer from [^{14}C]Phe-tRNA into proteins is inhibited by puromycin and cycloheximide, but not by coinjected large amounts of [^{12}C]phenylalanine (Gatica and Allende, 1977). This demonstrates that part of the amino acid is directly transferred from the tRNA to nascent proteins. This fact, and the observation that foreign mRNAs are readily accepted by the translation apparatus of the oocytes (see Chapter 17), allow the formulation of two questions. What is the response of a specific tRNA to, first, amino acid codons, and second, to termination codons (suppression efficiency)?

(1) Decoding

In the following paragraph one experiment will be discussed in some detail which addresses the first type of question. One of the characteristics of tRNA is its high degree of modification (Dirheimer, 1983; Björk, 1984). The modified bases in the anticodon loop have received special attention, since their location suggests an involvement in the decoding process. One of the most conspicuous modifications is the Q-base localized in the wobble position of four tRNAs: $tRNA^{Asp}$, $tRNA^{Asn}$, $tRNA^{His}$, and $tRNA^{Tyr}$ [Q = queuosine = 7-(4,5-*cis*, dihydroxy-1-cyclo-pentene-3-amino-methyl)-7-deaza-guanosine]. These tRNAs read the codons NA*U* and NA*C* (N = A, U, C or G) and the extent of their modifications varies considerably depending upon the physiological and developmental stage in many organisms (Nishimura, 1983). This fact, and the biased usage of the NA^{C}_{U} codons in highly expressed mRNAs (Grosjean and Fiers, 1982) suggest a role for the Q-base on the decoding properties of the four Q-containing tRNAs. Thus, the codon response of four $tRNA^{His}$ isoacceptors, two from *Drosophila melanogaster* and two from brewer's yeast, were studied in the *Xenopus* oocyte (Meier *et al.*, 1985). The *Drosophila* isoacceptors are identical except for having either a guanosine (G) or the hypermodified nucleoside Q in the wobble positions. The brewer's yeast isoacceptors differ

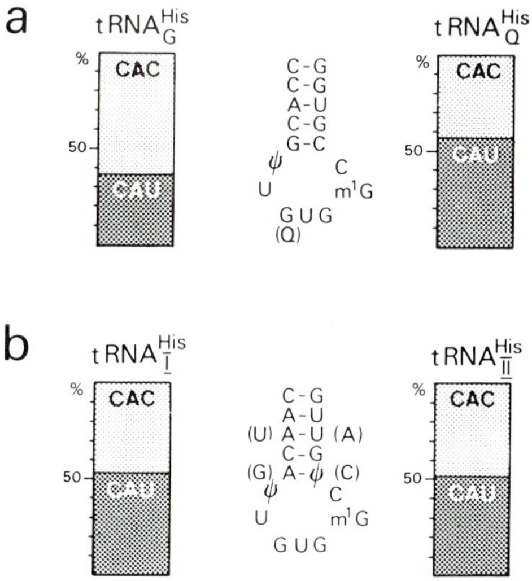

Fig. 4. Codon preferences under *in vivo* competing conditions of (a) *Drosophila* and (b) brewer's yeast tRNA^{His} isoacceptors injected into *Xenopus* oocytes. The percentage of histidine incorporation per codon for each isoacceptor shows clearly that *Drosophila* His-tRNA^{His}-G$_{34}$ prefers the CA*C* codon, whereas the His-tRNA^{His}-Q$_{34}$ shows a slight preference for the CA*U* codon and the two yeast tRNAs do not prefer either of the two codons. Anticodon loops and stems are shown for the two *Drosophila* and the two yeast tRNA^{His} isoacceptors. The two *Drosophila* tRNAs differ only by the presence/absence of the hypermodified base Q in the wobble base, the two yeast isoacceptors by five bases outside the anticodon loop (one is located in the amino acid acceptor stem, not shown). Sequence of the brewer's yeast tRNA$^{His}_{II}$ in brackets. Reproduced with permission from Meier *et al.* (1985).

by five bases outside the anticodon loop. Equal amounts of pre-charged tRNA^{His} (one of them labelled with [^{3}H]histidine) of each species were injected, along with histidinol (an efficient inhibitor of the oocyte histidinyl-tRNA ligase), and Turnip yellow mosaic virus-coat protein mRNA into *X. laevis* oocytes. The TYMV-coat protein contains two CA*U* and one CA*C* coded histidines. Cyanogen bromide cleavage of the coat protein yields peptides containing the CA*U* and CA*C* coded histidines in separate portions. Thus, the incorporation of histidine derived from each isoacceptor in response to each histidine codon can be studied after isolation and cleavage of the synthesized protein and determination of the cpm's accumulated in the corresponding peptides.

Figures 4a and b clearly show that, under competing *in vivo* conditions, the *Drosophila* tRNA^{His} with the anticodon *G*UG prefers the histidine codon CA*C* to the codon CA*U*, whereas little preference is observed for the tRNA^{His} with the anticodon *Q*UG for the codon CA*U*, and no preference for either codon by the two yeast isoacceptors. Hence, it can be concluded that the presence of the Q-base clearly affects the choice of the codon, and that one function of the Q-base modification is at the translational level. This

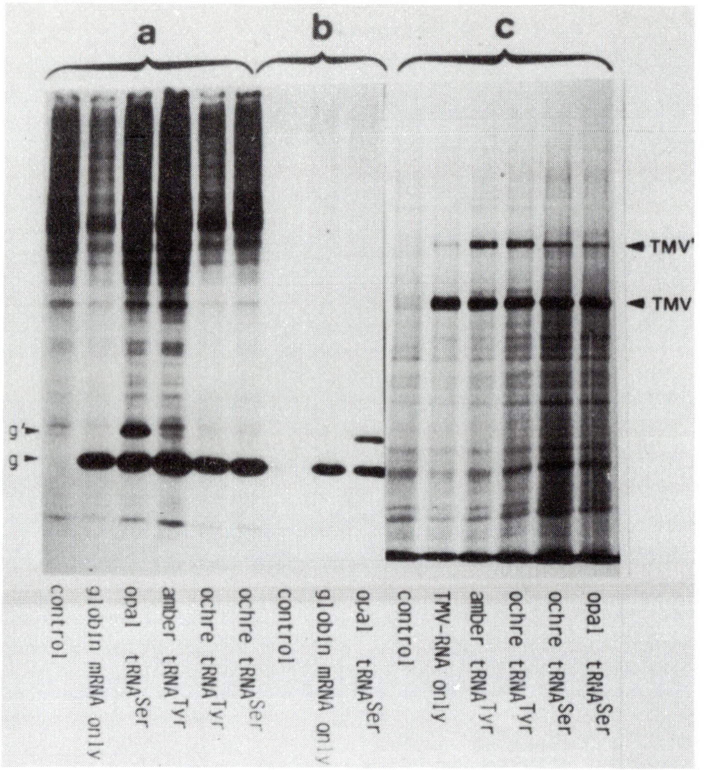

Fig. 5. Autoradiographs of labelled translational products of *X. laevis* oocytes under the direction of various microinjected macromolecules: (a) after rabbit globin mRNA; (b) after rabbit globin mRNA and subsequent immunoprecipitation with corresponding goat antiglobin; or (c) TMV-RNA injection and concomitant cytoplasmic yeast suppressor tRNA injection (about 5 ng/oocyte). (d) Shows the results with *X. laevis* oocytes coinjected with rabbit globin mRNA, *E. coli* tryptophanyl-tRNA synthetase and various amounts of yeast *mitochondrial* $tRNA^{Trp}$, 0.11, 0.55, 2.2, 11, 110 and 220 ng/oocyte (lanes 1 to 6, respectively). The gel patterns shown in (a), (b), (c) and (d) originate from different sets of experiments and were run on gels of different concentrations. Arrows in (a) and (d) point to the 16 × kDa globin (g) and to the 18.5 kDa globin read-through product (g′); to the 126 kDa TMV and to the 183 kDa TMV′ = read-through product protein in (c). Opal $tRNA^{Ser}$ and mitochondrial $tRNA^{Trp}$ induce read-through of the globin UGA stop codon, amber and ochre $tRNA^{Tyr}$ enhance read-through of the leaky UAG TMV-RNA stop codon. Hence, all three types of nonsense suppressors can be screened for in the *Xenopus* oocyte using either rabbit globin mRNA or TMV-RNA as a messenger. Reproduced with permission from Bienz *et al.* (1980) and Martin *et al.* (1981).

experiment demonstrates that decoding properties of tRNA isoacceptors can be studied using the *Xenopus* oocytes as a translation system. Thus, studies concerned with tRNA structure–function relationships during translation, effects of biased mRNA codon usage, and mRNA codon context can be approached under *in vivo* conditions. In this connection, it should be remembered that the oocyte segregates mRNAs to free and membrane-

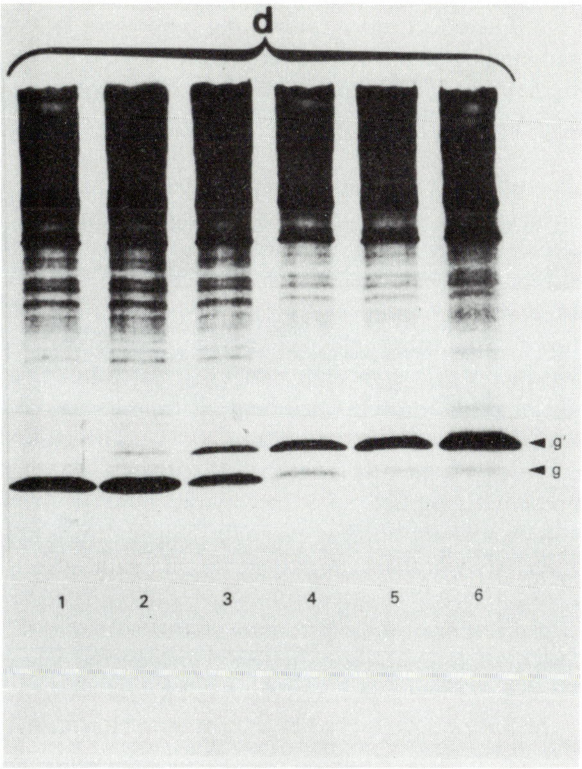

bound polysomes, dependent on the type of protein synthesized (Richter and Smith, 1981). The oocyte seems to contain a differential translation capacity localized in two compartments. No competition is observed between mRNAs translated in the two compartments.

(2) Suppression and related problems.
Nonsense mutations and their suppressors have played a key role in the study of gene expression in bacteria and yeast (Celis and Smith, 1979; Steege and Söll, 1979). Considering the complexity of higher eukaryotes, great efforts have been made to identify these important mutations in several higher organisms. As pointed out by Kaltoft *et al.* (1976), a crucial part in the search for nonsense suppressors is the assay system employed for screening. Bienz *et al.* (1980) have successfully introduced the *Xenopus* oocyte as a sensitive screening system for UAG (amber), UAA (Ochre), and UGA (opal) suppressors. The principle rests on the observation that stop codons of eukaryotic messengers injected into the oocytes can be suppressed by their cognate suppressor tRNAs isolated from yeast. The suppression effects are detected as a read-through protein on SDS-polyacrylamide gels (Fig. 5).

The system is very sensitive. The effect of 1 ng yeast opal suppressor tRNA per oocyte can be detected, and even unfractionated tRNA isolated from a *Schizosaccharomyces pombe* opal suppressor stock induces a clear read-through of the β-globin UGA stop codon (Bienz *et al.*, 1980). An additional advantage of this *in vivo* screening system is its insensitivity to Mg^{2+} concentration and to polyamine addition, factors which affect the extent of read-through of termination codons in the *in vitro* systems (Pelham, 1978; Morch and Benicourt, 1980). Bienz (1981) has used this system for the screening of 21 genetically characterized *D. melanogaster* suppressor stocks for putative amber, ochre, and opal nonsense suppressors. In the process of screening RPC-5 fractions for read-through of amber and ochre codons using tobacco mosaic virus (TMV) RNA as a messenger, it was found that one fraction of every RPC-5 profile tested (including the wild-type) contained strong read-through activity (Bienz and Kubli, 1981). The tRNA inducing this read-through was subsequently identified as a $tRNA^{Tyr}$ with the anticodon GψA (Suter and Kubli, unpubl. res.). Interestingly the $tRNA^{Tyr}$ with the anticodon QψA does not support read-through. This finding is not an artifact of the *Drosophila* tRNA or the *Xenopus* oocyte. The same effects were obtained using the two $tRNA^{Tyr}$ isoacceptors isolated from tobacco plants with TMV-RNA as a messenger in a wheat germ system (Beier *et al.*, 1984). These results show that the amount of read-through of the leaky UAG TMV-RNA stop codon (Goelet *et al.*, 1982) is determined by the presence or absence of the Q-base in the wobble position. Hence, the synthesis of the 183 kDa read-through protein is regulated by the extent of modification of the $tRNA^{Tyr}$. This supports the conclusion drawn from the experiments described in the preceding paragraph, that the modified nucleoside queuosine influence the decoding properties of tRNAs.

The *Xenopus* oocyte translation system does also accept tRNAs isolated from organelles, provided an appropriate cognate acylating enzyme is coinjected (Martin *et al.*, 1981). Yeast mitochondrial $tRNA^{Trp}$, if coinjected with *E. coli* tryptophanyl-tRNA ligase, suppresses the β-globin UGA stop codon five times more efficiently than a *S. pombe* opal suppressor $tRNA^{Ser}$ (sup-3e). This shows convincingly that yeast mt-$tRNA^{Trp}$, once it has been properly aminoacylated, is functional in *all* steps of protein synthesis in the *cytoplasm* of a living cell, i.e. codon recognition on the ribosome, interaction with elongation factors, transpeptidation, and competition with the UGA termination factor(s). The fact that the oocyte cannot aminoacylate the mt-$tRNA^{Trp}$ could be the only barrier to the use of this UGA-suppressing tRNA in the cytoplasmic compartment of a cell. Thus, the *Xenopus* oocyte microinjection method provides not only a simple and sensitive system to assay for the coding properties of eukaryotic tRNAs *in vivo*, but also for tRNAs of organellar and possibly prokaryotic origin. Such an approach could be used to determine other coding changes in the mitochondrial and other codes, and to evaluate the influence of the reduced number of tRNA isoacceptors operating in mitochondria.

Transfer RNA suppressor efficiency is dependent upon the sequence and modification of a tRNA. RNA engineering techniques allow the replacement of nucleotides in the anticodon loop at specific sites in a systematic way and the constructed molecules can be tested subsequently for suppression efficiency (Bruce and Gesteland, 1982; Bruce *et al.*, 1982; Uhlenbeck *et al.*, 1984). A yeast $tRNA^{Cys}$ suppressor was constructed by replacing the first base of GCA anticodon by an uracil (Vacher *et al.*, 1984) and the biological activity of this molecule tested by injection into oocytes. Interestingly the level of aminoacylation was similar to that of the parent molecule. However, suppression of the UGA β-globin stop codon was much less efficient than with other suppressors. This might be due to the fact that the uracil at the wobble position in yeast $tRNA^{Cys}$ is not modified in the oocyte. Although other interpretations can be imagined, this experiment demonstrates unambiguously that the UCA anticodon is not the only determinant for suppression activity. Thus, again, this approach offers the opportunity to study the functional relationships between anticodon and other parts of the tRNA molecule.

A very elegant approach using the *Xenopus* oocyte as a transcription–translation system has been employed to demonstrate the suppressor activity of a tRNA transcribed from a human $tRNA^{Lys}$ gene converted by *in vitro* mutagenesis into an amber suppressor (Temple *et al.*, 1982). The mutated gene was injected into the germinal vesicles of oocytes, and 20 h later poly (A^+) reticulocyte RNA from a β^0-thalassaemia patient (the β^0-thalassaemia mRNA used has a $\beta^{17\ \mathrm{Lys\ (AAG)} \rightarrow \mathrm{UAG}}$ mutation). The translation products analysed after 48 h of incubation with [^{3}H]histidine, and subsequent purification with monoclonal antibodies against human globin, show unambiguously that the UAG codon has been suppressed, i.e. that the mutated $tRNA^{Lys}$ gene codes for an active amber suppressor.

It has been proposed that stop codons, besides serving as terminators in protein synthesis, might have additional separate functions and meanings. Although it can be concluded from determined sequences of mRNAs and genes that all stop codons are used in a eukaryotic cell, it is of interest to study the stop codons used in the population of a *single* cell. Bienz *et al.* (1981) have addressed this question by injecting *Xenopus* oocytes with purified amber, ochre and opal suppressor tRNAs from yeast. The radioactive labelled proteins were then separated on two-dimensional gels, and the changes induced by the injected suppressor tRNAs in comparison to the control determined. All three termination codons are used. But a surprisingly low number of read-through polypeptides were observed from the 600 mRNAs studied in comparison to uninjected oocytes. This result suggested that the stop codons of the oocyte mRNAs are very well *protected* against read-through. These studies led to a statistical analysis of stop codon contexts in mRNAs and genes of various origin (Kohli and Grosjean, 1981). It could be demonstrated that specific contexts exist for viral, phage, prokaryotic, and eukaryotic stop codons, supporting the idea that the neighbouring nucleotides determine the leakyness or tightness of the termination codon.

Two other eukaryotic systems have been used to assay and screen *in vivo* for tRNA suppressors and nonsense mutants: the nematode *C. elegans* (Kimble *et al.*, 1982; Wills *et al.*, 1983), and mammalian cells in culture (Capecchi *et al.*, 1977; Hudziak *et al.*, 1982; Laski *et al.*, 1982, 1984). In comparison with the oocyte it seems that these systems should be especially suited for the search of nonsense mutants and their suppressors created by mutagenesis. Whereas this approach has been successful for *Caenorhabditis* (Wills *et al.*, 1983) it has not worked so far for the selection of mammalian cell lines with suppressor activity by conventional methods of reversion of the phenotype of nonsense mutants. However, as an alternative, transformation of cells with tRNA genes with suppressor activity created by site-specific mutagenesis is feasible (Laski *et al.*, 1982, 1984). When introduced into the cells, the suppressor activity is expressed and not toxic, and the genes are integrated into the chromosomes (Hudziak *et al.*, 1982; Laski *et al.*, 1982, 1984). Thus, at least in principle, it should be possible to induce nonsense suppressors by mutagenesis, and it is not clear why this approach has not worked so far.

(3) Factors affecting protein synthesis

The *Xenopus* oocyte is less sensitive to many factors affecting protein synthesis than *in vitro* systems. However, using the oocyte for the purpose of protein synthesis, a few characteristic features of this cell should be taken into account.

Isolated oocytes are able to take up radioactive amino acids from the exogenous medium (Bravo *et al.*, 1976). The uptake mechanisms are specific for groups of amino acids sharing similar chemical characteristics. Aspartic acid and glutamic acid are very poorly incorporated into the oocyte proteins. This effect is due to two factors: first the uptake is very low, and second, the internal pool is very high for these two amino acids (Eppig and Dumont, 1972; Bravo and Allende, 1976). Thus, the labelled amino acid has to be chosen carefully and adapted to the experiment to be performed. There are also indications of a non-homogenous intracellular distribution of amino acids in amphibians. In *Rana pipiens*, after two hours of labelling with a mixture of radioactive amino acids, the vegetal pole of the oocyte contains almost no radioactivity, whereas high concentrations of amino acids were found in the germinal vesicle, the perinuclear cytoplasm, the cortex, and in the animal pole cytoplasm (Merriam, 1969).

Finally, an important point is the fact that the oocyte is able to perform a wide variety of secondary modifications on the synthesized proteins, e.g. phosphorylation, hydroxylation, glycosylation, signal sequence removal, cleavage of polypeptides, and assembly of multimeric proteins (Lane, 1981). In general, the oocyte processes foreign proteins faithfully. This is probably due to the fact that the processing is substrate-determined. Furthermore, the oocyte possesses functional secretory pathways. Proteins can be secreted into the medium at intrinsic different rates or sequestered in oocyte compartments. Although all these factors impose restrictions upon the experimenter they can also be of great advantage for the study of these very processes in a giant living cell.

III. CONCLUSIONS AND PERSPECTIVES

The review presented here summarizes the research based on microinjection of tRNA into the *Xenopus* oocyte with emphasis on protein synthesis. This choice reflects the interests and experience of the authors. However, it should be realized that many other aspects of the molecular biology of tRNA have not been covered, e.g. the very important analysis of tRNA biosynthesis. A short summary of this field seems justified, since here again the application of the oocyte system has been especially fruitful and its potential is clearly evident.

Formally, the biosynthesis of tRNA can be subdivided into four parts: transcription, removal and addition of nucleotides (5′ and 3′ nucleotides, introns), transport, and modification. In reality all these processes are highly interwoven and interdependent.

The transcription of tRNA genes is a complex process involving polymerase III and other protein factors (Ciliberto *et al.*, 1983; Sharp *et al.*, 1985). As also observed with other primary transcription products, the tRNA transcribed initially, has additional nucleotides at both the 5′ and 3′ ends and (for some tRNA genes) an intron localized adjacent to the 3′ end of the anticodon sequence. The removal of those nucleotides is a process ordered in time and space (Melton *et al.*, 1980; Nishikura *et al.*, 1982). Due to the large size of the oocyte and its germinal vesicle it has been possible to localize the splicing activity in the nucleoplasm (De Robertis *et al.*, 1981). Transfer RNA maturation does not only involve the removal of 5′, and 3′, and eventually internal nucleotides, but also the subsequent addition of nucleotides at the 3′ and in some instances at the 5′ end. In eukaryotes the 3′

CCA-end present in all tRNAs is not encoded but added post-transcriptionally by the enzyme nucleotidyl transferase, an enzyme also present in the *Xenopus* oocyte (Solari *et al.*, 1977). Similarly all $tRNA^{His}$ sequenced so far have an additional nucleotide at the 5′ end not encoded in their genes. The 5′ guanylate residue of *D. melanogaster* and *S. pombe* are added post-transcriptionally (Cooley *et al.*, 1982). The intimate connection of the processing steps with other maturation events has been impressively demonstrated by the fact that a yeast $tRNA^{Tyr}$ intron is essential for the correct modification of its tRNA product (Johnson and Abelson, 1983). All these steps require many enzymes which are only poorly characterized so far and new activities are still being discovered (Deutscher *et al.*, 1984). The *Xenopus* oocyte seems to be a system especially suited to study these kinds of problems.

The *Xenopus* oocyte has also served to study the processes involved in the transport of tRNA from the nucleus into the cytoplasm (Zasloff, 1983). It could be shown that the transport resembles a carrier-mediated translocation process and it has been proposed that ribosome-like particles surrounding the nuclear pores may function as a tRNA translocation device. Here again the suitable size of this cell makes it particularly feasible for an approach to these intriguing problems.

In this paragraph we tried to stress and exemplify that modification is an important and puzzling aspect of tRNA maturation. Not only do more than 60 enzymes participate in this process, but curiously enough it does involve the *active replacement* of G_{34} in the wobble position by queuosine (Nishimura, 1983), and the insertion of hypoxanthin at the place of guanine at the same site (Elliot and Trewyn, 1984). The combination of site-directed replacement of nucleotides in the tRNA anticodon together with post-labelling techniques has already allowed us to gain insight into the processes responsible for the modification of the wobble base in *Xenopus* oocytes (Carbon *et al.*, 1983; Fournier *et al.*, 1983; Haumont *et al.*, 1984). This approach could certainly lead to the elucidation of the rules and constraints which govern the modification of this important part of the tRNA molecule.

The attractiveness of the *Xenopus laevis* oocyte as a living test tube has been demonstrated convincingly also by its many applications outside the field covered in this article (see Chapters 15 and 17). Despite some drawbacks (e.g. lack of genetic data, biological constraints) we believe that the advantages of the oocyte will become increasingly recognized as a means of studying in a living cell complex processes such as gene expression and regulation, transport, compartmentation and other important biological phenomena.

ACKNOWLEDGEMENTS

The work described in this chapter has been supported by grants from the Belgian Government (Actions Concertées) and by the "Fonds National de la Recherche Scientifique" to HG, and by the Swiss National Science Foundation, the Julius Klaus-Stiftung, and the Hescheler-Stiftung to EK. We gratefully acknowledge the help of many collaborators and friends which contributed to this work. We thank our collaborators, Professors H. Chantrenne, J. Brachet, R. Cedergren, and Dr E. Stumm for critically reading the manuscript. We thank A. Holström and S. Schlegel for typing the manuscript.

REFERENCES

Abelson, H. T., Johnson, L. F., Penman, S. and Green, H. (1974). *Cell* **1**, 161–165.

Agris, P. F., Playl, T., Goldman, L., Horton, E., Woolverton, D., Setzer, D. and Rodi, C. (1983). *In* "Recent Results in Cancer Research" (G. Nass, ed.) Vol. 84, pp. 237–254. Springer-Verlag, Berlin.

Allende, C. C., Allende, J. E. and Firtel, R. E. (1974). *Cell* **2**, 189–196.

Allende, C. C., Errazuriz, R., Gatica, M., Bravo, R. and Allende, C. (1981). *In* "Molecular Approaches to Gene Expression and Protein Structure", pp. 173–195. Academic Press, London and New York.

Barrett, P., Kloetzel, P. M. and Sommerville, J. (1983). *Biochim. Biophys. Acta* **740**, 347–354.

Beier, H., Barciszewska, M. and Sickinger, H. D. (1984). *EMBO J.* **3**, 1091–1096.

Bienz, M. (1981). Ph.D. Thesis, Universität Zürich, Zürich, Switzerland.

Bienz, M. and Kubli, E. (1981). *Nature* **294**, 188–190.

Bienz, M., Kubli, E., Kohli, J., de Henau, S. and Grosjean, H. (1980). *Nucl. Acids Res.* **8**, 5169–5178.

Bienz, M., Kubli, E., Kohli, J., Huez, G., Marbaix, G. and Grosjean, H. (1981). *Nucl. Acids Res.* **9**, 3835–3850.

Björk, G. R. (1984). *In* "Processing of RNA" (D. Apirion, ed.) pp. 291–330. CRC Press, Boca Raton.

Borek, E., Baliga, B. S., Gehrke, Ch. W., Kuo, C. W., Belman, S., Troll, W. and Waalkes, T. P. (1977). *Cancer Res.* **37**, 3362–3366.

Borek, E., Sharma, O. K. and Waalkes, T. P. (1983). *In* "Recent Results in Cancer Research" (G. Nass, ed.) Vol. 84, pp. 301–316. Springer-Verlag, Berlin.

Bravo, R. and Allende, J. E. (1976). *Arch. Biochem. Biophys.* **172**, 648–653.

Bravo, R., Salazar, I. and Allende, J. E. (1976). *Exp. Cell Res.* **103**, 169–174.

Bruce, A. G. and Gesteland, R. F. (1982). "Interaction of Translational and Transcriptional Controls in the Regulation of Gene Expression" (M. Grunberg-Manago and B. Safer, eds) pp. 203–213. Elsevier, Amsterdam.

Bruce, A. G., Atkins, J. F., Ulhenbeck, O. and Gesteland, R. F. (1982). *Proc. Natl. Acad. Sci. USA* **79**, 7127–7131.

Capecchi, M. R., Von der Haar, R. A., Capecchi, N. E. and Sveda, M. M. (1977). *Cell* **12**, 371–381.

Carbon, P., Haumont, E., de Henau, S., Keith, G. and Grosjean, H. (1982). *Nucl. Acids Res.* **10**, 3715–3730.

Carbon, P., Haumont, E., Fournier, M., de Henau, S. and Grosjean, H. (1983). *EMBO J.* **2**, 1093–1097.

Celis, J. E. and Smith, J. D. (1979). "Nonsense Mutations and tRNA Suppressors." Academic Press, London, New York and San Francisco.

Ciliberto, G., Castagnoli, L. and Cortese, R. (1983). *Curr. Topics Devel. Biol.* **18**, 59–88.

Clarkson, S. G., Birnstiel, M. L. and Serra, V. (1973). *J. Mol. Biol.* **79**, 391–410.

Clarkson, S. G. (1983). *In* "Eukaryotic Genes, Their Structure, Activity and Regulation" (N. Maclean, S. P. Gregory and R. A. Flavell, eds) pp. 239–261. Butterworth, London.

Cooley, L., Appel, B. and Söll, D. (1982). *Proc. Natl. Acad. Sci. USA* **79**, 6475–6479.

Corbo, L., Ciliberto, G., Traboni, C., Santamaria, R., Cimino, F., Cortese, R. and Salvatore, F. (1982). *Nucl. Acids Res.* **10**, 7363–7371.

Cortese, R. (1979). *In* "Biological Regulation and Development" (R. F. Goldberger, ed.) Vol. 1, pp. 401–432. Plenum Press, New York.

Denis, H. and Lemaire, M. (1983). *Subcell. Biochem.* **9**, 263–297.

Denis, H. and Lemaire, M. (1985). *Eur. J. Biochem.*, **149**, 549–556.

Denis, H. and Mairy, M. (1972). *Eur. J. Biochem.* **25**, 424–534.

Denis, H., Mazabraud, A. and Wegnez, M. (1975). *Eur. J. Biochem.* **58**, 43–50.

De Robertis, E. M., Black, P. and Nishikura, K. (1981). *Cell* **23**, 89–93.

Deutscher, M. P. (1984). *J. Cell Biol.* **99**, 373–377.

Deutscher, M., Marlor, C. W. and Zaniewski, R. (1984). *Proc. Natl. Acad. Sci. USA* **81**, 4290–4293.

Dirheimer, G. (1983). *In* "Recent Results in Cancer Research" (G. Nass, ed.) pp. 15–46. Springer-Verlag, Berlin.

Dixon, L. and Ford, P. J. (1982). *Devel. Biol.* **91**, 474–477.

Elliot, M. S. and Trewyn, R. W. (1984). *J. Biol. Chem.* **259**, 2407–2410.

Eppig, J. J. and Dumont, J. N. (1972). *Devel. Biol.* **28**, 531–536.

Ford, P. J. (1971). *Nature* **233**, 561–564.

Fournier, M., Haumont, E., de Henau, S., Gangloff, J. and Grosjean, H. (1983). *Nucl. Acids Res.* **11**, 707–718.

Gatica, M. and Allende, J. E. (1977). *Biochem. Biophys. Res. Commun.* **79**, 352–356.

Gatica, M., Tarrago, A., Allende, C. C. and Allende, J. E. (1975). *Nature* **256**, 675–677.

Gatica, M., Solari, A., Aranciabia, M. and Allende, J. E. (1979). *Arch. Biol. Med. Exp.* **12**, 427–432.

Gatica, M., Allende, C. C. and Allende, J. E. (1980). *Arch. Biochem. Biophys.* **202**, 653–656.

Ghosh, R. K. and Deutscher, M. P. (1978). *J. Biol. Chem.* **253**, 997–1000.

Giégé, R., Kern, D., Ebel, J. P., Grosjean, H., de Henau, S. and Chantrenne, H. (1974). *Eur. J. Biochem.* **45**, 351–362.

Gillam, I. C. and Tener, G. M. (1971). *Methods Enzymol.* **20**, 55–71.

Ginzburg, I., Cornelis, P., Giveon, D. and Littauer, U. Z. (1979). *Nucl. Acids Res.* **6**, 657–672.

Goelet, P., Lomonosoff, G. P., Butler, P. J. G., Akam, M. E., Gait, M. J. and Karn, J. (1982). *Proc. Natl. Acad. Sci. USA* **79**, 5818–5822.

Grosjean, H. and Fiers, W. (1982). *Gene* **18**, 199–209.

Grosjean, H., Charlier, J., de Henau, S., Takada, C., Parfait, R., Darte, C., Keith, G., Dirheimer, G., and Giégé, R. (1976). *Experientia*, Suppl. 26, 347–361.
Grosjean, H., de Henau, S., Sibler, A. P., Martin, R., Dirheimer, G., Keith, G. and Kohli, J. (1981). *Arch. Int. Physiol. Biochim.* **89**, B58–B59.
Gurevitz, M. and Apirion, D. (1983). *Biochem.* **22**, 4000–4005.
Haumont, E., Fournier, M., de Henau, S. and Grosjean, H. (1984). *Nucl. Acids Res.* **12**, 2705–2715.
Hudziak, R. M., Laski, F. A., RajBandary, U. L., Sharp, P. A. and Capecchi, M. (1982). *Cell* **31**, 137–146.
Johnson, P. F. and Abelson, J. (1983). *Nature* **302**, 681–687.
Joshi, S., Haenni, A. L., Hubert, E., Huez, G. and Marbaix, G. (1978). *Nature* **257**, 339–341.
Kaltoft, K., Zeuthen, J., Engbaek, F., Piper, P. W. and Celis, J. E. (1976). *Proc. Natl. Acad. Sci. USA* **73**, 2793–2797.
Kimble, J., Hodgkin, J., Smith, R. and Smith, J. (1982). *Nature* **299**, 456–458.
Kleiman, L., Peters, S., Woodward, J. J., Myers, J. (1980). *Exp. Cell Res.* **129**, 415–424.
Kleiman, L., Heron, R., Essagian, C., Nicoghosian, K. and Cedergren, R. J. (1983). *Nucl. Acids Res.* **11**, 2585–2598.
Kohli, J. and Grosjean, H. (1981). *Mol. Gen. Genet.* **182**, 430–439.
La Rossa, R. and Söll, D. (1978). *In* "Transfer RNA" (S. Altman, ed.) pp. 136–167. M.I.T. Press.
Lane, C. D. (1981). *Cell* **24**, 281–282.
Laski, F. A., Belagaje, R., RajBandary, U. L. and Sharp, P. A. (1982). *Proc. Natl. Acad. Sci. USA* **79**, 5813–5817.
Laski, F. A., Belagaje, R., Hudziak, R. M., Capecchi, M. R., Norton, G. P., Palese, P., RajBandary, U. L. and Sharp, P. A. (1984). *EMBO J.* **3**, 2445–2452.
Mairy, M. and Denis, H. (1971). *Devel. Biol.* **24**, 143–165.
Martin, R. P., Sibler, A. P., Dirheimer, G., de Henau, S. and Grosjean, H. (1981). *Nature* **293**, 235–237.
Meier, F., Suter, B., Grosjean, H., Keith, G. and Kubli, E. (1985). *EMBO J.* **4**, 823–827.
Melton, D. A., De Robertis, E. and Cortese, R. (1980). *Nature* **284**, 143–148.
Merriam, R. W. (1969). *Exp. Cell. Res.* **56**, 259–264.
Morch, M. D. and Benicourt, C. (1980). *Eur. J. Biochem.* **105**, 445–451.
Nishikura, K., Kurjan, J., Hall, B. D. and De Robertis, E. M. (1982). *EMBO J.* **1**, 263–268.
Nishimura, S. (1983). *Progr. Nucl. Acids Res.* **28**, 49–73.
Pelham, H. R. B. (1978). *Nature* **272**, 469–471.
Picard, B., Lemaire, M., Wegnez, M. and Denis, H. (1980). *Eur. J. Biochem.* **109**, 359–368.
Randerath, K., Tseng, W. C., Harris, J. S. and Lu, L. J. W. (1983). *In* "Recent Results in Cancer Research" (G. Nass, ed.) Vol. 84, pp. 283–297. Springer-Verlag, Berlin.
Richter, J. D. and Smith, D. L. (1981). *Cell* **27**, 183–191.
Schlegel, R. A., Iversen, P. and Rechsteiner, M. (1978). *Nucl. Acids Res.* **5**, 3715–3729.
Sharp, S., Cooley, L., Schaack, J., Burke, D. J. and Söll, D. (1985). *In* "Critical Reviews in Biochemistry", Vol. 19, 107–144.
Solari, A., Gatica, M. and Allende, J. E. (1977). *Nucl. Acids Res.* **6**, 1873–1880.

Sprinzl, M., Moll, J., Meissner, F. and Hartmann, T. (1985). *Nucl. Acids Res.* **13**, r1–r49; r51–r104.

Steege, D. A. and Söll, D. G. (1979). *In* "Biological Regulation and Development" (R. F. Goldberger, ed.) Vol. 1, pp. 433–485. Plenum Press, New York.

Temple, G. F., Dozy, A. M., Roy, K. L. and Kan, Y. W. (1982). *Nature* **296**, 537–540.

Traboni, C., Ciliberto, G. and Cortese, R. (1984). *Cell* **36**, 179–187.

Uhlenbeck, O. C., Bare, L., Bruce, A. G. (1984). *In* "Gene Expression, the Translational Step and its Control" (B. F. C. Clark and H. U. Petersen, eds) pp. 163–175. Munksgaard, Copenhagen.

Vacher, J., Grosjean, H., de Henau, S., Finelli, J. and Buckingham, R. H. (1984). *Eur. J. Biochem.* **138**, 77–81.

Wegnez, M. and Denis, H. (1979). *Eur. J. Biochem.* **98**, 67–75.

Wegnez, M., Mazabrand, A., Denis, H., Petrissant, G. and Boisnard, M. (1975). *Eur. J. Biochem.* **60**, 295–302.

Wills, N., Gesteland, R. F., Karn, J., Barnett, L., Bolten, S. and Waterston, R. H. (1983). *Cell* **33**, 575–583.

Zasloff, M. (1983). *Proc. Natl. Acad. Sci. USA* **80**, 6436–6440.

17

Microinjection of mRNAs into Xenopus *Oocytes*

G. Huez and G. Marbaix

I. INTRODUCTION

Cell-free systems and intact cells can both be used to translate the genetic information carried by isolated messenger RNA. Reticulocyte lysate (Pelham and Jackson, 1976) and wheat-germ (Marcus *et al.*, 1974) extract are two well known examples of *in vitro* translation systems. They both allow a rapid and convenient estimation of the translational capacity of mRNA preparations. These cell-free systems are efficient and capable of translating messengers from various origins. However, they suffer from three main limitations: (1) they are short lived — the translation is linear only for a limited period of time (usually 90–120 m); (2) these systems are also relatively poor in performing post-translational modifications of the newly synthesized polypeptides; and (3) due to their very nature, these extracts are unsuitable for the study of the cellular compartmentalization of the polypeptides synthesized.

Most of these limitations do not apply to *in vivo* translation systems, where the mRNA is directly injected into the cytoplasm of intact cells. As the translation machinery continues to work as long as the recipient cell is in good condition, the translation of the injected mRNA may last for several hours or days. In practice it is very often limited by the stability of the mRNA molecules themselves. Since the complex organization of the cell is preserved, most of the post-translational modifications of the foreign polypeptide synthesized on the injected mRNA normally occur. Moreover, it is often observed that cell compartmentalization or secretion of the exogenous protein also takes place as in the cell from which the injected mRNA is isolated.

Microinjection and Organelle Transplantation Techniques

ISBN: 0-12-164722-6
ISBN: 0-12-164723-4 Pbk

In 1971, almost simultaneously, two reports were published demonstrating the translation of messenger RNAs after microinjection into living cells. In one experiment, the mRNA was injected into somatic cells in culture (Graessmann and Graessmann, 1971) while in the other, the messenger was introduced into frog *Xenopus* oocytes (Gurdon *et al.*, 1971; Lane *et al.*, 1971).

Microinjection of RNA into somatic cells is described elsewhere in this book (see Chapter 12) and we will focus here on microinjection of mRNA into frog oocytes. It was quite a surprise when Gurdon and coworkers showed that frog oocytes are able to translate, over several hours, a mixture of α- and β-mRNAs isolated from rabbit reticulocytes. Since these initial experiments, a great number of different mRNAs isolated from a variety of origins has been translated into these cells. As those experiments are numerous, it is not possible in this chapter to describe all of them. We will rather only consider here the general properties of the system and show some examples of its utilization.

II. SOME TECHNICAL ASPECTS OF mRNA MICROINJECTION INTO *XENOPUS* OOCYTES

Since fully grown (stage 6; Dumont, 1978) oocytes used in these experiments are huge cells, the injection of RNA can be performed very easily using a simple micromanipulator and a low power magnification binocular (see also Chapter 15). The pipettes can be conveniently made with an automatic puller from 2 μl "microcap" (Drumont) capillaries. As the mRNA preparation is usually injected into the cytoplasm, the size of the needle is not critical; the diameter at the tip should be in the range of 10–30 μm. The use of needles with tips wider than 30 μm may damage the oocytes. The size of the *Xenopus* oocytes is such that usually only a few cells are needed for the analysis of the translation products. It is however good practice to inject 10 or more oocytes in a given experiment in order to decrease the influence of individual variations in their response.

In a typical experiment, the volume injected in each oocyte is 50 nl. The RNA concentration is usually adjusted to between 0.2 and 1 mg/ml. For a complete translation experiment, it is rarely necessary to use more than a few hundred oocytes. These are easily obtained without killing the animal. After anaesthesia, a part of the ovary is removed through a small incision in the ventral side of the animal (see also Chapter 15). The process may be repeated two or three times on the same animal.

III. GENERAL PROPERTIES OF THE OOCYTE TRANSLATION SYSTEM

A. Translation efficiency

As mentioned above, rabbit globin mRNAs were the first messengers to be successfully translated after injection into frog oocytes (Gurdon *et al.*, 1971; Lane *et al.*, 1971). Several of the principal virtues of this system were revealed in these original experiments.

The high translational efficiency is one of these virtues. Figure 1, reproduced from the initial publication of Gurdon and his colleages (Gurdon *et al.*, 1971) shows the elution profiles from a G100 Sephadex column of labelled homogenates from oocytes injected or not injected with rabbit globin mRNA. After injection of the mixture of α- and β-globin mRNAs, the oocytes were incubated in Barth medium (see Chapter 15) containing [^{3}H]histidine. Histidine was chosen as it is one of the most abundant amino acids in the globin chains. At the end of the incubation period (15 h), the oocytes were washed and homogenized in a buffer containing unlabelled carrier haemoglobin.

Control oocytes injected with the medium alone were incubated in parallel. Figure 1 shows that, in oocytes injected with globin mRNA, a large proportion (more than 60%) of the radioactivity incorporated into proteins is recovered as a peak comigrating with the carrier haemoglobin. It was further demonstrated by peptide mapping analysis that this material is indistinguishable from genuine rabbit haemoglobin (Marbaix and Lane, 1972). Time-course experiments performed with globin and several other messengers have shown that the maximum level of translation of the foreign mRNA is reached several (7–20) hours after injection (Gurdon *et al.*, 1971; Huez *et al.*, 1974; Berridge and Lane, 1976; Zehavi-Willner and Lane, 1977; Asselbergs *et al.*, 1979). This delay is probably at least partially due to the time needed for diffusion of the injected mRNA molecules into oocyte cytoplasm and appears to be more or less linked to the size of the mRNA (unpubl. obs.). The injected mRNA most probably diffused into all parts of the oocyte cytoplasm. This is suggested by the fact that the injection of an antisense RNA complementary to globin mRNA inhibits almost completely the synthesis of this protein in oocytes previously injected with the corresponding mRNA. This inhibition takes place even when the antisense mRNA is injected 5 h after the injection of the normal globin messenger and regardless of the point of injection (Krug and Melton, 1984).

As suggested by the results presented in Fig. 1, the efficiency of globin mRNA translation appears to be very high. From these results, Gurdon *et*

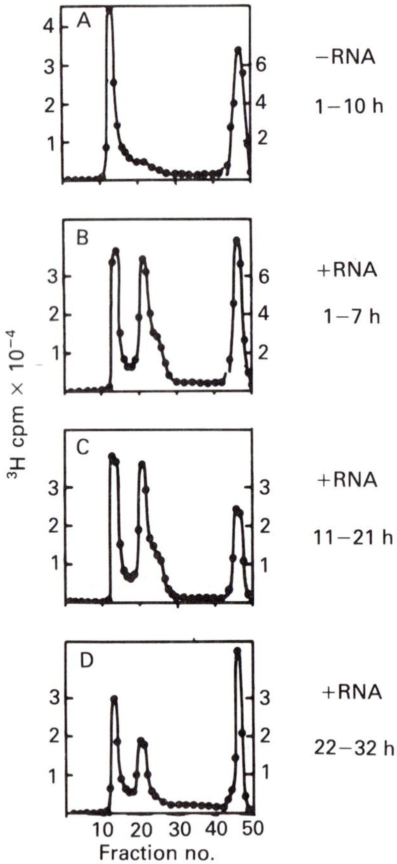

Fig. 1. Oocytes were injected with rabbit globin mRNA (B, C and D) or the injection medium (A) and incubated with [^{3}H]histidine for the time period indicated. The homogenates were subjected to Sephadex G100 filtration. The first peak corresponds to oocyte endogenous proteins. The second, to haemoglobin. From Gurdon *et al.* (1971) with permission.

al. (1971) have computed that each β-globin mRNA molecule is translated 30 times every hour at 19°C (the normal incubation temperature for the oocytes). This is half the rate of synthesis of the globin mRNA in a reticulocyte lysate at the same temperature. However, it must be considered that in this lysate, the high translation efficiency is only maintained over a period of 90–120 min. Consequently, the same molecule of messenger is translated on average not more than 50 times. In contrast, one can estimate that, in an oocyte which is incubated for several days, a globin messenger molecule is translated 2000–6000 times. This makes the oocyte system a good choice when, for instance, the presence of a very scarce mRNA has to be detected in a given population of total poly A+ molecules. Of course, this only holds true if the corresponding protein is stable enough and able to accumulate in the oocyte during the prolonged incubation period. It has been demonstrated, for example, that enzymatic activities corresponding to acetylcholine esterase from Torpedo electric organ can be detected in oocytes injected with as low as 1.2×10^{-4} ng of the corresponding mRNA (Soreq *et al.*, 1982).

B. Injected mRNA competes with endogenous messengers

It was initially thought that an injected mRNA was translated on a spare translational machinery different from that engaged in endogenous protein synthesis. This was based on the observation that injected globin mRNA does not decrease $[^3H]$histidine incorporation into endogenous oocyte proteins (Gurdon *et al.*, 1971; Lane *et al.*, 1971). Subsequently, it appeared that this was a false impression due to the labelling conditions (Laskey *et al.*, 1977). This problem comes from the fact that the content of histidine in globin is high while the pool for this amino acid is relatively low in the oocytes. When a large amount of globin is made, the pool of unlabelled histidine is rapidly exhausted and thus the specific activity of the amino acid inside the oocyte increases. Accordingly, the incorporation of radioactivity in the endogenous proteins, and thus the synthesis, appears to be higher than it really is.

Using different labelled amino acids in similar experiments, it was demonstrated that there is competition for translation between the injected globin mRNA and the endogenous mRNA. The globin mRNA seems to have an advantage over the endogenous messenger in this competition. Indeed, the amount of globin made in the oocytes is roughly proportional to the concentration of mRNA injected up to at least 100 ng/oocyte. With this concentration of globin mRNA, one notes a 44% decrease in the amount of endogenous proteins made by the oocytes (Laskey *et al.*, 1977). The capacity of the oocyte to translate other messengers can be markedly different. For instance, 20 ng of Zein mRNA saturate the translational capacity of the cell. It appears that some components of the protein synthetic apparatus other than the ribosomes themselves are limiting factors. This experiment also implies that these unidentified factors are different for the globin and the Zein mRNAs. When the two messengers are injected in the same oocytes, no competition is observed and both messengers are translated as if they were alone in the cell. This lack of competition suggests that they are translated on different classes of polyribosomes, i.e. globin mRNA on "free" and Zein mRNA on "membrane-bound" ribosomes (Richter and Smith, 1981).

It should be mentioned, however, that this idea is not supported by an experiment showing strong competition between globin and EMC RNA, which is believed to be translated on the rough endoplasmic reticulum (Laskey *et al.*, 1977). From the practical point of view, due to the existence of competition between the injected mRNA and the endogenous mRNA, it is not worth injecting a huge amount of mRNA into the oocyte in the hope of detecting more easily the corresponding protein. Usually it is not profitable to inject more than 20–50 ng per oocyte — injecting a larger amount of RNA is just a waste of material.

IV. *XENOPUS* OOCYTES: AN ALMOST UNIVERSAL TRANSLATION SYSTEM

mRNAs from several different origins (vertebrates, invertebrates, plants, animal and plant viruses; see Table I) are successfully translated in *Xenopus* oocytes. The translation efficiency varies from one messenger to the other for reasons which are most of the time not understood. For instance, the two mRNAs for α- and β- rabbit globin are not translated at the same rate when injected into oocytes. α is translated 5–10 times less efficiently than β. This unbalanced translation of the two messengers disappears when haemin is injected together with the mixture of mRNAs (Gianni *et al.*, 1972). The increase in α translation observed in these conditions is still unexplained (Fig. 2).

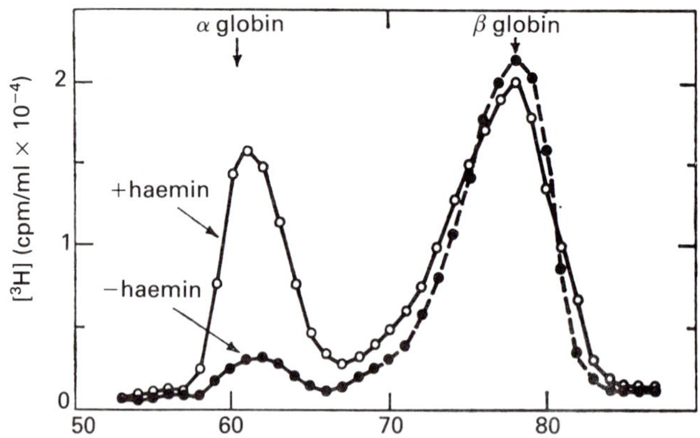

Fig. 2. Relative synthesis of α- and β- rabbit globin chains in oocytes injected with native globin mRNA (●) in the absence of haemin; (○) in the presence of haemin. Following injection, oocytes were incubated for 15 h. Globin chains were separated on carboxymethylcellulose columns. From Huez *et al.* (1977) with permission.

Table I. RNAs translated after microinjection into *Xenopus* oocytes.

Source of mRNA	Reference
Animal cells	
Ascidian acetylcholine esterase	Perry and Melton (1983)
Bovine lens α- and β-crystallins	Asselbergs *et al.* (1978)
Bovine thyroglobulin	Vassart *et al.* (1975)
Carp proinsulin	Rapoport *et al.* (1978)
Cat acetylcholine receptor	Miledi *et al.* (1982)
Chick conalbumin	Colman *et al.* (1981)
Chick GABA benzoadiazepine barbiturate receptors	Smart *et al.* (1983)
Chick lysozyme	Colman *et al.* (1981)
Chick ovalbumin	Chan *et al.* (1976); Colman *et al.*, (1981)
Chick ovomucoid	Colman *et al.* (1981)
Cuttlefish haemocyanin	Vanderbeke *et al.* (1982)
Duck globin	Lane *et al.* (1973)
Frog albumin	Lane *et al.* (1980)
Frog collagen	Rollins and Flickinger (1972)
Frog vitellogenin	Lane *et al.* (1980, 1983)
Gibbon interleukin	Lin *et al.* (1982)
Guinea pig caseins	Lane *et al.* (1979)
Guinea pig α-lactalbumin	Lane *et al.* (1979)
Honey bee promelittin	Lane *et al.* (1981)
Human acetylcholine receptors	Sumikawa *et al.* (1981)
Human brain proteins involved in drug and voltage operated channels formation	Gunderson *et al.* (1984)
Human chorionic gonadotropin	Mous *et al.* (1980)
Human erythropoietin	Farber and Zanjani (1983)
Human histones	Huez *et al.* (1978)
Human interferon	Reynolds *et al.* (1975); Sehgal *et al.* (1978a); Soreq *et al.* (1981); Devos *et al.* (1982)
Human interleukin 1	Windle *et al.* (1984)
Human interleukin 2	Hinuma *et al.* (1982)
Human 2–5 oligo adenylate synthetase	Shulman and Revel (1980); Hinuma *et al.* (1982); St-Laurent *et al.* (1983)
Human plasminogen activator	Miskin and Soreq (1981)
Locust vitellogenin	Lane *et al.* (1983)
Mouse albumin	Teraoka *et al.* (1982)
Mouse collagen	Lane and Knowland (1975)
Mouse colony stimulating factor	Bleackley *et al.* (1983)
Mouse pro EGF	Burmeister *et al.* (1984)
Mouse globin	
Mouse β-glucuronidase	Labarca and Paigen (1977)

Continued overleaf

Table I. Continued.

Source of mRNA	Reference
Mouse immunoglobulin	Jilka *et al.* (1979); Valle *et al.* (1981, 1983); Colman *et al.* (1982)
Mouse interferon	Lebleu *et al.* (1978)
Mouse interleukin 2	Labarca and Paigen (1977)
Mouse thyrotropin	Kourides and Weintraub (1979)
Paramecium surface antigen	Sommerville (1983)
Pig immunoglobulins	Kortbeek-Jacobs and van der Donk (1978)
Rabbit globin	Gurdon *et al.* (1971); Lane *et al.* (1971); Zehavi-Willner and Lane (1977)
Rabbit uteroglobulin	Beato and Rungger (1975)
Rat albumin	Lane *et al.* (1980)
Rat brain acetylcholine esterase	Soreq *et al.* (1982)
Rat cytochrome P450	Ohlsson *et al.* (1981)
Rat epoxide hydratase	Ohlsson *et al.* (1981)
Rat immunoglobulin	Deacon and Ebringer (1979)
Rat prostatic steroid binding protein	Mous *et al.* (1977, 1979, 1982)
Rat seminal vesicle proteins	Higgins *et al.* (1981)
Sea urchin histones	Higgins *et al.* (1981)
Squib haemocyanin	Vanderbeke *et al.* (1982)
Torpedo acetylcholine	Gundersen *et al.* (1985)
Torpedo acetylcholine esterase	Soreq *et al.* (1982)
Torpedo acetylcholine receptor	Sumikawa *et al.* (1984)
Torpedo proteins responsible for chloride channel formation	Sumikawa *et al.* (1984)
Torpedo choline acetyltransferase	Sumikawa *et al.* (1984)
Trout protamine	Gedamu *et al.* (1978)
Xenopus globin	Krug and Melton (1984)
Xenopus vitellogenin	Lane *et al.* (1983)
Xenopus laevis lipovitellin	Berridge and Lane (1976)
Xenopus laevis phosvitin	Berridge and Lane (1976)
Plant cells	
Barley secretory proteins	Lane *et al.* (1980)
Plant storage protein	Hurkman *et al.* (1981); Bassuner *et al.* (1983)
Viruses	
Adenovirus	De Robertis *et al.* (1977)
Alfalfa mosaic	Huez *et al.* (1983)
Avian myeloblastosis	Salden *et al.* (1976); Ghysdael *et al.* (1977)
Avian sarcoma	Katz *et al.* (1979)
Bovine leukemia	Ghysdael *et al.* (1979)

Table I. Continued.

Source of mRNA	Reference
Brome mosaic	Huez *et al.* (1983)
Citrus exocortis	Semancik *et al.* (1977)
Cowpea mosaic	Huez *et al.* (1983)
Cucumber mosaic	Schwinghamer and Symons (1977)
Encephalomyocarditis	Laskey *et al.* (1972)
Herpes simplex glycoprotein D	Watson *et al.* (1983)
Mengovirus	Littauer and Soreq (1982)
Moloney	Hesselink *et al.* (1981)
Mouse leukemia	Asselbergs *et al.* (1980)
Mouse mammary tumour	Nusse *et al.* (1978)
Polyoma	Lane *et al.* (1980)
Rabies	Wunner *et al.*, (1980)
Reovirus	McCrae and Woodland (1981)
Semliki forest envelope protein	Huth *et al.* (1984)
Simian virus 40	Lane *et al.* (1980)
Tobacco mosaic	Knowland (1974)
Bacteria	
E. coli β-lactamase	Wiedmann *et al.* (1984)

For the messengers mentioned in Table I, the detection of the corresponding protein was performed either by some physical identification (i.e. usually after labelling of the oocytes with radioactive precursors) or directly by measurement of the biological activity of the molecules.

Some RNAs from organelles like mitochondria or chloroplasts are apparently not translated in oocytes. It has been suggested, however, that the lack of translation may sometimes be only apparent and may simply be the result of difficulties in detecting very low amounts of the corresponding protein (Colman, 1984). The proteins encoded for by these organelle mRNAs may be very unstable in oocytes since they cannot associate rapidly with the corresponding organelar structure not present in oocytes.

Until recently, it was thought that oocytes could not be programmed with bacterial mRNAs. This is no longer true. Indeed, the translation of a β-lactamase mRNA from *Escherichia coli* has been reported (Mohun *et al.*, 1981). However, this mRNA is not a "natural" molecule directly extracted from bacteria. It is the result of an *in vitro* transcription of the corresponding gene and moreover this mRNA is capped *in vitro*. Nevertheless, these results confirm that eukaryotic ribosomes can cope with prokaryotic messengers even in a normal cellular environment.

V. *XENOPUS* OOCYTE IS A VERY GOOD SYSTEM IN WHICH TO STUDY THE TRANSLATION OF LONG mRNAs

While successful translations of long mRNAs have been reported in acellular systems, the yield of complete protein made in these systems may be quite low. Very often, the picture is confused by the presence of several other smaller polypeptides which are the result of incomplete translation. Apart from the degradation of the mRNA by nucleases, incomplete translation may also be explained in these *in vitro* systems by the fact that they are short lived. They simply do not work long enough to allow several rounds of translation of a very long mRNA. Indeed, the translation of mRNA corresponding to a 3000 kDa protein takes about 20 min at 37°C, the same order of magnitude as the life-time of the *in vitro* system itself.

This problem, of course, does not exist in oocytes which can be incubated for several days after injection of the mRNA. Moreover, incomplete proteins are usually not detected in oocytes. It is possible that the enzymes responsible for the elimination of incomplete or abnormal endogenous proteins are somehow also able to recognize and degrade the foreign incomplete polypeptides.

Translation of large proteins like thyroglobulin (Vassart *et al.*, 1975), fibroin (G. Chavancy, unpubl. obs.), haemocyanin (Vanderbeke *et al.*, 1982) and a high molecular mass antigen from paramecium (Vanderbeke *et al.*, 1982) can be cited as examples of the capacity of the oocytes to handle very long mRNAs. Translation in oocytes has even been used to ascertain the real size of the corresponding protein (Vassart *et al.*, 1975).

VI. POST-TRANSLATIONAL MODIFICATIONS OF PROTEINS TRANSLATED ON FOREIGN MESSENGERS

The capacity of the oocytes to perform post-translational modifications of the proteins translated on foreign messengers is probably one of the most interesting aspects of this system (Table II).

One class of modifications concerns the addition of chemical groups to the protein. *N*-acetylation, glycosylation, hydroxylation or phosphorylation of foreign proteins have been reported to occur in these cells. The modification takes place even if a purified mRNA for a given protein is injected into the oocytes. This means that these cells possess the enzymes which are able to modify the foreign protein in a similar way as in the original cell. However, some modifications, like the glycosylation, are not as extended as in the normal cell. For the chorionic gonadotropin and rat prostatic binding

Table II. Examples of post-translational modifications of foreign proteins.

Type of modification	Protein	Reference
N-acetylation	α2-crystallin	Asselbergs *et al.* (1978)
	Histones	Woodland and Wilt (1980)
N-glycosylation	Ovalbumin	Colman *et al.* (1981)
	Prostatic binding proteins	Mous *et al.* (1979)
	Immunoglobulin	Jilka *et al.* (1979); Deacon and Ebringer (1979)
	Chorionic gonadotropin	Mous *et al.* (1980)
Hydroxylation	Fibroblast collagen	Lane and Knowland (1975)
Poly protein cleavage	Viral proteins (various)	Laskey *et al.* (1972); Salden *et al.* (1976); Ghysdael *et al.* (1977, 1979); Nusse *et al.* (1978); Asselbergs *et al.* (1980)
	Vitellogenin	Berridge and Lane (1976)
Covalent subunit assembly	Uteroglobulin	Beato and Rungger (1975)
	Immunoglobulins	Deacon and Ebringer (1979); Jilka *et al.* (1979); Valle *et al.* (1983)
Non-covalent subunit assembly	Acetylcholin receptor	Sumikawa *et al.* (1981)
	β-glucuronidase	Labarca and Paigen (1977)
	α- and β-crystallins	Asselbergs *et al.* (1978)
Removal of "signal" sequence	Insulin	Rapoport *et al.* (1978)
	Immunoglobulin	Deacon and Ebringer (1979
	Honey bee promelittin	Lane *et al.* (1981)
	EGF	Burmeister *et al.* (1984)
	Uteroglobulin	Beato and Rungger (1975)
	Ovalbumin	Colman *et al.* (1981)
	Lysozyme	Colman *et al.* (1981)
	Seminal vesicle proteins	Higgins *et al.* (1981)
	β-lactamase	Wiedmann *et al.* (1984)
Haeme addition	Haemoglobin	Gurdon *et al.* (1971)
Phosphorylation	Protamine	Gedami *et al.* (1978)

protein, for instance, the carbohydrate composition found in oocytes is different from that of the genuine hormone (Mous *et al.*, 1979, 1980).

Another kind of post-translational modification observed in oocytes is the cleavage of high relative molecular mass precursors into the mature proteins. Fig. 3 shows an example of such processing. In this experiment, [^{35}S]RNA from an avian retrovirus (AMV) was injected into the oocytes and a pulse-chase experiment was performed (see Fig. 3). As can be observed, the 76 kDa polyprotein is progressively processed to give the mature structural protein of the virus. Similarly, precursor proteins made on a variety of virus EMC (Laskey *et al.*, 1972), BLV (Ghysdael *et al.*, 1979), MMTV (Nusse *et*

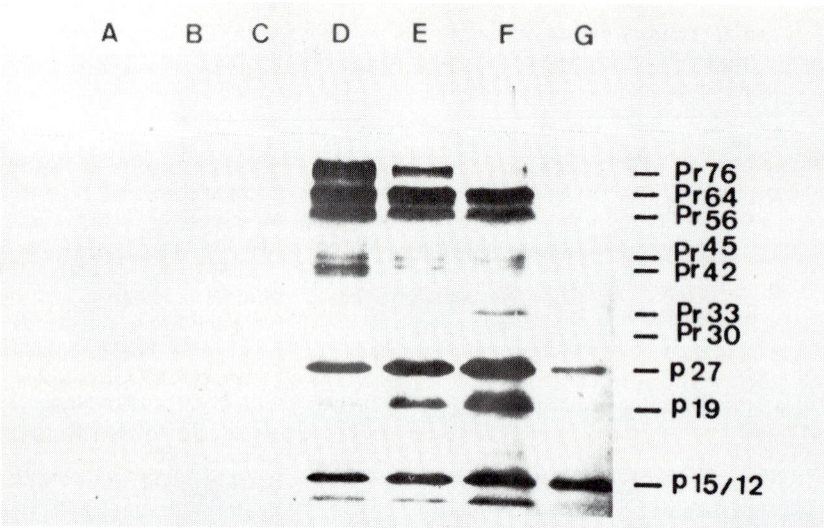

Fig. 3. Oocytes injected with AMV-RNA were labelled for 20 h with [^{35}S]methionine. Homogenates were prepared and immunoprecipitations performed with polyvalent antiserum against AMV. The immunoprecipitates were subjected to electrophoresis on 15% polyacrylamide gel. (A) Non-injected oocytes labelled for 20 h. (B) As (A) but chased for 24 h. (C) As (A) but chased for 72 h. (D) Oocytes injected with AMV-RNA and labelled for 20 h. (E) As (D) but chased for 24 h. (F) As (D) but chased for 72 h. From Ghysdael *et al.* (1977) with permission.

al., 1978), MLV (Asselbergs *et al.*, 1980) are processed in oocytes. The same is true for other polyproteins like vitellogenin (Berridge and Lane, 1976).

Apart from the cleavages of large precursor proteins, there are numerous examples of the cleavage of the so-called "signal" peptides involved in the secretion of the proteins (see Ch. 18). The removal of "pro" sequence from a precursor protein is also observed but appears to vary with the type of protein. Oocytes injected with mouse liver mRNA are able to synthesize and correctly process albumin (Teraoka *et al.*, 1982). The initial product of translation of liver albumin mRNA is pre-proalbumin, a protein which contains a pre-segment of 18 amino acids. This pre-segment is first cleaved, proalbumin is then converted into albumin just before secretion. Oocytes apparently perform all these steps since the albumin found outside the oocytes is indistinguishable from the authentic mouse proteins when analysed by two-dimensional electrophoresis gels. However, the oocytes are unable to perform correctly some form of processing of precursor "pre-pro" proteins. This has been demonstrated for pre-proinsulin, which can be transformed into proinsulin by the cleavage of the signal peptide, but cannot be converted into insulin (Rapoport *et al.*, 1978). The same is true for epidermal growth factor (EGF) which is processed to pro-EGF (Burmeister *et al.*, 1984) only, and promelittin which is not transformed into melittin (Lane *et al.*, 1981).

These processings are tissue specific and it is assumed that the oocytes lack the enzymes needed for such modifications. It remains to be seen if injection of mRNAs for the specific enzymes involved in these cleavages, together with the mRNA for the precursor protein, would allow these processings to occur, or if a special structure, only present in the original cells and probably missing in the oocytes, is also necessary.

VII. SECRETION OF PROTEINS ENCODED BY FOREIGN MESSENGERS INJECTED INTO OOCYTES

When mRNAs directing the synthesis of secretory proteins are injected into frog oocytes, in most cases the corresponding proteins are secreted in the incubation medium. Interferon was the first protein to be detected outside oocytes microinjected with a total poly A+ messenger preparation isolated from interferon-producing cells (Lebleu *et al.*, 1978). Subsequent detailed studies have proved that only those proteins which are normally secreted in the original cells are exported outside the oocytes. Colman and Morser (1979) have shown that this process is highly specific: even if guinea pig, casein and rabbit globin mRNAs are injected together into the oocytes, only casein is exported from the cells. Globin made from the injected mRNA is found in the cytosol and can barely be detected in the surrounding medium. The export of proteins made under the direction of injected messenger is not species specific. Indeed, proteins from diverse animals and plants are secreted from oocytes (see Table III). This process appears to lack cell-type specificity since proteins from different tissues are equally well secreted. The secretion of proteins appears to be unaffected by the presence or the absence of follicular cells surrounding the oocyte (Mohun *et al.*, 1981).

Interesting conclusions concerning the conditions for foreign protein excretion come from experiments where chick oviduct mRNA is injected into oocytes. In this case, ovalbumin, conalbumin, ovomucoid and lysozyme are made and secreted. It is observed that ovalbumin is mainly confined inside the oocyte within the endoplasmic reticulum (Colman *et al.*, 1981). However, a small amount is found in the cytosol. This cytosolic fraction (not secreted) is different from the secreted form: it is not glycosylated. Treatment of the injected oocytes with tunicamycin, which prevents the glycosylation of the form found in the endoplasmic reticulum (which is now identical to the cytosolic form), does not stop its secretion. It thus appears that the key event in the secretion of the protein by the oocytes is the

Table III. Segregation of foreign proteins made after mRNA injection.

Protein	Reference
Proteins found associated with oocyte membranes	
Cat muscle acetylcholine receptors	Miledi *et al*. (1982)
Chick GABA benzoadiazepine barbiturate receptors	Smart *et al*. (1983)
Common bean storage proteins	Matthews *et al*. (1981)
Human acetylcholine receptors	Sumikawa *et al*. (1981)
Human brain proteins responsible for voltage operated channels formation	Gundersen *et al*. (1984)
Maize storage proteins	Hurkman *et al*. (1981)
Mouse non-secretory immunoglobulin	Valle *et al*. (1983)
Rat liver cytochrome P450	Ohlsson *et al*. (1981)
Rat liver epoxide hydratase	Ohlsson *et al*. (1981)
Semliki forest envelope proteins	Huth *et al*. (1984)
Torpedo acetylcholine receptors	Sumikawa *et al*. (1984)
Torpedo proteins responsible for chloride channel formation	Sumikawa *et al*. (1984)
Proteins associated with yolk platelets	
Xenopus liver lipovitellin	Berridge and Lane (1976)
Xenopus liver phosvitin	Berridge and Lane (1976)
Proteins exported from the oocyte	
Barley seed low rel. mol. mass proteins	Lane *et al*. (1980)
Carp proinsulin	Rapoport *et al*. (1978)
Chick conalhaemin	Colman *et al*. (1981)
Chick lysozyme	Colman *et al*. (1981)
Chick ovalbumin	Chan *et al*. (1986); Colman *et al*. (1981)
Chick ovomucoid	Colman *et al*. (1981)
Guinea pig caseins	Lane *et al*. (1979)
Human interferons	Reynolds *et al*. (1975); Devos *et al*. (1982)
Human interleukins 1 and 2	Hinuma *et al*. (1982); Windle *et al*. (1984)
Human plasminogen activator	Miskin and Soreq (1981)
Locust vitellin polypeptides	Lane *et al*. (1983)
Mouse albumin	Teraoka *et al*. (1982)
Mouse colony stimulating factor	Bleackley *et al*. (1983)
Mouse immunoglobulins	Valle *et al*. (1981, 1983)
Mouse interferons	Lebleu *et al*. (1978)
Mouse pro-EGF	Burmeister *et al*. (1984)
Mouse thyrotropin	Kourides and Weintraub (1979)
Parmecium surface antigen	Sommerville (1983)
Plant storage globulins	Bassuner *et al*. (1983)
Rat albumin	Lane *et al*. (1980)
Rat brain acetylcholinesterase	Soreq *et al*. (1982)
Rat regulatory proteins from spinal cord cells	D. Schmid (pers. commun.)
Rat seminal vesicle proteins	Higgins *et al*. (1981)
Bacterial β-lactamase	Wiedmann *et al*. (1984)

possibility of reaching the endoplasmic reticulum, and not the glycosylation process.

Several arguments suggest that the signal peptide plays a role in protein secretion in oocytes, as it does in other cells. Thc "signal" hypothesis implies a cotranslational transfer of the newly made protein across the endoplasmic reticulum. One should thus expect that the export of protein will be linked to translation. Results obtained with oocytes confirm this hypothesis. If labelled proteins, previously exported from oocytes injected with liver mRNA, are reintroduced into fresh oocytes, no secretion is observed (Lane *et al.*, 1980). This is also observed with other proteins like ovalbumin or the oocytes' own proteins (Lane *et al.*, 1980).

There is also evidence that, in *Xenopus* oocytes, the leader peptide is involved in both translocation and some of the later steps in the secretory pathway. This is suggested by the results of an experiment where a small peptide corresponding to the NH_2 terminal leader sequence of mouse immunoglobulin light chain precursor is injected into oocytes. This results in a competitive inhibition of secretory proteins synthesis and also in a rapid acceleration in the rate of export of these proteins from the oocytes (Koren *et al.*, 1983).

Secretory proteins from prokaryotic origins are also exported from the oocytes. This was shown using an *E. coli* β-lactamase mRNA synthesized *in vitro* by transcription of a plasmid DNA with *E. coli* RNA polymerase (Wiedmann *et al.*, 1984). Injection of this *in vitro* capped mRNA into oocytes promotes the secretion of mature β-lactamase which can be identified either by immunoprecipitation or enzymatic activity.

It is estimated that 10^{10} molecules of β-lactamase are exported per oocyte in 24 h. These values are similar to those observed for eukaryotic proteins exported from oocytes (Huth *et al.*, 1984). This confirms previous observations (Müller *et al.*, 1982) that the signal peptide present in a prokaryotic pre-protein is recognized by mammalian signal recognition particle (SRP) and is cleaved by eukaryotic signal peptidase. The presence of the signal peptide is not always sufficient in itself to ensure the secretion of proteins from oocytes. For the immunoglobulin the correct association of heavy and light chains into functional tetrameric (H_2L_2) structure is necessary for their secretion. Injection of heavy and light chain mRNAs separately leads to the synthesis, but not the secretion, of the corresponding chains (Valle *et al.*, 1981). Secretion of the proteins is only observed when the two messengers are injected into the same oocyte simultaneously, or even days apart.

As mentioned in the preceding section, oocytes are in some cases unable to perform the complete processing of the precursor proteins: this is true for Carp proinsulin, Honey bee promelittin and mouse pro-EGF. While proinsulin and pro-EGF are secreted by the oocyte (Rapoport *et al.*, 1978;

Burmeister *et al.*, 1984), promelittin is not (Lane *et al.*, 1981). Complete processing is thus not necessary for secretion. Cellular localization of promelittin in oocytes revealed that the protein remains confined in the vesicle fraction for several days. The lack of secretion of this protein may be due to its hydrophobic nature, which causes the trapping of the molecules in the intracellular membrane of these vesicles (Lane *et al.*, 1981).

The experiments mentioned above are only a few among the numerous examples in which oocytes have been used to study protein secretion. Other examples are given in Table III. It should be stressed here that oocytes apparently also export proteases in the incubation medium. It is thus good practice to add some protease inhibitors to the incubation medium in order to protect the foreign mRNA directed secretory protein against degradation. Various mixtures of inhibitors have been successfully used (Soreq and Miskin, 1981). We have observed that the addition to the incubation medium of 1% bovine serum albumin and 1% Trasylol is effective in preventing, for instance, the degradation of interferon exported from oocytes (unpubl. obs.).

VIII. CELLULAR COMPARTMENTALIZATION OF EXOGENOUS mRNA ENCODED PROTEINS IN OOCYTES

Secretion of foreign protein outside the oocytes upon injection of the corresponding mRNA is only one aspect of the ability of these cells to perform the correct compartmentalization of the exogenous proteins. In most cases, these proteins segregate in the oocytes to the same cellular compartments as in the original cells.

Some proteins are found inside membrane vesicles. This occurs with secretory proteins which are subsequently released, with the few exceptions mentioned above, into the surrounding medium. Other proteins associate with intracellular membranes of the oocyte. This has been clearly demonstrated for cytochrome P450 and the rat liver epoxide hydratase (Ohlsson *et al.*, 1981). This process of membrane integration is highly specific: for cytochrome P450, the biological activity of the protein is direct evidence for its correct orientation into the oocyte membranes. Segregation of the proteins into membranes is highly selective.

When oocytes are programmed with rat liver RNA, rat albumin is clearly exported to the incubation medium whilst cytochrome P450 and epoxide hydratase are not found outside the cells (Ohlsson *et al.*, 1981). Several other foreign proteins were shown to migrate into the oocyte membranes (see Table III). For instance, acetylcholine receptors from tissues as different as

Torpedo electric organ and cat muscle are detected on the surface of oocytes injected with total poly A^+ isolated from the corresponding cells.

Direct biochemical evidence for the ability of foreign transmembrane proteins to appear on the oocyte surface comes from experiments where RNAs coding for the Semliki forest virus envelope glycoproteins are injected into oocytes. Specific antibodies raised against these viral proteins are indeed able to bond to the surface of the injected cells. This fixation is specific since it increases with the amount of viral mRNA injected and is minimal in oocytes injected with water (Huth *et al.*, 1984).

IX. STABILITY OF INJECTED mRNA

mRNA stability is, of course, of utmost importance for the success of any translation experiment performed in oocytes. So far, there is relatively little understanding of the structural features responsible for the observed diversity in mRNA stability in eukaryotic cells in general. In oocytes, however, at least two elements of the mRNA structure are important for the mRNA stability: the presence of (1) a poly A segment at its 3′ end and (2) an intact cap structure at its 5′ end. Some of the most informative experiments leading to the understanding of the role of these structures have been performed using *Xenopus* oocytes as a test system. These experiments represent good examples of the use of oocytes as a model to elucidate some of the mechanisms operative in normal somatic cells.

A. Role of poly A in mRNA stability

A clear demonstration that poly A sequences play a role in mRNA stability was obtained by comparing the translational capacity of native and enzymatically deadenylated globin mRNA in frog oocytes. When a native globin messenger is injected in these cells, the molecule is translated over several days (Gurdon *et al.*, 1973). On the contrary, in oocytes injected with the deadenylated molecules, globin synthesis only last for a few hours (Huez *et al.*, 1974).

During the first few hours, however, the translation efficiency of both messenger RNAs is similar. Thus, the removal of poly A does not impair the capacity of the mRNA to be translated but clearly affects its stability. The lower translational stability of the molecules lacking poly A is solely due to the absence of poly A. Indeed, when previously deadenylated globin mRNA molecules are readenylated *in vitro*, they recover the same stability within the oocytes as that of the native mRNA molecules (Huez *et al.*, 1975). It is clear that the rapid decline in globin synthesis observed with mRNA lacking poly A is due to a real degradation of the messenger molecule. This is shown by measuring, with a specific cDNA probe, the amount of hybridizable mRNA molecules remaining in the oocytes at different times after injection.

In oocytes injected with native molecules, the amount of globin mRNA sequences remains constant, at least for 48 h after injection. In oocytes injected with deadenylated messenger, almost all the globin mRNA sequences have disappeared by that time (Huez *et al.*, 1977). The observation that poly A plays a role in mRNA stability is not restricted to the globin messengers. HeLa cell histone mRNAs coding for H_{2A}, H_{2B}, H_3 and H_4 naturally lack poly A. When injected into oocytes, these RNAs exhibit a short translational half-life similar to that of deadenylated rabbit globin mRNA (Huez *et al.*, 1978; Woodland and Wilt, 1980). If these histone mRNAs are adenylated *in vitro* prior to injection, their stability is markedly increased and becomes comparable to that of native globin mRNA (Huez *et al.*, 1978).

Similar observations have been made with plant viral RNA. For three of them — the alfalfa, the brome grass and the cowpea mosaic viruses — the presence of a poly A segment, either added *in vitro* or occurring naturally, also confers to these RNAs a higher translational stability in oocytes (Huez *et al.*, 1983). The degree of stability of the injected mRNA does not appear to be proportional to the length of the poly A segment. It is rather observed that there exists a minimal length of the poly A track necessary to ensure the stabilization of the molecules in oocytes.

When the poly A segment is shorter than about 20 nucleotides, the injected messenger molecules are rapidly degraded (Fig. 4; Nudel *et al.*, 1976). In contrast, mRNAs with poly A segments longer than this are equally stable in oocytes regardless of the number of A residues. These results may be explained if one assumes that the poly A segment must have a certain minimum length to allow the formation of some structural organization which protects the mRNA against degradation. These results also imply that the mechanism of poly A shortening, which is present in other cells (Nokin *et al.*, 1976), is not, or is very poorly, active in oocytes.

While the above-mentioned experiments strongly suggest that poly A plays an important role in mRNA stability, it is not the only factor which influences messenger half-life in oocytes. Indeed, some RNAs lacking poly A exhibit a higher stability in oocytes than either deadenylated globin mRNA or HeLa cell histone mRNAs. This is the case for the RNA isolated from the reovirus (McCrae and Woodland, 1981), brome grass mosaic virus (Huez *et al.*, 1983) and alfalfa mosaic virus (Huez *et al.*, 1983). It should be noted, however, that for the two latter messengers at least, the addition of a poly A segment further increases their half-life in oocytes (Huez *et al.*, 1983). These relatively stable poly A-lacking messengers are all of viral origin. This

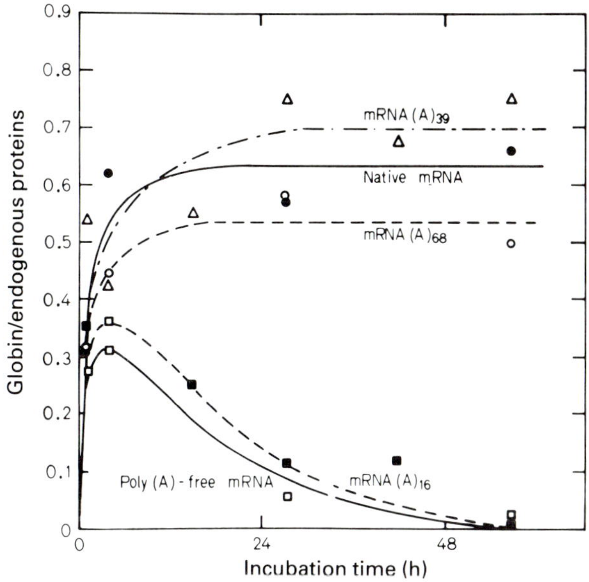

Fig. 4. Xenopus oocytes were injected with globin mRNA having different lengths of poly A (as indicated). The cells were incubated with labelled histidine for different time intervals and the extent of globin synthesis measured. The rate of globin synthesis relative to endogenous proteins is given versus the time of incubation. From Nudel *et al.* (1976) with permission.

class of RNAs may possess some unknown structural feature which stabilizes them almost in the same way as the poly A for the bulk of the normal cellular messengers.

The case of the interferon β messenger is in this respect very interesting since it is, so far, a unique example of a non-viral mRNA whose stability in frog oocytes is not affected by the removal of its terminal poly A. Soreq and collaborators have shown that native or deadenylated interferon mRNAs have a similar half-life of about 8 h in frog oocytes (Sehgal *et al.*, 1978b; Soreq *et al.*, 1981). However, it should be mentioned here that this result contrasts with that of Colman and Morser. These authors have observed, in apparently similar experimental conditions, that oocytes injected with poly A + RNA secrete interferon at the same rate for more than 48 h (Colman and Morser, 1979). The reason for this discrepancy has not yet been explained satisfactorily.

B. Influence of the cap structure

The so-called "cap" structure is found at the 5′ end of most eukaryotic mRNAs. The absence or alteration of this structure seems to impair markedly the translational capacity of messengers when injected in oocytes (Furuichi *et al.*, 1977). This is observed with natural globin mRNA from which the cap is either removed or modified (Lockard and Lane, 1978). In both cases, the ability of the messenger to direct globin synthesis is reduced to less than 5% of its original value. Similar results are obtained with "synthetic" *Xenopus* globin or human β interferon mRNA synthesized *in vitro* from plasmid DNA using Sp6 polymerase (Krug and Melton, 1984). It is, in this case, very easy to obtain molecules which are either capped or not since this structure is added *in vitro* after transcription.

The synthetic capped mRNAs are almost as efficiently translated in oocytes as the genuine messengers. The uncapped molecules are, on the contrary, apparently not translated. Even a 10-fold increase in the amount of mRNA injected is not sufficient to allow the synthesis of a detectable amount of the proteins (Krug and Melton, 1984). The absence of cap structure not only impairs translation, but also influences the stability of the messenger molecules, as demonstrated with reovirus RNA (McCrae and Woodland, 1981). Some mRNAs naturally lack the normal cap structure. Satellite necrosis virus and cowpea mosaic virus are two examples. These RNAs are translated efficiently in the oocytes and are also quite stable (Huez *et al.*, 1983; Lane, 1983).

It thus appears that the stability of a messenger RNA in the oocytes is influenced by more than one parameter. Very little is known concerning the mechanism involved in mRNA degradation either in normal cells or in oocytes. While it is clear that structures like poly A or the "cap" play a role in this mechanism, this does not seem to apply to all mRNA.

X. CONCLUSION

As we have seen in the preceding sections, the oocytes have many special merits. They constitute a highly efficient system which can be used to test the translational capacity of a great variety of messengers since they lack species specificity. This system is very useful for the study of the role played by the different structural constituents of the mRNA molecules in their translational capacity or their stability.

Moreover, it is possible with this system to analyse the behaviour of the products of translation. This is especially helpful in the study of the mechanisms of cellular compartmentalization or secretion. Since a total population of RNA can be injected without previous purification, this system has also proved very useful for the identification and the molecular cloning of some messengers coding certain proteins.

A promising new field is now being developed with the injection of antisense mRNA which can be used to inhibit the expression of a given mRNA. It is possible that in the future, this will lead to a new example of utilization of this amazing and ubiquitous "cellular test tube".

REFERENCES

Asselbergs, F. A. M., Koopmans, M., Van Venrooij, W. J. and Bloemendal, H. (1978). *Eur. J. Biochem.* **91**, 65–72.

Asselbergs, F. A. M., Van Venrooij, W. J. and Bloemendal, H. (1979). *Eur. J. Biochem.* **94**, 249–254.

Asselbergs, F. A. M., Salden, M. H. L. and Bloemendal, H. (1980). *Eur. J. Biochem.* **109**, 395–403.

Bassuner, R., Huth, A., Manteuffel, R. and Rapoport, T. A. (1983). *Eur. J. Biochem.* **133**, 321–326.

Beato, M. and Rungger, D. (1975). *FEBS Lett.* **59**, 305–309.

Berridge, M. and Lane, C. (1976). *Cell* **8**, 283–297.

Bleackley, R. C., Horak, H., Elhamey, J. M., Havele, C., Shaw, A. R., Turner, A. R. and Petkau, V. H. (1983). *Nucl. Acids Res.* **11**, 3027–3032.

Burmeister, M., Avivi, A., Schlessinger, J. and Soreq, H. (1984). *EMBO J.* **3**, 1499–1505.

Chan, L., Kohler, P. O. and O'Malley, B. W. (1976). *J. Clin. Invest.* **57**, 576.

Colman, A. (1984). *In* "Transcription and Translation: A Practical Approach" (B. D. Hames and S. J. Higgins, eds). IRL Press.

Colman, A. and Morser, J. (1979). *Cell* **17**, 517–526.

Colman, A., Lane, C. D., Craig, R., Boulton, A., Mohun, T. and Morser, J. (1981). *Eur. J. Biochem.* **113**, 339–348.

Colman, A., Besley, J. and Valle, G. (1982). *J. Mol. Biol.* **160**, 459–474.

Deacon, N. J. and Ebringer, A. (1979). *FEBS Lett.* **79**, 191–194.

De Robertis, E. M., Partington, G. A., Longthorne, R. F. and Gurdon, J. B. (1977). *J. Embryol. Exp. Morphol.* **40**, 199–214.

Devos, R., Cheroutre, H., Taya, Y. and Fiers, W. (1982). *J. Interferon. Res.* **2**, 409–420.

Dumont, J. N. (1978). *J. Morphol.* **136**, 153.

Farber, N. M. and Zanjani, E. D. (1983). *J. Lab. Clin. Med.* **102**, 681.

Furuichi, Y., Lafiandra, A. and Shatkin, A. L. (1977). *Nature* **266**, 235–239.

Gedamu, L., Dixon, G. H. and Gurdon, J. B. (1978). *Exp. Cell Res.* **117**, 325–334.

Ghysdael, J., Hubert, E., Travnicek, M., Bolognesi, D. P., Burny, A., Cleuter, Y., Huez, G., Kettmann, R., Marbaix, G., Portetelle, D. and Chantrenne, H. (1977). *Proc. Natl. Acad. Sci. USA* **74**, 3230–3234.

Ghysdael, J., Kettmann, R. and Burny, A. (1979). *J. Virol.* **29**, 1987–1998.

Gianni, A. M., Giglioni, B., Ottolenghi, S., Comi, P. and Guidotti, G. G. (1972). *Nature New Biol.* **240**, 183–185.

Graessmann, A. and Graessmann, M. (1971). *Hoppe-Seyler's Z. Physiol. Chem.* **352**, 527–532.

Gundersen, C. G., Miledi, R. and Parker, I. (1984). *Nature* **308**, 421–424.

Gundersen, C. B., Jenden, D. J. and Miledi, R. (1985). *Proc. Natl. Acad. Sci. USA* **82**, 608–611.

Gurdon, J. B., Lane, C. D., Woodland, H. R. and Marbaix, G. (1971). *Nature* **233**, 177–182.

Gurdon, J. B., Lingrel, J. B. and Marbaix, G. (1973). *J. Mol. Biol.* **80**, 539–543.

Hesselink, W. G., Van der Kemp, A. and Bloemers, H. (1981). *Virology* **110**, 375–384.

Higgins, S., Colman, A., Fuller, F. and Jackson, P. (1981). *Mol. Cell. Endocrinol.* **21**, 255–262.

Hinuma, S., Onda, H., Naruo, K., Ichimori, Y., Koyama, M. and Tsukamoto, K. (1982). *Biochem. Biophys. Res. Commun.* **109**, 363–369.

Huez, G., Marbaix, G., Hubert, E., Leclercq, M., Nudel, U., Soreq, H., Salomon, R., Lebleu, B., Revel, M. and Littauer, U. Z. (1974). *Proc. Natl. Acad. Sci. USA* **71**, 3143–3146.

Huez, G., Marbaix, G., Hubert, E., Cleuter, Y., Leclercq, M., Chantrenne, H., Devos, R., Soreq, H., Nudel, U. and Littauer, U. Z. (1975). *Eur. J. Biochem.* **59**, 589–592.

Huez, G., Marbaix, G., Burny, A., Hubert, E., Leclercq, M., Cleuter, Y., Chantrenne, H., Soreq, H. and Littauer, U. Z. (1977). *Nature* **266**, 472–473.

Huez, G., Marbaix, G., Gallwitz, D., Weinberg, E., Devos, R., Hubert, E. and Cleuter, Y. (1978). *Nature* **271**, 572–573.

Huez, G., Cleuter, Y., Bruck, C., Van Vloten-Doting, L., Goldbach, R. and Verduin, B. (1983). *Eur. J. Biochem.* **130**, 205–209.

Hurkman, W. J., Smith, L. D., Richter, J. and Larkins, B. A. (1981). *J. Cell. Biol.* **89**, 292–299.

Huth, A., Rapoport, T. A. and Kääriäinen, L. (1984). *EMBO J.* **3**, 767–771.

Jilka, R. L., Familletti, P. and Pestka, S. (1979). *Arch. Biochem. Biophys.* **192**, 290–295.

Katz, R. A., Maniatis, E. M. and Guntaka, R. V. (1979). *Biochem. Biophys. Res. Commun.* **86**, 447–453.

Knowland, J. (1974). *Genetics* **78**, 383–394.

Koren, R., Burnstein, Y. and Soreq, H. (1983). *Proc. Natl. Acad. Sci. USA* **80**, 7205–7209.

Kortbeek-Jacobs, N. and van der Donk, H. (1978). *J. Immunol. Methods* **24**, 195–199.

Kourides, I. and Weintraub, B. (1979). *Proc. Natl. Acad. Sci. USA* **76**, 298–302.

Krug, P. A. and Melton, D. A. (1984). *Nucl. Acids Res.* **12**, 7057–7062.

Labarca, C. and Paigen, K. (1977). *Proc. Natl. Acad. Sci. USA* **74**, 4462–4465.

Lane, C. D. (1983). *In* "Current Topics in Developmental Biology" (A. A. Moscona and A. Monroy, eds) Vol. 18, pp. 89–115. Academic Press, New York and London.

Lane, C. D. and Knowland, J. S. (1975). *In* "The Biochemistry of Animal Development" (R. A. Weber, ed.) Vol. 3, pp. 145–181. Academic Press, New York and London.

Lane, C. D., Marbaix, G. and Gurdon, J. B. (1971). *J. Mol. Biol.* **61**, 73–91.

Lane, C. D., Gregory, C. M. and Morel, C. (1973). *Eur. J. Biochem.* **34**, 219–227.

Lane, C. D., Shannon, S. and Craig, R. (1979). *Eur. J. Biochem.* **101**, 485–495.

Lane, C. D., Colman, A., Mohun, T., Morser, J., Champion, J., Kourides, I., Craig, R., Higgins, S., James, T. C., Applebaum, S. W., Ohlsson, R. I., Pancha, E., Houghton, M., Matthews, J. and Miflim, B. J. (1980). *Eur. J. Biochem.* **111**, 225–235.

Lane, C. D., Champion, J., Haiml, Z. and Kreil, G. (1981). *Eur. J. Biochem.* **113**, 273–281.

Lane, C. D., Champion, J., Colman, A., James, T. C. and Applebaum, S. W. (1983). *Eur. J. Biochem.* **130**, 529–535.

Laskey, R. A., Gurdon, J. B. and Crawford, L. V. (1972). *Proc. Natl. Acad. Sci. USA* **69**, 3665–3669.

Laskey, R. A., Mills, A. D., Gurdon, J. B. and Partington, G. A. (1977). *Cell* **11**, 345–352.

Lebleu, B., Hubert, E., Content, J., Dewit, L., Brande, I. A. and De Clercq, E. (1978). *Biochem. Biophys. Res. Commun.* **82**, 665–673.

Lin, Y., Stadler, B. M. and Rabin, H. (1982). *J. Biol. Chem.* **257**, 1587–1590.

Littauer, U. Z. and Soreq, H. (1982). *Prog. Nucl. Acid. Res. Mol. Biol.* **27**, 53–83.

Lockard, R. E. and Lane, C. D. (1978). *Nucl. Acids Res.* **5**, 3237–3247.

Marbaix, G. and Lane, C. D. (1972). *J. Mol. Biol.* **67**, 517–524.

Marcus, A., Efron, D. and Weeks, D. P. (1974). *Methods Enzymol.* **30**, 749–754.

Matthews, J., Brown, J. and Hall, T. (1981). *Nature* **294**, 175–176.

McCrae, M. A. and Woodland, H. R. (1981). *Eur. J. Biochem.* **116**, 467–470.

Miledi, R., Parker, I. and Sumikawa, K. (1982). *EMBO J.* **1**, 1207–1312.

Miskin, R. and Soreq, H. (1981). *Nucl. Acids Res.* **9**, 3355–3363.

Mohun, T. J., Lane, C. D., Colman, A. and Wylie, C. (1981). *J. Embryol. Exp. Morphol.* **61**, 367–383.

Mous, J., Peeters, B. and Rombauts, W. (1977). *Biochem. Biophys. Res. Commun.* **79**, 1111–1116.

Mous, J., Peeters, B., Rombauts, W. and Heyns, W. (1979). *FEBS Lett.* **103**, 81–84.

Mous, J., Peeters, B. and Rombauts, W. (1980). *FEBS Lett.* **122**, 105–108.

Mous, J. M., Peeters, B. L., Heyns, W. J. and Rombauts, W. A. (1982). *J. Biol. Chem.* **257**, 11 822–11 828.

Müller, M., Ibrahim, I., Chang, C. N., Walter, P. and Blobel, G. (1982). *J. Biol. Chem.* **257**, 11 860–11 863.

Nokin, P., Burny, A., Huez, G. and Marbaix, G. (1976). *Eur. J. Biochem.* **68**, 431–436.

Nudel, U., Soreq, H., Littauer, U. Z., Marbaix, G., Huez, G., Leclercq, M., Hubert, E. and Chantrenne, H. (1976). *Eur. J. Biochem.* **64**, 115–121.

Nusse, R., Asselbergs, F. A. M., Salden, M. H. L., Michalides, R. J. A. M. and Bloemendal, H. (1978). *Virology* **91**, 106–115.

Ohlsson, I., Lane, D. and Guengerich, F. (1981). *Eur. J. Biochem.* **115**, 367–373.

Pelham, H. R. and Jackson, R. J. (1976). *Eur. J. Biochem.* **67**, 247–256.

Perry, H. E. and Melton, D. A. (1983). *Cell Differentiation* **13**, 233–238.

Rapoport, T. A., Thiele, B. J., Prehn, S., Marbaix, G., Cleuter, Y., Hubert, E. and Huez, G. (1978). *Eur. J. Biochem.* **87**, 229–233.

Reynolds., F. H. Jr, Premkumar, E. and Pitha, P. M. (1975). *Proc. Natl. Acad. Sci. USA* **72**, 4881–4885.

Richter, J. D. and Smith, L. D. (1981). *Cell* **27**, 183–191.

Rollins, J. W. and Flickinger, R. (1972). *Science* **178**, 1204.

Salden, M., Asselbergs, F. A. M. and Bloemendal, H. (1976). *Nature* **259**, 696–699.

Schwinghamer, M. and Symons, R. (1977). *Virology* **79**, 88–108.

Sehgal, P. B., Lyles, D. S. and Tamm, I. (1978a). *Virology* **89**, 186–198.

Sehgal, P. B., Soreq, H. and Tamm, I. (1978b). *Proc. Natl. Acad. Sci. USA* **75**, 5030–5033.

Semancik, J. S., Conejero, V. and Gerhart, J. (1977). *Virology* **80**, 218–221.

Shulman, L. and Revel, M. (1980). *Nature* **288**, 98–100.

Smart, T. G., Constanti, A., Bilbe, G., Brown, D. A. and Barnard, E. A. (1983). *Neurosci. Lett.* **40**, 55–59.

Sommerville, J. (1983). *Nucl. Acids Res.* **11**, 7375–7380.

Soreq, H. and Miskin, R. (1981). *FEBS Lett.* **128**, 305–310.

Soreq, H., Sagar, H. and Sehgal, P. B. (1981). *Proc. Natl. Acad. Sci. USA* **78**, 1741–1745.

Soreq, H., Parvari, R. and Silman, I. (1982). *Proc. Natl. Acad. Sci. USA* **79**, 830–834.

St-Laurent, G., Yoshie, O., Floyd-Smith, G., Samanta, H. and Sehgal, P. B. (1983). *Cell* **33**, 95–102.

Sumikawa, K., Houghton, M., Emtage, J. S., Richards, B. M. and Barnard, E. A. (1981). *Nature* **292**, 862–864.

Sumikawa, K., Parker, I., Amano, T. and Miledi, R. (1984). *EMBO J.* **3**, 2291–2294.

Teraoka, H., Arita, H., Tamaki, M., Fuji, Y. and Tanaka, K. (1982). *J. Biochem.* **91**, 933–938.

Valle, G., Besley, J. and Colman, A. (1981). *Nature* **291**, 338–340.

Valle, G., Besley, J., Williamson, A. R., Mosmann, T. R. and Colman, A. (1983). *Eur. J. Biochem.* **132**, 131–138.

Vanderbeke, E., Cleuter, Y., Marbaix, G., Préaux, G. and Lontie, R. (1982). *Biochem. Int.* **5**, 23–29.

Vassart, G., Refetoff, S., Brocas, H., Dinsart, C. and Dumont, J. E. (1975). *Proc. Natl. Acad. Sci. USA* **72**, 3839–3843.

Watson, R. J., Colberg-Poley, A. M., Marcus-Sekura, C. J., Carter, B. J. and Enquist, L. W. (1983). *Nucl. Acids Res.* **11**, 1507–1522.

Wiedmann, M., Huth, A. and Rapoport, T. A. (1984). *Nature* **309**, 637–639.

Windle, J., Shin, H. S. and Morrow, J. F. (1984). *J. Immunol.* **132**, 1317–1322.

Woodland, H. R. and Wilt, F. H. (1980). *Develop. Biol.* **75**, 199–213.

Wunner, W., Curtis, P. and Wiktor, T. J. (1980). *J. Virol.* **36**, 133–142.

Zehavi-Willner, T. and Lane, C. D. (1977). *Cell* **11**, 683–693.

18

Gene Transfer in Mouse Eggs

J. W. Gordon

I. INTRODUCTION

Efforts to transfer genes into mouse embryos have only recently achieved success (Gordon *et al.*, 1980). In the few years since its development, however, this technique has gained central importance in the investigation of problems in mammalian development and genetics. The ability to introduce cloned DNA sequences from any source into the developing mouse has made possible studies of gene regulation which far exceed in their sophistication those which could previously be performed. Studies undertaken thus far have shown that tissue specificity of gene expression resides in the promoter sequences of eukaryotic genes (Brinster *et al.*, 1981; Palmiter *et al.*, 1983). In addition, enhancer sequences may also exist which augment expression of mammalian genes (Brinster *et al.*, 1983). Endogenous human counterparts of retroviral oncogenes of human can cause cancer in mice if linked to an inappropriate promoter (Stewart *et al.*, 1984) and oncogenic sequences of SV40 virus can cause cancer in specific mouse tissues (Brinster *et al.*, 1984). Thus the technique of gene transfer has opened the door to the delineation of specific sequences in and around eukaryotic genes which regulate expression. In addition, insertion of foreign genetic material to the mouse genome has the potential of disrupting host sequences. Such "insertional mutants" can manifest themselves as lethal recessives (Wagner *et al.*, 1981). The production of insertional mutants by integration of foreign DNA allows for recovery of the affected gene by construction of genomic libraries and utilization of the microinjected DNA as a probe for screening. Gene transfer therefore also affords the opportunity to assemble a panel of genes whose action is necessary for the completion of normal development.

Although the potential of this gene transfer system is clear, several aspects of it remain poorly understood. Foreign DNA may be integrated as a single copy or as a gigantic concatameric structure composed of multimers of the

Microinjection and Organelle Transplantation Techniques

ISBN: 0-12-164722-6
ISBN: 0-12-164723-4 Pbk

injected sequence. Factors determining which of these two pathways to integration will be observed in each individual case remain to be clarified. At present integration appears to occur randomly throughout the host genome. However, in other organisms (Hinnen *et al.*, 1978; Struhl *et al.*, 1979) site specific integration based on an apparent homologous recombination event is observed. We do not yet know whether the potential for this mode of integration exists in mammals. As a consequence, expression of foreign material integrated into the mouse genome is difficult to predict. Frequently expression is not observed.

There is also great variability in rates of success reported for this gene transfer approach. While in some experiments as many as 30% of embryos which survive microinjection are positive by screening, in other cases, as few as 3% may be positive. A number of possible explanations exist for this variability. Experimental technique may vary slightly between laboratories, or the DNA sequences themselves may vary in their intrinsic capacities for integration. One study has compared various gene constructs for their relative frequency of integration (Palmiter *et al.*, 1982). These investigators reported no apparent difference in integration rates between supercoiled circular molecules, blunt-ended linearized molecules, molecules with restriction enzyme staggered ends, or molecules which had been ligated to an excess of mouse DNA. However, it is generally accepted that linearized molecules are integrated with greater frequency. There is also substantial variability in the length of time between injection of the foreign DNA sequence and its ultimate integration into the host genome. Many transgenic mice have been found to contain foreign DNA in all of their cells and transmit this DNA to 50% of progeny, results indicative of integration very early in development. On the other hand, a number of reports of mosaic animals exist. These findings indicate that at least in some cases foreign DNA remains unintegrated for several cleavage divisions. Finally, neither the structure nor the characteristics of expression of foreign DNA inserted into transgenic mice is entirely predictable. Loss of sequences during their transmission through the germ line has been reported (Palmiter *et al.*, 1982). In addition, alterations of the structure of the integrated material have been found (Gordon, 1983). Where expression is concerned, three major patterns have been described. Genes may be stably expressed at a high, reproducible level within individual lines (Brinster *et al.*, 1983; Storb *et al.*, 1984); they may be reproducibly expressed but at a low level (Lacy *et al.*, 1983); or their expression may vary dramatically between individuals within single transgenic mouse lines (Palmiter *et al.*, 1984).

Before embarking on the production of transgenic mice, therefore, these observations should be taken into account. It is recommended that convenient restriction sites be utilized to produce linear fragments for microinjection. Parallel experiments in which the genes of interest are linked to promoters known to function efficiently after transfer into mice should also be considered. Screening of litters for transgenic offspring should always be initially conducted by Southern blot analysis rather than by dot blotting, as transformants carrying single copies of a foreign gene may be indistinguishable from negative mice by dot blotting. Once transformants have been identified, they should be immediately bred for screening of a number of progeny. Positive offspring should be heterozygotes which subsequently transmit foreign sequences to 50% of offspring, while initial transformants may be mosaics which only rarely transmit the sequence. When transgenic mice carrying large concatamers of DNA are identified their offspring can easily be screened by dot blotting. When dot blotting is performed, it is strongly recommended that DNA be visualized by an ethidium bromide staining on agarose gels prior to blotting to nitrocellulose. In this way, changes in the number of copies of the genes after transmission in the germ line will not be missed. Of course, it must be recognized that dot blotting will always miss changes in structure of a foreign sequences that can only be identified by restriction enzyme analysis.

With these issues in mind, we will now proceed to describe the method for producing transgenic mice. A very detailed technically oriented publication describing this protocol already exists (Gordon and Ruddle, 1983). Therefore, in the present chapter, a more general discussion of techniques will be made. Here, however, emphasis on the various pitfalls of these techniques as well as the subsequent analyses will be given greater emphasis. It is hoped that this approach will maximize the efficiency with which the new investigator achieves positive results. The overall approach for producing transgenic mice is depicted in Fig. 1.

II. PRODUCTION OF TRANSGENIC MICE

A. Selection and maintenance of mice

There are several factors to be considered when selecting mouse strains for production of transgenic mice. When first attempting this procedure, it is particularly important that strains be used which yield a large number of embryos after superovulation. Unfortunately, a good response to superovulation is not characteristic of many inbred strains. This presents a problem when one wishes to produce transgenic mice whose evaluation depends upon the presence of foreign genes on an inbred background. When this is the case it is of course recommended to attempt superovulation of the inbred strain one wishes to use. If sufficient numbers of embryos are not obtained

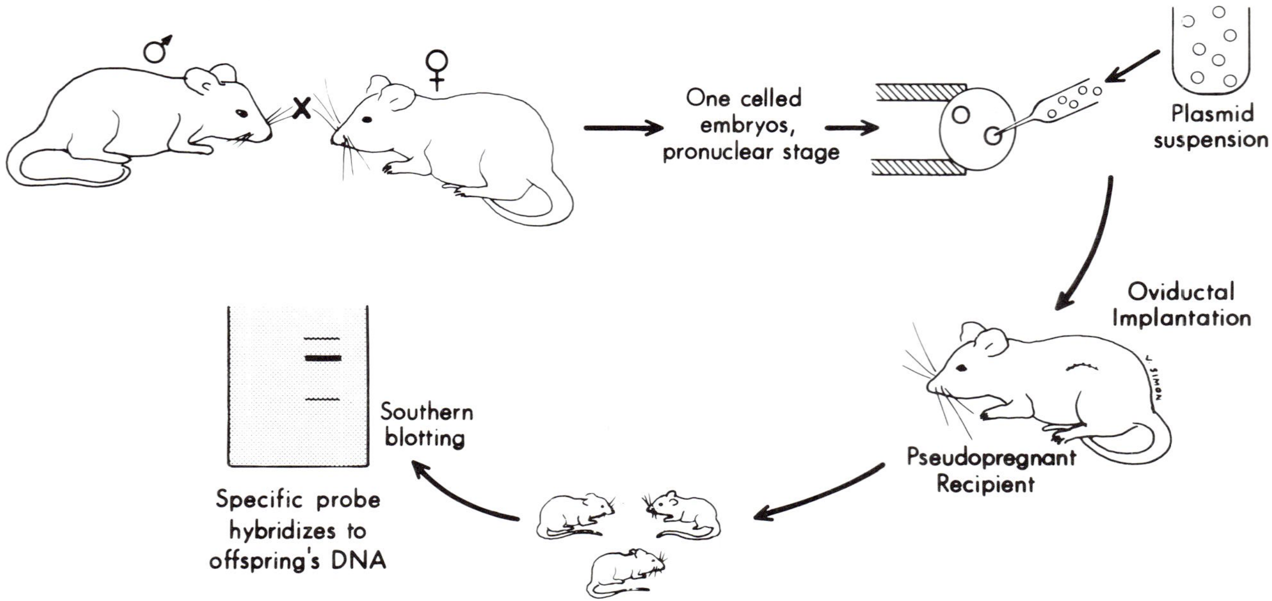

Fig. 1. Summary of transformation procedure.

the following strategy is suggested: select a hybrid mouse, one of whose parents belongs to the strain desired. Then superovulate the hybrid females and cross them back to males of the same inbred strain desired. Once transgenic mice are born they can then be rapidly back-crossed to the inbred strain of choice. This strategy has the obvious difficulty that genetic crossing-over may complicate the evaluation. However, particularly when first learning the microinjection procedure, it is very important that large numbers of embryos be available for practice.

When inbred strains are not needed the choice of mice should depend upon several factors. An outbred strain with particularly good response to superovulation should be chosen. In addition, in our laboratory, we choose males heterozygous at a number of pigment loci. A good example is the B62D2F_1 mouse, which is heterozygous at the black locus for the recessive allele brown, and is also heterozygous for the recessive gene dilute. Transgenic mice can then be back-crossed to B6D2F_1 mice and the offspring obtained will have a variety of pigment phenotypes. Variable pigment phenotypes produced by back-crossing greatly facilitate record keeping.

B. Housing and superovulation procedures

Mice should be housed and maintained in such a way as to maximize their reproductive efficiency. The light:dark cycle in the animal room should be adjusted such that the animals experience 14 hours of light and 10 hours dark in each 24 hour day. The precise time in which the lights turn on and off can be adjusted to suit the needs of the investigator. We routinely employ a schedule where lights go off at 10.00 p.m. and come on at 8.00 a.m. When this schedule is used mice are superovulated at 4.00 p.m. and placed with males to mate. The following day embryos with prominent pronuclei can be obtained in mid-afternoon.

Males to be used as studs for fertilizing the embryos should be housed individually. The same is true for vasectomized males, which are needed for obtaining pseudo-pregnant foster females. Mice which are superovulated are usually immature and therefore have not begun their own oestrous cycle. They can accordingly be conveniently housed in large cages. Mice to be used as pseudo-pregnant foster females, on the other hand, should be mature and should be not induced to mate by superovulation. Although hormone injections will induce mating in these mice, a relatively large percentage of them will not maintain a pregnancy after embryo transfer. Therefore, it is most efficient to maintain large numbers of mature females which are randomly cycling, and to mate these females each night with vasectomized males. When housing mature females, it is important to recognize that cohabitation often results in synchronization of the oestrous cycle. If 20 mature female mice are housed together for a long period, they will gradually become completely synchronized. If one wishes to use the mice every day for transfer of microinjected embryos, the synchronization phenomenon will result in the failure to obtain pseudo-pregnant mice on most days, while more mice than can possibly be used will be plugged on every fourth or fifth day. To overcome this problem, our laboratory houses our mature females in groups of five. These randomly cycling females, after placement with vasectomized males are always returned to the same cage from which they were obtained. The females within each cage of 5 may become synchronized, but separate lots of 5 will not be synchronized with each other. With this protocol, one cage of 5 mature females may yield no plugs on a given day, but another cage may yield 2 or 3 plugs. Therefore, if one maintains 4 or 5 cages, each of which contains 5 mature mice, it is rare to fail to obtain plugged foster mice.

Because pseudo-pregnant mice used as recipients for embryo transfer cannot be reused, it is necessary to slowly replenish the population of mature foster females. Our laboratory does not purchase mice for this purpose. Instead, we maintain this population by adding female mice which failed to mate after superovulation. Such mice are kept in the laboratory for a 2 week period. After this time, their period of pseudo-pregnancy induced by superovulation will have ended, and the mice have also reached a sufficient age to begin random cycling. Thus, when immature mice are not plugged, we place them in cages and note the date on which they will be ready for use as foster females. When the pseudo-pregnancy period has ended, the mice are also weighed prior to use as foster females. We have found that outbred mice weighing less than 30 g do not become pregnant after an embryo transfer with the same frequency as heavier animals. We maintain an inexpensive pan balance in the animal facility and weigh all mice prior to mating with vasectomized males.

Immature mice as young as 21 days of age may be used for superovulation. However, mice which are immature but nearly old enough to begin an endogenous oestrous cycle respond better to superovulation protocols. Accordingly, we order outbred mice 5 to 6 weeks of age for superovulation. When inbred strains of mice are used, endogenous oestrous cycling may not begin until the animals are somewhat older. Therfore, particularly if difficulty is encountered in superovulation, inbred mice may be injected at a great age.

Immature female mice are superovulated by administration of 5 IU of pregnant mares serum (PMS) by intraperitoneal injection at 4.00 p.m., followed 48 h later by 2.5 IU of human chorionic gonadotropin (HCG), also administered at 4.00 p.m. by introperitoneal injection. Immediately after administration of HCG, the females are placed with fertile males to mate. At

Table I. Schedule for producing transgenic mice. This schedule assumes a light cycle in the animal facility in which lights go off at 10.00 p.m. and on at 8.00 a.m.

Day	Time	Procedure
−3	4.00 p.m.	Inject 10 immature female mice with 5 IU PMS
−1	4.00 p.m.	Inject immature mice with 2.5 IU HCG, place males to mate Place 15 randomly cycling mature females with 15 vasectomized males
0	10.00 a.m.	Examine immature and mature female mice for vaginal plugs
0	2.00 p.m.	Prepare media and glassware for microinjection
2	2.30 p.m.	Sacrifice immature females and obtain embryos for microinjection Prepare micromanipulation system
0	3.00–5.00 p.m.	Microinject DNA
0	6.00 p.m.	Implant surviving microinjected embryos into plugged pseudo-pregnant females
18–21	9.00 a.m.	Check animals for birth of transgenic mice Deliver animals by Caesarian section if not born by day 21

the same time mature, randomly cycling females are placed with vasectomized males. The following morning all mice are examined for the presence of vaginal plugs. Superovulated mice with plugs are separated off for sacrifice later in the day, while mature females are reserved for embryo transfer. As stated above, immature females which have not mated are saved for 2 weeks for subsequent use as foster females. The same day that plugs are observed, immature mice are sacrificed for pronuclear injections and transferred to the plugged foster females. The schedule for the experiments as described above are outlined in Table I.

C. Vasectomy of the male

Vasectomy is readily performed by making a midline vertical abdominal incision. The incision should be sufficiently high in the abdomen so as not to violate the preputial gland, which is situated subcutaneously in the lower abdomen. The scrotal sac is then squeezed so that the testes can be moved toward the incision. The testicular fat pad is identified and both testes and associated vasa deferentia are exposed. A loop of each vas is isolated in a hemostat and the hemostat is closed fully, crushing the structure. While being held in place in the hemostat, the intervening loop of vas is then torn away leaving crushed, widely separated ends. This method of vasectomy is quite reliable and ligation of the vas with suture material is not required.

When mature males are vasectomized, it is necessary to mate them at least once with females in order to clear the distal vas of residual speramotozoa. This procedure can be omitted if males are vasectomized at a sufficiently young age such that sperm have not yet reached the distal vas deferens. Regardless of which procedure is used, there is always a possibility that vasectomized males will regain their fertility. Occasionally, the vas will reconstruct itself such that spermatozoa get through and are able to fertilize oocytes. Because of this possibility, it is recommended that a genetic marking system be employed to assure that all microinjected embryos are of different genotypes from those resulting from fertilization by the vasectomized male. A simple genetic marking system would include the use of the albino mutation. We routinely use albino vasectomized males and albino females as foster mothers. However, the embryos we inject are heterozygous for albino and thus are normally pigmented. The birth of albino mice indicates that a vasectomized male is fertile. This system assures that mice which have not developed from microinjected embryos are not evaluated by DNA blotting procedures. Careful record keeping also assures that when vasectomized males are fertile they can quickly be identified and eliminated from the colony.

D. Preparation and handling of embryos

Production of transgenic mice requires that mouse embryos be removed and maintained for several hours *in vitro*. During the period of microinjection the embryos must be on a microscope stage and therefore not in controlled incubator conditions.

Several culture media are routinely employed for maintenance of mouse embryos. We have successfully produced transgenic mice using the medium of Mullen and Witten (1971) for all procedures. However, recently we have employed media devised by Whittingham and his colleagues (Whittingham, 1971; Quinn *et al.*, 1982). This system consists of two culture media. The first, M16, is used for isolation of mouse embryos, treatment with hyaluronidase, and culture following microinjection. The second medium, M2, is buffered with Hepes and maintains an appropriate pH in atmospheric air. This medium is used to prepare the microdrop in which the embryos are injected. All other media are composed of M16. Because M2 is used only for microinjection, 50 ml lots are more than sufficient for injecting every day for the two week period in which the medium lasts, while 100 ml of M16 may be required for the same number of experiments. Additionally, a small amount of M16 supplemented with hyaluronidase, 1 mg/ml, is also needed. Embryos must be placed in this latter medium for removal of follicle cells. Because the embryos are treated only briefly with hyaluronidase, their exposure to decayed medium components is very brief. Accordingly, we do not replace the M16 with hyaluronidase every two weeks. Instead this medium is used until its supply is exhausted, frequently for periods of up to 2 months.

For each experiment the following materials are needed:

1. Six 35 mm tissue culture dishes, each containing 2 ml of M16.

2. One small depression slide containing 0.1–0.2 ml of M16 medium + 1 mg/ml hyaluronidase.

3. One 100 mm tissue culture dish containing a long rectangular microdrop of M2 medium covered with mineral oil. These materials should all be placed in an incubator providing an atmosphere of 5% CO_2 in air or 90% N_2, 5% CO_2, 5% O_2. Humidity should be at least 95%.

4. Two embryo transfer pipettes fashioned from 9″ Pasteur pipettes as previously described (Gordon and Ruddle, 1983). One of these transfer pipettes should be fire polished in a microburner so that when the microdrop of M2 medium is placed on the 100 mm tissue culture dish, the pipette will not scratch the surface of the dish.

5. One implantation pipette, also made as previously described (Gordon and Ruddle, 1983). According to the schedule shown in Table I, immature, plugged mice are sacrificed at 2.30 p.m. Their oviducts are removed to one 35 mm tissue culture dish containing M16 medium. From there, each oviduct is placed in the depression slide containing M16 with hyaluronidase. The ampulla of the oviduct, identified by its relative transparency to transmitted light, is opened with watchmaker's forceps and the eggs with associated follicle cells expressed into the depression slide. This procedure is continued until all oocytes have been removed to the depression slide. After 2–5 min of incubation in the depression slide, the embryos are washed with a transfer pipette and removed to another dish with M16. Here the embryos are washed and transferred again to a fresh dish of M16, this time taking care to transfer only the oocytes and to leave most of the debris behind. This procedure is repeated until embryos are free of all accompanying debris. The embryos should be sufficiently cleaned by three successive transfers, such that two unused dishes of M16 remain in the incubator when washing has been completed. The embryos are stored in a dish of M16 until just prior to microinjection. At this point, if optical conditions are optimized, it is possible to identify those eggs which have two pronuclei. Thus, when loading the microdrop of M2 medium, it is possible to avoid loading abnormal or unfertilized oocytes.

The construction of holding pipettes and microneedles for microinjection have been described in detail elsewhere (Gordon and Ruddle, 1983). However, several additional points should be made. With regard to the holding pipettc, it is advisablc that the outside diameter at the tip be approximately the same as that of a fertilized egg with its zona pellucida. When the diameter is too small the oocyte may be lost when the pipette is lowered to the floor of the dish for microinjection. When it is too large, the aperture of the holding pipette is situated high off the floor of the dish. Consequently, excessive amounts of medium are drawn into the holding pipette before sufficient suction is created to drawn an embryo onto the holding pipette. It should be noted that a certain amount of leeway exists here. When the outside diameter of the holding pipette is somewhat large, it is advisable that the aperture itself be relatively small. Contrariwise, a thin holding pipette should have a relatively large aperture. These adjustments prevent excessive suction from drawing oocytes into the holding pipette and thus killing them while at the same time providing for sufficient suction to hold the oocyte in place during microinjection.

Production of microneedles varies according to several factors. Some DNA preparations are more difficult to microinject and therefore require a microneedle with a relatively large opening at the tip. Very clean preparations, on the other hand, can be microinjected through a much finer needle. Fine needles have the advantage that they are able to pierce the pronuclear membrane with ease, while larger microneedles are not as sharp. However, the flow of DNA across the tip of a larger microneedle is smoother and more easily controlled. As noted in our initial publication (Gordon *et al.*, 1980), microneedles may be fashioned from tubing which has a fine capillary tube fused to the inside wall. This allows for DNA solution to climb directly to the tip of the needle. It is also possible to draw DNA through the tip for microneedle loading. This is done by placing the microneedle on the micromanipulator apparatus, dipping the microneedle into the DNA solution, and applying suction. This latter technique has the advantage that particulate matter too large to cross the tip of the microneedle will not be contained in the loaded solution. Its disadvantage that it is cumbersome and difficult. Regardless of the method used, all air should be purged from both the holding pipette and the microneedle system prior to microinjection. It is also advisable to arrange the micromanipulator apparatus such that the manipulation system for the microneedle is on the opposite side of the microscope from the injecting syringe itself. This allows one to manipulate the microneedle and hold it in position while applying pressure for microinjection.

Microinjection is performed by loading the cleaned, sorted embryos into one end of the long and rectangular microdrop of M2 medium. When the holding pipette is lowered through the oil and into the medium, care should be taken that a slight positive pressure is present in the holding pipette system. This pressure prevents mineral oil from being drawn into the holding pipette. If the latter takes place, the holding pipette will not respond as sensitively to changes in pressure. The holding pipette may be quickly lowered through the oil into the medium and to the floor of the tissue culture dish. The holding pipette is sufficiently thin such that pressure against the bottom of the dish is usually not sufficient to break the relatively flexible tip. The holding pipette is then located in the microscope field, and an embryo is drawn onto it to stop continued flow of culture medium into the pipette due to capillary action. At this point it is wise to test the system and assure oneself that embryos can be expelled and fixed on the holding pipette with ease. If the holding pipette does not function properly it should be changed immediately. With an embryo held in place, the microneedle is then lowered into the microdrop. It is usually necessary to lower the microneedle with a substantial angle such that the tip of the needle is far lower than the heel. This angle allows one to clear the edge of the tissue culture dish. Before proceeding to microinject, one should make certain that the microneedle tip may be lowered to the floor of the tissue culture dish without interference by the edge of the dish.

Microinjection is then accomplished by rotating the embryo on the holding pipette in such a way that one of the two pronuclei is positioned well for microinjection. Although some investigators take care to assure themselves that they are injecting the male pronucleus (Brinster *et al.*, 1981), we do not do so. Instead, we choose the pronucleus that is most readily positioned for access to the microneedle. If the circular embryo is imagined to be the face of a clock, we like to inject a pronucleus which is at the 2.00–4.00 position, with the holding pipette fixed at the embryo at the 9.00 position. The vertical distance between the floor of the tissue culture dish and the pronucleus is then gauged by gently probing the embryo with the microneedle. When the microneedle tip is at the same depth in the medium as the pronucleus to be injected, the pronuclear membrane will recoil quite sensitively when the embryo is probed. If the microneedle is either too high or too low such a sensitive response will not be observed. The microneedle is then inserted into the pronucleus and microinjection is attempted. Successful microinjection may be confirmed by observing a lightening of the colour of the pronuclear contents and/or a swelling of the pronucleus. If neither of these is observed, it is probable that the microneedle is not in the pronucleus or that flow across the microneedle tip is not taking place. When the microneedle is malfunctioning it should not be possible to observe the flow of DNA into the ooplasm; on the other hand, failure to enter the pronucleus with a functioning microneedle results in the observable flow of

DNA solution into the ooplasm. It is quite common that microneedles initially do not function well. If flow is not observed after significant pressure has been applied to the microneedle system, the microneedle may be removed from the embryo and adjusted so as to initiatc flow. Flow can be frequently started by gently wiping the tip of the microneedle along the wall of the holding pipette. This clears the tip or causes minor breaks in the tip which free obstructions. This usually results in observable flow across the microneedle. It may be necessary to wait for this flow to subside before injecting the first embryo, as the rate of flow secondary to build-up of pressure during previous attempts to microinject may be so great that embryos will be killed if the microneedle is inserted into them. When flow has been established, the microinjection procedure is attempted again. Embryos which have been successfully injected can be lifted off the floor of the dish and carried to the opposite end of the rectangular microdrop by moving the vertical access of the microscope stage. There the embryos are deposited and thus separated from the uninjected embryos. This procedure is repeated until all embryos have been injected. Under optimal conditions, one may inject as many as 100 embryos in a single afternoon. However, it is far more common to inject 30–40 embryos with survival of 10–20.

It is frequently necessary to force the microneedle completely beyond the opposite wall of the pronucleus and then to draw the microneedle back into the nucleoplasm before injecting. This contingency is created by the fact that the pronuclear membrane is very elastic and is often difficult to breach. This problem is more common in large pronuclei which are observed if mice are sacrificed later in the afternoon. When pronuclei are pierced in this way, it is also more common to withdraw nuclear DNA upon removal of the microneedle. Obviously, this results in death of the embryo. Both of these problems may be circumvented by microinjecting somewhat earlier in the day ($\frac{1}{2}$ to $1\frac{1}{2}$ hours). Younger pronuclei are smaller and therefore more difficult to target. However, as already stated, they are more easily pierced. In addition, they are somewhat more resistant to destruction by the addition of DNA solution. This latter phenomenon may relate to the fact that addition of a given volume of solution to a smaller container will result in a relatively small increase in wall tension. When first attempting to microinject, these various factors should be adjusted to suit the individual's preference. It is not uncommon that regardless of the steps taken, microinjection is very difficult. For this reason, particularly in the beginning, it is advisable to make several microneedles for each day's work. When one microneedle fails to function to one's satisfaction, it should be changed. We do not change the microneedle, however, if 50% of embryos or more survive microinjection. It is often better to accept embryonic mortality rather than to change a functioning microneedle for one which may function even more poorly.

Changing equipment during the microinjection procedure may also be time consuming and distracting.

When all new embryos have been microinjected, they should be removed to a dish of M16 medium, washed well, and transferred a second time to a fresh dish of M16. Here they may be scored for success. Dead embryos can easily be recognized as pale diffuse objects with a very small or absent perivitelline space. We normally incubate the embryos for an hour or more in order to allow severely damaged embryos to manifest the signs of demise.

E. Embryo reimplantation

After microinjection the surviving embryos must be returned to pseudo-pregnant foster mice for continued development. This is accomplished by transfer of the embryos into the oviduct. When fewer than 10 embryos have survived microinjection, transfer into a single oviduct is suitable; 10–30 embryos may be transferred into a single female using both oviducts. When we have more than 40 surviving embryos, we transfer them back to two pseudo-pregnant mice. If only one pseudo-pregnant mouse is available and more than 40 embryos have survived microinjection, it is not contraindicated to transfer all back to a single animal. It is probable that many of the embryos which appear viable at the time of transfer in fact will subsequently die. Therefore it is unlikely that a pseudo-pregnant mouse will give birth to more embryos than she can effectively rear. Our laboratory has on one occasion transferred 50 microinjected embryos into one mouse, with the resultant birth of 17 mice. However, these mice were effectively reared by the female. The advantage of using more than one pseudo-pregnant mouse as recipient for microinjected embryos numbering more than 40 is that the pregnancy rate in normally cycling mice is about 90%. Thus, the chances of transferring embryos into a mouse that is unable to become pregnant are 10%. If two mice are used, the chances that neither will be capable of maintaining a pregnancy is only 1%.

The tip of the embryo transfer pipette, fashioned as previously described (Gordon and Ruddle, 1983), should have an inside diameter of approximately 1.5 times that of the embryo with its zona pellicuda. Larger pipettes may be difficult to insert into the ostium of the oviduct, while with smaller pipettes difficulty may be encountered in collecting the embryos. Obviously there is a considerable margin for error. In general, it is advisable that a smaller transfer pipette be used if the recipient female is small, while larger pipettes can be used for larger mice. When the embryo transfer pipette is properly constructed and used, as many as 20 embryos can be transferred into the oviduct in less than 3 μl of medium.

The ostium, or opening of the oviduct, can be located just adjacent to the ovary. It should be isolated through a vertical incision about 0.5 cm lateral to the dorsal midline. In the mouse the ovary is covered by a bursal layer which must be opened for access to the ostium. When opening the bursa care should be taken not to violatc major blood vessels, as such violation will obscure the field with blood. The ostium can be approached on both sides from the caudal direction and can be identified as a somewhat enlarged region of the oviduct. The holding pipette should be inserted until resistance is met. The oviduct should not be distorted or manipulated in such a way as to advance the pipette beyond the distance which it readily attains. We normally collect the embryos in a small volume of medium distal to a small air bubble which is used as a marker. When the embryos are expelled into the oviduct, the appearance of the air bubble marker at the ostium indicates that the embryos have all been transferred. We usually expel the contents of the transfer pipette until the air bubble marker enters the lumen of the oviduct. This assures us that all embryos have left the surgical pipette, and in addition, the air bubble serves as a plug, preventing the back flow of medium.

Pseudo-pregnant females should deliver approximately 18 to 21 days after transfer. If animals have not been born by the morning of the 21st day, and if the appearance and weight gain of the pseudo-pregnant mouse indicate a pregnancy has been achieved, the mouse is sacrificed and the embryos are delivered by Caesarean section. Clearly this cannot be done unless another animal in the colony has delivered within the previous 24–48 hours. However, if another mouse in the colony is available to receive sectioned mice, the addition of a new animal to the previous litter is usually successful. When fetuses are removed by Caesearan section, it is also possible to save the placenta for DNA analysis.

III. PREPARATION OF DNA FOR MICROINJECTION

When preparing DNA for microinjection, two major factors should be considered. First, is the quality and cleanliness of the preparation; second, the form in which the material is injected may be of importance.

While the mechanism by which exogenous DNA gains access to cultured cells during gene transfer experiments is becoming well understood, this is not the case with embryo transfer. Specifically, it is not known whether cotransfer of unlinked molecules is universally observed, while in microinjected cultured cells such cotransfer appears to occur invariably (Anderson *et al.*, 1983). In addition, when large concatamers are integrated into transgenic mice, it is not clear whether such concatamers are derived from single molecules which have undergone replication or from the linkage of independent fragments to form a single giant transgenome. In addition, while it has been suggested that linear molecules are integrated with a greater frequency than circular ones, success in the transfer of supercoiled circular molecules has also been observed. Finally, it is not clear whether DNA sequences in and of themselves can affect either the rate of success in producing transgenic mice or the likelihood that transferred sequences will be expressed. The balance of the data suggest to us that when designing molecules for microinjection, a linearized molecule should be injected and vector sequences into which the desired genes have been cloned should be eliminated to as great an extent as possible. With recombinant plasmids this can readily be done by double-digesting the DNA at unique restrictions sites within the plasmid sequences. The fragments desired can then be purified by agarose gel electrophoresis. The disadvantage of this approach is that fine particulate matter within the agarose matrix invariably accompanies the DNA through subsequent purification. We have attempted to remove such material by several methods, none of which have been successful. However, while this material can complicate the microinjection procedure, it does not appear to affect the rate of gene transfer. When two unique restriction sites cannot be found in a plasmid, a single site may be utilized to linearize the molecule. This latter approach has the advantage that agarose gel purification is not required, but has the disadvantage that all plasmid sequences accompany the desired genes into the recipient genome. When recombinant bacteriophage are used it is of course more difficult to remove vector sequences. The length and complexity of such recombinant molecules makes the specific excision of vector molecules difficult. However, a high rate of success in producing transgenic mice has been reported with the transfer of intact recombinant phage (Costantini and Lacy, 1981). However, it should be pointed out that animals carrying such sequences manifested very low levels of expression of donor molecules (Lacy *et al.*, 1983).

DNA should be cleaned as much as possible before microinjection. Regardless of the type of molecule injected, caesium chloride (CsCl) gradient centrifugation is recommended. In addition, the DNA should be extensively dialysed. We routinely dialyse our DNA in 10 mM Tris HCl, pH 7.5; 0.1 mM EDTA, pH 7.5. When DNA is isolated from CsCl gradients, care should be taken to avoid contamination with bacterial DNA. In one line of mice previously described (Gordon and Ruddle, 1982) cotransfer of *Escherichia coli* chromosomal DNA has been discovered (unpubl. obs.). Therefore, it is advisable to sacrifice the yield of recombinant DNA from gradients in order to assure purity. When DNA is isolated from agarose gels, it should be extracted once with phenol, once with phenol:chloroform-isoamyl alcohol (25:1), and once with chloroform-isoamyl alcohol prior to dialysis. For such extractions we always use ultra-pure phenol. DNA which is linearized with restriction enzymes and not purified through agarose is likewise extracted, precipitated, redissolved, and extensively dialysed. While such procedures reduce the yield of DNA, very little DNA is actually needed for microinjection experiments. As few as 200 copies of recombinant molecule may be injected into a mouse embryo with significant success in producing transgenic mice (Brinster *et al.*, 1981; Costantini and Lacy, 1981). Once dialysed the DNA should be centrifuged for 10–15 min in a microfuge prior to use. We frequently centrifuge 200–300 μl and remove the top 100–150 μl after centrifugation. This assures that particulate matter at the bottom of the centrifuge tube will not contaminate the microinjection solution. Although 1 μl of solution is sufficient under ideal conditions to inject 10^6 embryos, it is advisable to prepare at least 100 μl of solution. Smaller volumes evaporate over the course of several experiments, and such evaporation concentrates contaminants and particulate matter that interfere with microinjection.

We have estimated that a mouse pronucleus will accommodate approximately 1 pl of microinjection solution (Gordon *et al.*, 1980). Therefore, DNA solutions may be adjusted to a concentration of as little as 200 DNA copies/pl. However, we have also observed that as many as 30 000 copies of a recombinant molecule per cell does not injure the embryo (Gordon *et al.*, 1980). Therefore, we recommend that when initiating attempts to produce transgenic mice, greater concentrations of DNA be employed. We routinely microinject 2000–10 000 molecules per cell. The utilization of higher concentrations of DNA assures the experimenter that even when a minimal volume is microinjected, a significant number of DNA molecules will be inserted.

The relative efficiency with which various heterologous genes may function in mouse tissues is as yet unknown. The promoter for mouse metallothionein one strongly stimulates the expression of a number of genes (Brinster *et al.*, 1981; Palmiter *et al.*, 1982). A variety of other promoters including that associated with the chicken transferrin gene (McKnight *et al.*, 1983), mouse immunoglobulin genes (Brinster *et al.*, 1983), the rat elastase 1 gene (Swift *et al.*, 1984), the SV40 T antigen promoter (Brinster *et al.*, 1984), and the long terminal repeat of mouse mammary tumour virus (Stewart *et al.*, 1984), all appear to work well in transgenic mice. However, the globin genes do not appear to be efficiently transcribed when associated with their own promoters (Lacy *et al.*, 1983). It is therefore difficult to predict how any specific sequence will behave after transfer. Accordingly, if doubt exists as to the performance of a given sequence after microinjection, the ligation of the sequence of interest to a promoter known to function efficiently in transgenic mice is recommended. It is also possible to coinject the sequence and the promoter without prior ligation. However, it is not clear that cotransfer of unlinked markers always occurs in transgenic mice. In fact, the cotransfer phenomenon has not been formally explored in this system. Therefore, if expression of the transferred sequence is desired, it is recommended that prior ligation at a convenient restriction site to a known potent promoter be carried out. Such preparations may well be unnecessary, however, due to the aforementioned fact that even promoters from other species will function effectively in transgenic mice. Therefore, it is reasonable to inject the sequence of interest alone provided that the recombinant clone contains all necessary promoter sequences.

IV. EVALUATION OF TRANSGENIC MICE

Evaluation of mice developed from microinjected embryos can be performed by several methods. DNA may be isolated from tail biopsies (Stewart *et al.*, 1984). However, in our experience, this DNA is frequently difficult to digest with restriction enzymes. Liver DNA may also be used (Costantini and Lacy, 1981). In this instance, caution should be taken to biopsy the liver only at the periphery of the lobe. Otherwise death by exsanguination is probable. Splenectomy is another method which we have used for DNA analysis (Gordon and Ruddle, 1981). This organ yields a large amount of DNA with little contaminating protein or RNA. However, if the genes injected are expected to alter the haematologic characteristics of mice, removal of the spleen may complicate the latter evaluation. Recently we have employed a technique of partial splenectomy for DNA analysis. This technique involves the exposure of the spleen with subsequent removal of the cardiac end. Cauterization of the cut end of the spleen is not necessary. We have not observed significant mortality with this technique. The only drawback of this approach is that if mice are very young the amount of DNA obtained from the spleen may be small. Whichever technique is employed, it is strongly recommended that restriction analysis and Southern blot hybridization be carried out in initial screening. This is because mice may contain only a single copy of foreign DNA per cell and this quantity of DNA may be difficult to distinguish from negative mice by dot blotting analysis. In addition, other mice may be produced which have more than one copy of DNA per cell but which are mosaics and consequently have an effective concentration of one or fewer copies of foreign DNA per cell. Therefore, dot blotting analysis may cause one to miss positive mice. Moreover, the mice which might be lost by dot blot screening may be those which are of particular interest. For example, evaluation of gene methylation and expression is complicated in transgenic mice carrying large concatamers of a foreign DNA sequence. However, when only one copy is present per cell, studies are greatly facilitated. Therefore, mice which carry one copy of foreign DNA per cell and which express the foreign gene are of particular value.

When mice are identified which carry large concatamers of foreign DNA sequence they and their offspring may be screened by dot blotting. In this case it is advisable to recall that some mice have been reported to lose large numbers of copies of DNA per cell during transmission of gene through the germ line (Palmiter *et al.*, 1982). This finding has been confirmed in studies in our own laboratory (J. W. Gordon, unpubl. obs.). In the aforementioned case increased expression of the foreign genes was associated with a loss in copy number. Accordingly, it may be of particular interest to identify those mice which have lost copies of the foreign gene. Because of this, our laboratory performs a modified version of Southern blot analysis. We load fixed volumes of DNA onto agarose gel slabs, electrophorese the DNA without restriction enzyme digestion overnight, and then visualize the DNA the following morning by ethidium bromide staining. In this way we can accurately assess the amounts of DNA in each slot. We then "flash" the film with short wave UV irradiation prior to performing a Southern blot. This technique allows us to quantify the relative amounts of DNA accurately and thereby determine if copies of the foreign gene have been lost during transmission through the germ line. Another approach is spectrophotometry of the DNA prior to dot blotting. The hazard here is that variable contamination with RNA or protein may make the spectrophotometric reading unreliable. This problem is particularly great when DNA isolated from tails is used. The problem may be largely circumvented by prior treatment of the DNA with RNase. However, when screening large numbers of animals such RNase treatment adds an additional step to an already high labour intensive enterprise.

V. CONCLUSION

For those without prior experience in handling mice or micromanipulation equipment the production of transgenic mice can be difficult. However, the evidence is increasingly great that once the minor technical problems are solved the production of such animals is relatively simple. As noted previously, the reasons why some molecules may be integrated with great frequency while others are very difficult to insert into mice are unknown. However, differences may well relate to the quality of the DNA preparation. Therefore, no expense should be spared in producing very high quality preparations. Because it is difficult to predict how one will fare in initial attempts to produce these mice, we recommend that microinjection experiments continue until a significant number of positive animals is produced. It is unwise to produce a few animals, screen them, and then return to microinjection if screening is negative. This approach incurs a significant delay in obtaining positive results, and may delay recognition of the fact that a particular sequence is difficult to insert. We also recommend that care be taken that all reimplanted embryos have actually been successfully microinjected. It is better to kill an embryo during microinjection than to screen a mouse which has not actually been injected. The cost in labour and supplies for maintaining mice is frequently the greatest expense in producing and maintaining transgenic mice.

Once facility is gained in this experimental technique, it will be observed that microinjection itself is the simplest part of the process. Maintenance, record keeping, and evaluation of positive mice is the most laborious process. Analyses may be further complicated if positive animals are in any way disturbed in their development or in their ability to survive the embryonic, fetal, or neonatal period. It is difficult to conceive of a DNA sequence whose injection into mouse embryos would be of no interest. This technique has such broad applicability that the insertion of any gene should yield interesting data. In addition, the production of transgenic mice carrying a greater variety of DNA sequences will expand our knowledge of the gene transfer mechanism itself. For these reasons we all look forward to the successful production of mice by a large number of laboratories.

REFERENCES

Anderson, W. F., Killos, L., Sanders-Haigh, L., Kretschmer, P. J. and Diacumakos, E. G. (1983). *Proc. Natl. Acad. Sci. USA* **77**, 5399–5403.

Brinster, R. L., Chen, H. Y., Trumbauer, M., Senear, A. W., Warren, R. and Palmiter, R. D. (1981). *Cell* **27**, 223–231.

Brinster, R. L., Ritchie, K. A., Hammer, R. E., O'Brien, R. L., Arp, B. and Storb, U. (1983). *Nature* **306**, 332–336.

Brinster, R. L., Chen, H. Y., Messing, A., van Dyke, T., Levine, A. J. and Palmiter, R. D. (1984). *Cell* **37**, 367–379.

Costantini, F. and Lacy, E. (1981). *Nature* **294**, 92–94.

Gordon, J. W. (1983). *J. Exp. Zool.* **32**, 313–324.

Gordon, J. W. and Ruddle, F. H. (1982). *In* "Embryonic Development", Part B: Cellular Aspects, pp. 112–124. Alan R. Liss, New York.

Gordon, J. W. and Ruddle, F. H. (1983). *Methods Enzymol.* **101**, 411–433.

Gordon, J. W., Scagnos, G. A., Plotkin, D. J., Barbosa, J. A. and Ruddle, F. H. (1980). *Proc. Natl. Acad. Sci. USA* **77**, 7380–7384.

Hinnen, A., Hicks, J. B. and Fink, G. R. (1978). *Proc. Natl. Acad. Sci. USA* **75**, 1929–1933.

Lacy, F., Roberts, S., Evans, E. P., Burtenshaw, M. D. and Costantini, F. E. (1983). *Cell* **34**, 343–358.

McKnight, G. S., Hammer, R. E., Kuenzel, E. A. and Brinster, R. L. (1983). *Cell* **34**, 335–341.

Mullen, R. J. and Whitten, W. K. (1971). *J. Exp. Zool.* **178**, 165–176.

Palmiter, R. D., Chen, H. Y. and Brinster, R. L. (1982). *Cell* **29**, 701–710.

Palmiter, R. D., Norstedt, G., Gelinas, R. E., Hammer, R. E. and Brinster, R. L. (1983). *Science* **222**, 809–814.

Palmiter, R. D., Wilkie, T. M., Chen, H. Y. and Brinster, R. L. (1984). *Cell* **36**, 869–877.

Quinn, P., Barros, C. and Whittingham, D. G. (1982). *J. Rep. Fertil.* **66**, 161–168.

Stewart, T. A., Pattengale, P. K., Leder, P. (1984). *Cell* **38**, 627–637.

Storb, U., O'Brien, R. L., McMullen, M. D., Gollahon, K. A. and Brinster, R. L. (1984). *Nature* **310**, 238–241.

Struhl, K., Stinchcomb, D. T., Scherer, S. and Davis, R. W. (1979). *Proc. Natl. Acad. Sci. USA* **76**, 1035–1039.

Swift, G. H., Craik, C. S., Stary, S. J., Quinto, C., Lahaie, R. G., Rutter, W. J. (1984). *J. Biol. Chem.* **259**, 14271–14278.

Wagner, T. E., Stewart, T. A. and Mintz, B. (1981). *Proc. Natl. Acad. Sci. USA* **78**, 5016–5020.

Whittingham, D. G. (1971). *J. Rep. Fertil. Suppl.* **14**, 7–21.

Index